THERMODYNAMICS OF
PHARMACEUTICAL
SYSTEMS

THERMODYNAMICS OF PHARMACEUTICAL SYSTEMS

An Introduction for Students of Pharmacy

Kenneth A. Connors

School of Pharmacy
University of Wisconsin—Madison

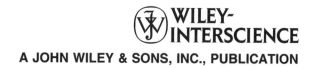

WILEY-
INTERSCIENCE

A JOHN WILEY & SONS, INC., PUBLICATION

For general information on our other products and services please contact our Customer Care Department
within the U.S. at 877-762-2974, outside the U.S. at 317-572-3993 or fax 317-572-4002.

Wiley also publishes its books in a variety of electronic formats. Some content that appears in print,
however, may not be available in electronic format.

Library of Congress Cataloging-in-Publication Data:

Connors, Kenneth A.
    Thermodynamics of pharmaceutical systems:
    An introduction for students of pharmacy

ISBN 0-471-20241-X

Printed in the United States of America.

10 9 8 7 6 5 4 3 2 1

To my brothers and sisters
Joy Connors Mojon, Lawrence M. Connors,
Peter G. Connors, Francis P. Connors,
and Kathleen Connors Hitchcock

CONTENTS

PREFACE

Classical thermodynamics, which was largely a nineteenth-century development, is a powerful descriptive treatment of the equilibrium macroscopic properties of matter. It is powerful because it is general, and it is general because it makes no assumptions about the fundamental structure of matter. There are no atoms or molecules in classical thermodynamics, so if our ideas about the atomic structure of matter should prove to be wrong (a very possible outcome to many nineteenth-century scientists), thermodynamics will stand unaltered. What thermodynamics does is to start with a few very general experimental observations expressed in mathematical form, and then develop logical relationships among macroscopic observables such as temperature, pressure, and volume. These relationships turn out to have great practical value.

Of course, we now have firm experimental and theoretical reasons to accept the existence of atoms and molecules, so the behavior of these entities has been absorbed into the content of thermodynamics, which thereby becomes even more useful to us. In the following we will encounter the most fundamental ideas of this important subject, as well as some applications of particular value in pharmacy. In keeping with our needs, the treatment will in places be less rigorous than that in many textbooks, and we may omit descriptions of detailed experimental conditions, subtleties in the arguments, or limits on the conclusions when such omissions do not concern our practical applications. But despite such shortcuts, the thermodynamics is sound, so if you later study thermodynamics at a deeper level you will not have to "unlearn" anything. Thermodynamics is a subject that benefits from, or may require, repeated study, and the treatment here is intended to be the introductory exposition.

Here are a few more specific matters that may interest readers. Throughout the text there will be citations to the Bibliography at the end of the book and the Notes sections that appear at the end of most chapters. Students will probably not find it necessary to consult the cited entries in the Bibliography, but I encourage you to glance at the Notes, which you may find to be interesting and helpful. Two of my practices in the text may be regarded by modern readers as somewhat old-fashioned, and perhaps they are, but here are my reasons. I make considerable use of certain units, such as the kilocalorie and the dyne, that are formally obsolete; not only is the older literature expressed in terms of these units, but they remain in active use, so the student must learn to use them. Appendix B treats the conversion of units. My second peculiar practice, which may seem quaint to students who have never used a table of logarithms, is often to express logarithmic relationships in terms of Briggsian (base 10) logarithms rather than natural logarithms. There are two reasons for the continued use of base 10 logarithms; one is that certain functions, such as pH and pK, are defined by base 10 logs, and these definitions can be taken as invariant components of chemical description; and the second reason, related to the first, is that order-of-magnitude comparisons are simple with base 10 logarithms, since we commonly operate with a base 10 arithmetic.

Obviously there is no new thermodynamics here, and I have drawn freely from several of the standard references, which are cited. Perhaps the only unusual feature of the text is my treatment of entropy. The usual development of the entropy concept follows historical lines, invoking heat engines and Carnot cycles. I agree with Guggenheim (1957, p. 7), however, that the idea of a Carnot cycle is at least as difficult as is that of entropy. Guggenheim then adopts a postulational attitude toward entropy [a method of approach given very systematic form in a well-known book by Callen (1960)], whereas I have developed a treatment aimed at establishing a stronger intuitive sense in my student readers [Nash (1974, p. 35) uses a similar strategy]. My approach consists of these three stages: (1) the basic postulates of statistical mechanics are introduced, along with Boltzmann's definition of entropy, and the concept is developed that spontaneous processes take place in the direction of greater probability and therefore of increased entropy; (2) with the statistical definition in hand, the entropy change is calculated for the isothermal expansion of an ideal gas; and (3) finally, we apply classical thermodynamic arguments to analyze the isothermal expansion of an ideal gas. By comparing the results of the statistical and the classical treatments of the same process, we find the classical definition of entropy, $dS = dq/T$, that will provide consistency between the two treatments.

Lectures based on this text might reasonably omit certain passages, only incidentally to save time; more importantly, the flow of ideas may be better served by making use of analogy or chemical intuition, rather than rigorous mathematics, to establish a result. For a good example of this practice, see Eq. (4.1) and the subsequent discussion; it seems to me to be more fruitful educationally to pass from Eq. (4.1), which says that, for a pure substance, the molar free energies in two phases at equilibrium are equal, to the conclusion for mixtures, by analogy, that the chemical potentials are equal, without indulging in the proof, embodied in Eqs. (4.2)–(4.6). But different instructors will doubtless have different views on this matter.

I thank my colleague George Zografi for providing the initial stimulus that led to the writing of this book. The manuscript was accurately typed by Tina Rundle. Any errors (there are always errors) are my responsibility.

KENNETH A. CONNORS

Madison, Wisconsin

THERMODYNAMICS OF PHARMACEUTICAL SYSTEMS

BASIC THERMODYNAMICS

1

ENERGY AND THE FIRST LAW OF THERMODYNAMICS

1.1. FUNDAMENTAL CONCEPTS

Temperature and the Zeroth Law. The concept of temperature is so familiar to us that we may not comprehend why scientists two centuries ago tended to confuse temperature with heat. We will start with the notion that temperature corresponds to "degree of hotness" experienced as a sensation. Next we assign a number to the temperature based on the observation that material objects (gases and liquids in particular) respond to "degree of hotness" through variations in their volumes. Thus we should be able to associate a number (its temperature) with the volume of a specified amount of material. We call the instrument designed for this purpose a thermometer.

The first requirement in setting up a scale of temperatures is to choose a zero point. In the common *Celsius* or *centigrade* scale we set the freezing point of water (which is also the melting point of ice) at 0°C [more precisely, 0°C corresponds to the freezing point of water (called the "ice point") in the presence of air at a pressure of 1 atmosphere (atm)]. The second requirement is that we must define the size of the degree, which is done for this scale by setting the boiling point of water (the "steam point") at 100°C. The intervening portion of the scale is then divided linearly into 100 segments. We will let t signify temperature on the Celsius scale.

Experience shows that different substances may give different temperature readings under identical conditions even though they agree perfectly at 0 and 100°C. For example, a mercury thermometer and an alcohol thermometer will not give precisely the same readings at (say) room temperature. In very careful work it would be advantageous to have available an "absolute" temperature scale that does not depend on the identity of the thermometer substance. Again we appeal to laboratory experience, which has shown that the dependence of the volume of a fixed amount of a gas on temperature, at very low pressures of the gas, is independent of the chemical nature of the gas. Later we will study the behavior of gases at low pressures in more detail; for the present we can call such gases "ideal gases" and use them to define an *absolute ideal-gas temperature scale*. We define the absolute temperature as directly proportional to the volume of a given mass of ideal gas at constant pressure (i.e., letting T be the absolute temperature and V the gas volume):

$$T \propto V$$

For convenience we define the size of the absolute temperature to be identical to the Celsius degree. If V_0 and V_{100} are the volumes of the ideal gas at the ice and steam points of water, respectively, the size of the degree is given by

$$\frac{V_{100} - V_0}{100}$$

Then our absolute temperature scale is defined by

$$T = \frac{V}{(V_{100} - V_0)/100} \tag{1.1}$$

Now suppose that we apply our ideal-gas thermometer to water at the ice point. In this special case Eq. (1.1) becomes

$$T_0 = \frac{V_0}{(V_{100} - V_0)/100}$$

Careful experimental work with numerous gases has revealed that $T_0 = 273.15\,\text{K}$. Thus the Celsius and absolute scales are related by

$$T = t + 273.15 \tag{1.2}$$

The absolute temperature scale is also called the *thermodynamic scale* or the *Kelvin scale*, and temperatures on this scale are denoted K (pronounced Kelvin, with no degree symbol or word).

According to Eq. (1.1), when $T = 0\,\text{K}$, $V = 0$; the volume of the ideal gas goes to zero at the *absolute zero*. Modern experimental techniques have achieved temperatures within microdegrees of the absolute zero, but $T = 0\,\text{K}$ appears to be an unattainable condition.

The concept and practical use of temperature scales and thermometers is based on the experimental fact that if two bodies are each in thermal equilibrium with a third body, they are in thermal equilibrium with each other. This is the *zeroth law of thermodynamics*.

Work and Energy. Let us begin with the mechanical concept of *work* as the product of a force and a displacement:

$$\text{Work} = \text{force} \times \text{displacement} \qquad (1.3)$$

The units of work are consequently those of force and length. Now from Newton's laws of motion,

$$\text{Force} = \text{mass} \times \text{acceleration} \qquad (1.4)$$

In SI units, force therefore has the units $kg\,m\,s^{-2}$, which is also called a newton, N. Hence the units of work are either $kg\,m^2\,s^{-2}$ or N m.

Energy is defined as any property that can be produced from or converted into work (including work itself). Therefore work and energy have the same dimensions, although different units may be used to describe different manifestations of energy and work. For example, $1\,Nm = 1\,J$ (joule), and energy is often given in joules or kilojoules. Here are relationships to earlier energy units:

$$1\,J = 10^7\,erg$$
$$4.184\,J = 1\,cal(calorie)$$

Note from the definition (1.3) that work is a product of an intensive property (force) and an extensive property (displacement). In general, work or energy can be expressed as this product:

$$\text{Work (energy)} = \text{intensity factor} \times \text{capacity factor} \qquad (1.5)$$

Here are several examples of Eq. (1.5):

Mechanical work = mechanical force × distance
Work of expansion = pressure × volume change
Electrical work = electric potential × charge
Surface work = surface tension × area change

All forms of work are, at least in principle, completely interconvertible. For example, one could use the electrical energy provided by a battery to drive a (frictionless) piston that converts the electrical work to an equivalent amount of work of expansion.

Heat and Energy. Heat has been described as *energy in transit* (Glasstone 1947, p. 7) or as a *mode of energy transfer* (Denbigh 1966, p. 18). Heat is that form of energy that is transferred from one place to another as a consequence of a difference in temperature between the two places. Numerically heat is expressed in joules (J) or calories (cal). Heat is not "degree of hotness," which, as we have seen, is measured by temperature.[1]

Table 1.1. The energy of a thermodynamic system

Total energy of a body			
Thermodynamic energy (U)		Mechanical energy	
Kinetic energy (translational energy)	Internal energy (vibrational, rotational, and electronic energy)	Kinetic energy as a result of the body's motion as a whole	Potential energy as a result of the body's position

Since both work and heat are forms of energy, they are closely connected. Work can be completely converted into an equivalent amount of heat (e.g., through friction). The converse is not possible, however; it is found experimentally that heat cannot be completely converted into an equivalent amount of work (without producing changes elsewhere in the surroundings). This point will be developed later; for the present we observe that this finding is the basis for the impossibility of a "perpetual-motion machine."

We find it convenient to divide energy into categories. This is arbitrary, but there is nothing wrong with it provided we are careful to leave nothing out. Now, we have seen that thermodynamics is not built on the atomic theory; nevertheless, we can very usefully invoke the atomic and molecular structure of matter in our interpretation of energy. In this manner we view heat as thermal energy, equivalent to, or manifesting itself as, motions of atoms and molecules. The scheme shown in Table 1.1 clarifies the several "kinds" of energy that a body (the "system") can possess.[2]

Chemical thermodynamics is concerned with the energy U. This energy is a consequence of the *electronic* distribution within the material, and of three types of atomic or molecular motion: (1) *translation*, the movement of individual molecules in space; (2) *vibration*, the movement of atoms or groups of atoms with respect to each other within a molecule; and (3) *rotation*, the revolution of molecules about an axis. If a material object is subjected to an external source of heat, so that the object absorbs heat and its temperature rises, the atoms and molecules increase their translational, vibrational, and rotational modes of motion. Energy is not a "thing"; it is rather one way of describing and measuring these molecular and atomic distributions and motions, as well as the electronic distribution within atoms and molecules.

Systems and States. In order to carry out experimental studies and to interpret the results, we must focus on some part of the universe that interests us. In thermodynamics this portion of the universe is called a *system*. The system typically consists of a specified amount of chemical substance or substances, such as a given mass of a gas, liquid, or solid. Whatever exists outside of the system is called the *surroundings*. Certain conditions give rise to several types of systems:

Isolated Systems. These systems are completely uninfluenced by their surroundings. This means that neither matter nor energy can flow into or out of the system.[3]

Closed Systems. Energy may be exchanged with the surroundings, but there can be no transfer of matter across the boundaries of the system.

Open Systems. Both energy and matter can enter or leave the system.

We can also speak of a *homogeneous* system, which is completely uniform in composition; or a *heterogeneous* system, which consists of two or more phases.

The *state* of a system, experiment has shown, can be completely defined by specifying four observable thermodynamic variables: the composition, temperature, pressure, and volume. If the system is homogeneous and consists of a single chemical substance, only three variables suffice. Moreover, it is known that these three variables are not all independent; if any two are known, the third is thereby fixed. Thus the thermodynamic state of a pure homogeneous system is completely defined by specifying any two of the variables pressure (P), volume (V), and temperature (T). The quantitative relationship, for a given system, among P, V, and T is called an *equation of state*. Generally the equation of state of a system must be established experimentally.

The fact that the state of a system can be completely defined by specifying so few (two or three) variables constitutes a vast simplification in the program of describing physicochemical systems, for this means that all the other macroscopic physical properties (density, viscosity, compressibility, etc.) are fixed. We don't know their values, but we know that they depend only on the thermodynamic variables, and therefore are not themselves independent. With this terminology we can now say that thermodynamics deals with changes in the energy U of a system as the system passes from one state to another state.

Thermodynamic Processes and Equilibrium. A system whose observable properties are not undergoing any changes with time is said to be in *thermodynamic equilibrium*. Thermodynamic equilibrium implies that three different kinds of equilibrium are established: (1) *thermal equilibrium* (all parts of the system are at the same temperature), (2) *chemical equilibrium* (the composition of the system is not changing), and (3) *mechanical equilibrium* (there are no macroscopic movements of material within the system).

Many kinds of processes can be carried out on thermodynamic systems, and some of these are of special theoretical or practical significance. *Isothermal processes* are those in which the system is maintained at a constant-temperature. (This is easy to do with a constant-temperature bath or oven.) Since it is conceivable that heat is given off or taken up by the system during the process, maintaining a constant temperature requires that the heat loss or gain be offset by heat absorbed from or given up to the surroundings. Thus an isothermal process requires either a closed or an open system, both of these allowing energy to be exchanged with the surroundings. An *adiabatic process* is one in which no heat enters or leaves the system. An adiabatic process requires an isolated system. Obviously if the process is adiabatic, the temperature of the system may change.

A *spontaneous process* is one that occurs "naturally"; it takes place without intervention. For example, if a filled balloon is punctured, much of the contained gas spontaneously expands into the surrounding atmosphere. In an equilibrium chemical reaction, which we may write as

$$A + B \rightleftharpoons M + N$$

it is conventional to consider the reaction as occurring from left to right as written. Thus if the position of equilibrium favors M + N (the products), the reaction is said to be spontaneous. If the reactants (A + B) are favored, the reaction is nonspontaneous as written. (Obviously we can change these designations simply by writing the reaction in the reverse direction.)

It is the business of thermodynamics to tell us whether a given process is spontaneous or nonspontaneous. However, thermodynamics, which deals solely with systems at equilibrium, cannot tell us how fast the process will be. For example, according to thermodynamic results, a mixture of hydrogen and oxygen gases will spontaneously react to yield water. This is undoubtedly correct—but it happens that (in the absence of a suitable catalyst) the process will take millions of years.

There is one more important type of thermodynamic process: the *reversible process*. Suppose we have a thermodynamic system at equilibrium. Now let an infinitesimal alteration be made in one of the thermodynamic variables (say, T or P). This will cause an infinitesimal change in the state of the system. If the alteration in the variable is reversed, the process will reverse itself exactly, and the original equilibrium will be restored. This situation is called *thermodynamic reversibility*. Reversibility in this sense requires that the system always be at, or infinitesimally close to, equilibrium, and that the infinitesimally small alterations in variables be carried out infinitesimally slowly. Because of this last factor, thermodynamically reversible processes constitute an idealization of real processes, but the concept is theoretically valuable. One feature of a reversible process is that it can yield the maximum amount of work; any other (irreversible) process would generate less work, because some energy would be irretrievably dissipated (e.g., by friction).

Now suppose that a system undergoes a process that takes it from state A to state B:

$$A \rightarrow B$$

We define a change in some property Q of the system by

$$\Delta Q = Q_B - Q_A \tag{1.6}$$

In other words, the incremental change in the property is equal to its value in the final state minus its value in the initial state.

Next consider this series of processes, which constitute a *thermodynamic cycle*:

$$
\begin{array}{ll}
\text{A} \xrightarrow{1} \text{B} & \Delta Q_1 = Q_{\text{B}} - Q_{\text{A}} \\
{}^4{\uparrow} \qquad {\downarrow}^2 & \Delta Q_2 = Q_{\text{C}} - Q_{\text{B}} \\
\text{D} \xleftarrow[3]{} \text{C} & \Delta Q_3 = Q_{\text{D}} - Q_{\text{C}} \\
& \underline{\Delta Q_4 = Q_{\text{A}} - Q_{\text{D}}} \\
& \text{Sum: } \Delta Q = 0
\end{array}
$$

In any cycle in which the system is restored exactly to its original state, the total incremental change is zero.

1.2. THE FIRST LAW OF THERMODYNAMICS

Statement of the First Law. To this point we have been establishing a vocabulary and some basic concepts, and now we are ready for the first powerful thermodynamic result. This result is solidly based on extensive experimentation, which tells us that although energy can be converted from one form to another, it cannot be created or destroyed [this statement is completely general in the energy regime characteristic of chemical processes; relativistic effects (i.e., the famous equation $E = mc^2$) do not intrude here]. This is the great *conservation of energy* principle, which is expressed mathematically as Eq. (1.7), the *first law of thermodynamics*.

$$\Delta U = q - w \tag{1.7}$$

Here ΔU is the change in thermodynamic energy of the system, q is the amount of energy gained by the system as heat, and w is the amount of energy lost by the system by doing work on its surroundings. These are the sign conventions that we will use:

> q is positive if the heat is taken up by the system (i.e., energy is gained by the system).
>
> w is positive if work is done by the system (i.e., energy is lost by the system).[4]

Equation (1.7) is the incremental form of the first law. The differential form is

$$dU = dq - dw \tag{1.8}$$

But now we must make a very clear distinction between the quantity dU and the quantities dq and dw. U is a *state function* and dU is an *exact differential*. This terminology means that the value of ΔU, which is obtained by integrating dU over the limits from the initial state to the final state, is independent of the path (i.e., the process or mechanism) by which the system gets from the initial state to the final state. A state function depends only on the values of the quantity in the initial and final states.

It is otherwise with q and w, for these quantities may be path-dependent. For example, the amount of work done depends on the path taken (e.g., whether the process is reversible or irreversible). Therefore dq and dw are not exact differentials, and some authors use different symbols to indicate this. Nevertheless, although q and w individually may be path-dependent, the combination $q-w$ is independent of path, for it is equal to ΔU.[5]

The Ideal Gas. Experimental measurements on gases have shown that, as the pressure is decreased, the volume of a definite amount of gas is proportional to the reciprocal of the pressure:

$$V \propto \frac{1}{P}$$

As P is decreased toward zero, all gases (at constant temperature) tend to behave in the same way, such that Eq. (1.9) is satisfied:

$$PV = \text{constant} \tag{1.9}$$

This result can be generalized as Eq. (1.10), which is called the *ideal-gas equation* (or the ideal-gas law):

$$PV = nRT \tag{1.10}$$

where P, V, and T have their usual meanings; n is the number of moles of gas; and R is a proportionality constant called the *gas constant*. Equation (1.10) is the equation of state for an ideal gas (sometimes called the "perfect gas"), and it constitutes a description of real-gas behavior in the limit of vanishingly low pressure.

Example 1.1. Experiment has shown that 1 mol of an ideal gas occupies a volume of 22.414 L at 1 atm pressure when $T = 273.15$ K. Calculate R:

$$R = \frac{PV}{nT} = \frac{(1\,\text{atm})(22.414\,\text{L})}{(1\,\text{mol})(273.15\,\text{K})}$$
$$= 0.082057\,\text{L atm mol}^{-1}\,\text{K}^{-1}$$

We can use a dimensional analysis treatment to convert to other energy units, as described in Appendix B:

$$R = \left(\frac{0.082057\,\text{L atm}}{\text{mol K}}\right)\left(\frac{101325\,\text{Pa}}{1\,\text{atm}}\right)\left(\frac{1\,\text{N m}^{-2}}{1\,\text{Pa}}\right)\left(\frac{10^3\,\text{cm}^3}{1\,\text{L}}\right)\left(\frac{1\,\text{J}}{1\,\text{N m}}\right)\left(\frac{1\,\text{m}}{10^2\,\text{cm}}\right)^3$$
$$= 8.3144\,\text{J mol}^{-1}\,\text{K}^{-1}$$

and since $1\,cal = 4.184\,J$, $R = 1.987\,cal\,mol^{-1}\,K^{-1}$. Notice that, in this calculation of R, its units are energy per mol per K. That is, since $R = PV/nT$, the units of the product PV are energy, which we expressed in the particular units L atm, J, or cal. These several values of R are widely tabulated, and they can serve as readily accessible conversion factors among these energy units.

We earlier mentioned a type of work called *work of expansion*. This is the work done by a gas when it expands against a resisting pressure, as happens when a piston moves in a cylinder. We can obtain a simple expression for work of expansion. Suppose a piston of cross-sectional area A moves against a constant pressure P. We know that mechanical work is the product of force (F) and distance, or

$$w = F(L_2 - L_1)$$

where L_1 is the initial position of the piston and L_2 is its final position. Pressure is force per unit area (A), so $F = PA$, giving

$$w = PA(L_2 - L_1)$$

But $A(L_2 - L_1) = V_2 - V_1$, where V_1 and V_2 are volumes, so

$$w = P(V_2 - V_1) = P\,\Delta V \tag{1.11}$$

where ΔV is the volume displaced. Thus work of expansion is the product of the (constant) pressure and the volume change; in fact, we often refer to work of expansion as $P\,\Delta V$ work.

Now, if the process is carried out reversibly, so that the pressure differs only infinitesimally from the equilibrium pressure, the volume change will be infinitesimal, and Eq. (1.11) can be written

$$dw = P\,dV \tag{1.12}$$

We can integrate this between limits:

$$w = \int_{V_1}^{V_2} P\,dV \tag{1.13}$$

(In the case of an isothermal, reversible expansion, w does not depend upon the path, but this is a special case.) Now suppose that the gas is ideal and that the process is carried out isothermally. From the ideal gas law, $P = nRT/V$, so

$$w = nRT \int_{V_1}^{V_2} \frac{dV}{V} \tag{1.14}$$

$$w = nRT \ln \frac{V_2}{V_1} \tag{1.15}$$

If $V_2 > V_1$, the system does work on the surroundings, and w is positive. If $V_1 > V_2$, the surroundings do work on the system, and w is negative.

In developing Eq. (1.15) we saw an example of thermodynamic reasoning, and we obtained a usable equation from very sparse premises. Here is another example, again based on the ideal gas. Suppose that such a gas expands into a vacuum. Since the resisting pressure is zero, Eq. (1.11) shows that $w = 0$; that is, no work is done. Careful experimental measurements by Joule and Kelvin in the nineteenth century showed that there is no heat exchange in this process, so $q = 0$. The first law therefore tells us that $\Delta U = 0$. Since the energy depends on just two variables, say, volume and temperature, we can express the result as

$$\left(\frac{\partial U}{\partial V}\right)_T = 0 \tag{1.16}$$

which says that the energy of an ideal gas is independent of its volume at constant temperature. We can interpret this thermodynamic result in molecular terms as follows. A gas behaves ideally when the intermolecular forces of attraction and repulsion are negligible. (This is why real gases approach ideality at very low pressures, for then the molecules are so far apart that they do not experience each others' force fields.) If there are no forces between the molecules, no energy is required to change the intermolecular distances, and so expansion (or compression) results in no energy change.

1.3. THE ENTHALPY

Definition of Enthalpy. In most chemical studies we work at constant pressure. (The reaction vessel is open to the atmosphere, and $P = 1$ atm, approximately.) Consequently the system is capable of doing work of expansion on the surroundings. From the first law we can write $q = \Delta U + w$, and since $w = P \Delta V$,

$$q = \Delta U + P \Delta V$$

at constant P. Writing out the increments, we obtain

$$q = (U_2 - U_1) + P(V_2 - V_1)$$

and rearranging, we have

$$q = (U_2 + PV_2) - (U_1 + PV_1) \tag{1.17}$$

where U, P, and V are all state functions. We define a new state function H, the *enthalpy*, by

$$H = U + PV \tag{1.18}$$

giving, from Eq. (1.17), the following:

$$q = \Delta H \tag{1.19}$$

Although Eq. (1.18) defines the enthalpy, it is usually interpreted according to Eq. (1.19), because we can only measure changes in enthalpy (as with all energy quantities). The enthalpy change is equal to the heat gained or lost in the process, at constant pressure (there is another restriction, viz., that work of expansion is the only work involved in the process). Since enthalpy is an energy, it is measured in the usual energy units.

From Eq. (1.18) we can write

$$\Delta H = \Delta U + P\,\Delta V \tag{1.20}$$

For chemical processes involving only solids and liquids, ΔV is usually quite small, so $\Delta H \approx \Delta U$, but for gases, where ΔV may be substantial, ΔH and ΔU are different. We can obtain an estimate of the difference by supposing that 1 mol of an ideal-gas is evolved in the process. From the ideal gas law we write

$$P\,\Delta V = (\Delta n)RT$$

For 1 mol, $\Delta n = 1$, so from Eq. (1.20), we have

$$\Delta H = \Delta U + RT$$

At 25°C, this gives

$$\Delta H = \Delta U + (1.987\,\text{cal mol}^{-1}\,\text{K}^{-1})(298.15\,\text{K})$$
$$= \Delta U + 592\,\text{cal mol}^{-1}$$

which is a very appreciable difference.

When a chemical process is carried out at constant pressure, the heat evolved or absorbed, per mole, can be identified as ΔH. Specific symbols and names have been devised to identify ΔH with particular processes. For example, the heat absorbed by a solid on melting is called the *heat of fusion* and is labeled ΔH_m or ΔH_f. The *heat of solution* is the enthalpy change per mole when a solute dissolves in a solvent. For a chemical reaction ΔH is called a *heat of reaction*. The heat of reaction may be positive (heat is absorbed) or negative (heat is evolved). By writing a reaction on paper in reverse direction its ΔH changes sign. For example, this reaction absorbs heat:

$$6C\ (s) + 3H_2\ (g) \rightarrow C_6H_6\ (l) \qquad \Delta H = +11.7\,\text{kcal mol}^{-1}$$

This reaction, its reverse, therefore evolves heat:

$$C_6H_6\ (l) \rightarrow 6C\ (s) + 3H_2\ (g) \qquad \Delta H = -11.7\,\text{kcal mol}^{-1}$$

We will later see how enthalpy changes for chemical processes can be measured.

Heat Capacity. A quantity C, called the *heat capacity*, is defined as

$$C = \frac{dq}{dT} \tag{1.21}$$

where C is a measure of the temperature change in a body produced by an increment of heat. The concept of the heat capacity is essential in appreciating the distinction between heat and temperature.

Chemical processes can be carried out at either constant volume or constant pressure. First consider constant volume. If only work of expansion is possible, at constant volume $\Delta V = 0$, so $w = 0$, and from the first law $dq = dU$. We therefore define the heat capacity at constant volume by

$$C_V = \left(\frac{\partial U}{\partial T}\right)_V \tag{1.22}$$

At constant pressure, on the other hand, we have, from Eq. (1.19), $dq = dH$, and we define the heat capacity at constant pressure by

$$C_P = \left(\frac{\partial H}{\partial T}\right)_P \tag{1.23}$$

In the preceding section we had obtained, for one mole of an ideal gas, Eq. (1.24).

$$\Delta H = \Delta U + RT \tag{1.24}$$

Let us differentiate this with respect to temperature. Using Eqs. (1.22) and (1.23), we get

$$C_P = C_V + R \tag{1.25}$$

For argon, at room temperature, $C_P = 20.8\,\text{J K}^{-1}\,\text{mol}^{-1}$ and $C_V = 12.5\,\text{J K}^{-1}\,\text{mol}^{-1}$; hence $C_P - C_V = 8.3\,\text{J K}^{-1}\,\text{mol}^{-1}$, which is R.

For most compounds only C_P has been measured. Values of C_P for typical organic compounds lie in the range 15–50 cal K^{-1} mol^{-1}. As seen here, heat capacity is expressed on a per mole basis, and is sometimes called the *molar heat capacity*. When the heat capacity is expressed on a per gram basis it is called the *specific heat*.

Taking the constant-pressure condition of Eq. (1.23) as understood, we can write $C_P = dH/dT$, or $dH = C_P\, dT$. If we suppose that C_P is essentially constant over the temperature range T_1 to T_2, integration gives

$$\Delta H = C_P\, \Delta T \tag{1.26}$$

Example 1.2. The mean specific heat of water is $1.00\,\text{cal g}^{-1}\,\text{K}^{-1}$. Calculate the heat required to increase the temperature of 1.5 L of water from 25°C to the boiling point.[6]

As a close approximation we may take the density of water as $1.00\,\text{g mL}^{-1}$ and the boiling point as 100°C, so, from Eq. (1.26), we obtain

$$\Delta H = \left(\frac{1.00\,\text{cal}}{\text{g K}}\right)(1500\,\text{g})(75\,\text{K}) = 112{,}500\,\text{cal}$$

or 112.5 kcal.

PROBLEMS

1.1. A piston 3.0 in. in diameter expands into a cylinder for a distance of 5.0 in. against a constant pressure of 1 atm. Calculate the work done in joules.

1.2. What is the work of expansion when the pressure on 0.5 mol of ideal gas is changed reversibly from 1 atm to 4 atm at 25°C? (*Hint*: For an ideal gas $P_1 V_1 = P_2 V_2$.)

1.3. Derive an equation giving the heat change in the isothermal reversible expansion of an ideal gas against an appreciable pressure. [*Hint*: Make use of Eq. (1.16) and the first law.]

1.4. What is the molar heat capacity of water? (See Example 1.2 for the specific heat.)

1.5. The molar heat capacity of liquid benzene is $136.1 \, \mathrm{J \, mol^{-1} \, K^{-1}}$. What is its specific heat?

1.6. The specific heat of solid aluminum is $0.215 \, \mathrm{cal \, g^{-1} \, K^{-1}}$. If a 100-g block of aluminum, initially at 25°C, absorbs 1.72 kcal of heat, what will be its final temperature?

1.7. A 500-g piece of iron, initially at 25°C, is plunged into 0.5 L of water at 75°C in a Dewar flask. When thermal equilibrium has been reached, what will the temperature be? The specific heat of iron is $0.106 \, \mathrm{cal \, g^{-1} \, K^{-1}}$.

1.8. In the following thermodynamic cycle, ΔH_f, ΔH_v, and ΔH_s are, respectively, molar heats of fusion, vaporization, and sublimation for a pure substance. Obtain an equation connecting these three quantities. (*Hint*: Pay careful attention to the directions of the arrows.)

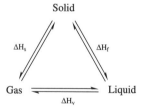

NOTES

1. Note that temperature is an intensive property, whereas heat is an extensive property. Two hot potatoes differing in size may have the same temperature, but the larger potato possesses more heat than the smaller one.

2. This scheme is consistent with the usage of most authors, but some variation is found in the literature. The thermodynamic energy U may also be symbolized E, and some authors label the thermodynamic energy the internal energy. The internal energy shown Table 1.1 may be identified with the potential energy of the molecules (to be distinguished from the potential energy of the body as a whole).

3. A truly isolated system is an idealization, but a very close approximation can be achieved inside a closed thermos (derived from the original trade name *Thermos* in 1907) bottle. (The laboratory version is called a *Dewar flask.*)

4. This is the sign convention used by most authors, but the International Union of Pure and Applied Chemistry (IUPAC) reverses the convention for w, giving as the first law $\Delta U = q + w$.

5. This analogy will clarify the difference between path-dependent and path-independent quantities. Suppose we wish to drive from Madison (WI) to Green Bay. Obviously there are numerous routes we might take. We could drive via Milwaukee, or via Oshkosh, or via Stevens Point, and so on. Graphically the possibilities can be represented on a map, as shown in the accompanying figure. Now, no matter which path we take, the changes in latitude, ΔLat, and in longitude, ΔLon, will be exactly the same for each route; for example, ΔLat = Lat(GB) − Lat(MAD), and this quantity is independent of the route. Thus latitude and longitude are state functions. But the amount of gasoline consumed, the time spent driving, and the number of miles driven all depend on the path taken; these are not state functions. This analogy is taken from Smith (1977).

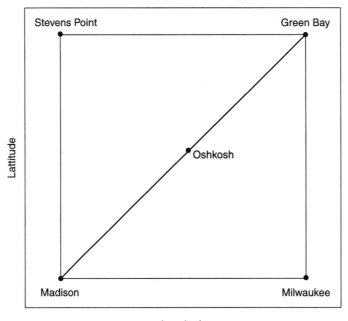

6. It is not a coincidence that the specific heat of water is $1.00 \, \text{cal} \, \text{g}^{-1} \, \text{K}^{-1}$, for this is how the calorie was originally defined: one calorie was the amount of heat required to raise the temperature of one gram of water by $1°C$. Actually the specific heat of water varies slightly with the temperature.

2

THE ENTROPY CONCEPT

2.1. THE ENTROPY DEFINED

Why Energy Alone Is Not a Sufficient Criterion for Equilibrium. Let us try to develop an analogy, based on what we know from classical mechanics, between a mechanical system and a chemical (thermodynamic) system. The position of equilibrium in a mechanical system is controlled by potential energy. Consider a rock poised near the top of a hill. It possesses potential (gravitational) energy as a consequence of its position. If it is released, its potential energy will be converted to heat (through friction) and to kinetic energy as it rolls down the hill. It will come to rest, having zero potential energy, at the foot of the hill (since we can measure only *changes* in energy, we mean that the potential energy is zero relative to some arbitrary reference value, which we are free to take as the value at the foot of the hill). It is now at mechanical equilibrium. Thus the criterion for a spontaneous mechanical process is that the change in potential energy be negative (it gets smaller), and the criterion for mechanical equilibrium is that the change in potential energy be zero.

Why don't we simply apply an analogous criterion to chemical systems? We might argue that ΔU (for a system at constant volume) or ΔH (for a system at constant pressure) play the role of potential energy in the mechanical system. But we find experimentally that this suggestion is inadequate to account for the observations. Consider first the following experiment (Smith 1977, p. 6):

1. Dissolve some solid NaOH in water. The solution becomes warm; that is, heat is liberated in the process. This means that ΔH is negative in the spontaneous process of NaOH dissolving in water. (The reaction is said to be *exothermic.*) This is entirely in accord with the proposal we are examining.

2. Dissolve some solid $NaNO_3$ in water. The solution becomes cool; that is, heat is absorbed as the dissolution occurs, and this cools the solution. Therefore ΔH is positive in this spontaneous process. (It is an *endothermic* reaction.) This behavior is in conflict with the proposal.

Here is another pertinent experiment. Suppose that we have two identical chambers connected by a stopcock. With the stopcock closed, we let one chamber contain a gas and the other chamber be evacuated (i.e., it "contains" a vacuum). Now we open the stopcock. We know what will happen—the gas will spontaneously distribute itself uniformly throughout the two chambers. If the gas is ideal (and most gases behave nearly ideally at low pressures), we know [see Eq. (1.16)] that $\Delta U = 0$ for this spontaneous process. Thus, with *no energy change at all* the system spontaneously underwent a change to an equilibrium position.

This inability to predict the direction of chemical change based on energy considerations alone was one of the great nineteenth-century scientific problems. Since energy minimization alone is not an adequate criterion for chemical equilibrium, *something else* must be involved. This is our next concern, and we are going to use an approach somewhat different from that taken in many textbooks, which adopt an argument based on the historical development of the ideas. We are going to sidestep classical thermodynamic history by turning to a description based on the particulate (i.e., atomic) nature of matter.

The Statistical Mechanical Entropy. We have seen that classical thermodynamics is based on macroscopic observations and makes no assumptions about the ultimate structure of matter. An alternative viewpoint, called *statistical mechanics* (or *statistical thermodynamics* when applied to thermodynamic problems), adopts the assumption that matter is composed of vast numbers of very small particles (which we now identify as electrons, atoms, molecules, etc.). In many circumstances this point of view provides physical insight not available from classical thermodynamics, and we will turn to it to illuminate our present problem.

Let us reconsider the example of the apparatus with two chambers, in one of which a gas was initially confined. Suppose that only a single molecule of gas had been present. After the stopcock is opened (and presuming that both chambers have equal volumes), evidently the probability that the molecule will be in one specified chamber (say, the left chamber) is $\frac{1}{2}$. Next suppose we were to start with two molecules, say, a and b, and ask for the probability that both will be found, at equilibrium, in the left chamber. These are the only possible distributions:

Left	Right
a	b
b	a
a,b	—
—	a,b

Thus of four possible distributions only one places both a and b in the left chamber, so the probability[1] of this distribution is $\frac{1}{4} = (\frac{1}{2})^2$. Generalizing to N molecules we get $(\frac{1}{2})^N$ for the probability that at equilibrium all N molecules will be found in the left chamber. Since for chemical systems N, the number of atoms or molecules, can be very large indeed, we see that the probability is extremely small that all of the molecules will end up in one chamber. On the other hand, the probability is extremely high that the molecules will be distributed equally between the two chambers.

This simple example (Glasstone 1947, p. 184) suggests a general statement, which in fact constitutes a basic premise of statistical mechanics, namely, that *all spontaneous processes represent changes from a less probable to a more probable state*. This postulate leads us to the next stage of our inquiry, which consists essentially of counting all possible distributions that are accessible to a system, for this is how the probability of a state is to be established.

In this next example the system is more complicated, although still artificially simple. We imagine that two crystals of different elements, A and B, are placed in contact, so that atoms of A may diffuse into the B crystal and vice versa [this example is given by Denbigh (1966, p. 49)]. In this simple example we suppose that crystal A contains four A atoms (4A), and likewise crystal B contains four B atoms (4B). We can distinguish between A and B atoms, but all A atoms are indistinguishable among themselves, and similarly for B. The sites that the atoms occupy in the crystals are distinguishable. Initially let all A atoms be in the left-hand crystal and all B atoms in the right-hand crystal.

We are going to count all possible configurations (called *microstates*) of our system. There are 4A and 4B to be distributed among eight sites. (We assume that the energies of interaction are identical no matter which type of atom is on which site.) Clearly there is only one microstate having 4A in the left crystal and 4B in the right crystal:

A	A	B	B
A	A	B	B

Similarly, there is only one microstate with 4B in the left and 4A in the right crystal.

But now consider the number of ways we can have $3A + 1B$ on the left and $3B + 1A$ on the right. We could argue in this way—the A atom on the right has any one of 4 right-hand sites available to it, and likewise the B atom on the left has 4 sites available, making $4 \times 4 = 16$ configurations. These 16 microstates are explicitly shown in Fig. 2.1 Obviously the symmetrical arrangement of $1A + 3B$ on the left and $3A + 1B$ on the right will also have 16 microstates.

The remaining arrangement of $2A + 2B$ (left) and $2A + 2B$ (right) is slightly more difficult. First consider the left crystal. The first B atom has 4 sites available, whereas the second B atom has only 3 accessible sites. Hence there appear to be 4×3 possible configurations. However, the two B atoms are indistinguishable, so we have double-counted, and must compensate, giving $(4 \times 3)/2$ as the number of

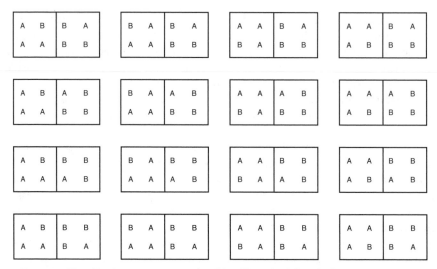

Figure 2.1. The 16 microstates possessing 3A +1B on the left and 3B + 1A on the right.

microstates. But an equal number is contributed by the right-hand side, making in all $(4 \times 3)/2 \times (4 \times 3)/2 = 36$ microstates. Here are the results summarized.[2]

Atoms to Left	Atoms to Right	Number of Microstates
4A	4B	1
3A + 1B	1A + 3B	16
2A + 2B	2A + 2B	36
1A + 3B	3A + 1B	16
4B	4A	1
		———
		70

In modern terminology, the microstates are called *quantum states*.

Now, another key premise of statistical mechanics is that the system is as likely to be in any one microstate as in another. That is, *all microstates are equally probable*. In our example above, there is a probability of $\frac{1}{35}$ that all of the A atoms will be found in a single crystal (either left or right); but there is a probability of $\frac{36}{70}$ that the atoms will be uniformly distributed. All the microstates are accessible, and the system is simply more likely to be found (at equilibrium) in the state possessing the largest number of microstates. (It can also be stated that the system spends an equal amount of time in each microstate, so it spends the most time in the system with the most microstates.)

For chemical systems the number of particles is extremely large (recall that Avogadro's number is about 6×10^{23}), so the number of microstates is vast, and the consequence is that the most probable state of the system is *so* probable that all other states (although possible in principle) may be disregarded in practice. The total number of microstates accessible to a system (which, we have just noted, is essentially equal to the number of microstates in the most probable state) we label W. (Some authors use Ω.) We now define a quantity S, called *entropy*, by Eq. (2.1), which is due to Boltzmann:

$$S = k \ln W \tag{2.1}$$

This is a definition. We will later establish the significance of the proportionality constant k. The equation says that the entropy S of a system increases logarithmically as W, the number of accessible microstates, increases.

We have noticed in our crystal diffusion example how W is composed of contributions from various configurations, and within each configuration the contributions are multiplicative; for example, for the $3A + 1B$ (left) and $1A + BB$ (right) state we had $4 \times 4 = 16$ microstates. Supposing, more generally, that we write $W = W_L \times W_R$, Eq. (2.1) gives us

$$S = k \ln W_L W_R = k \ln W_L + k \ln W_R = S_L + S_R$$

Thus, entropy is additive. (This is one reason why Boltzmann used a logarithmic function in his definition.)

Another point is to be made here. Our crystal diffusion example involved microstates all having the same energy, and we calculated all possible configurations. The resulting entropy is known as the *configurational entropy*. More generally, in chemical systems we must also consider a very large number of quantum states, most of which occupy different energy levels. The total entropy receives contributions from both sources: the microstates counting all configurations and those counting all energies.

Summarizing to this point, we conclude that spontaneous processes occur in a direction of increasing probability, and that entropy as calculated by the statistical mechanical definition is a quantitative measure of this probability. Therefore *spontaneous processes occur with an increase in entropy.*[3]

Before leaving the statistical mechanical treatment, let us apply our results to the calculation of the entropy change accompanying the isothermal expansion of an ideal gas from volume V_1 to volume V_2 (Glasstone 1947, p. 186; Denbigh 1966, p. 55; Rossini 1950, p. 73). (We will shortly see the point of this particular calculation.) Recall that $\Delta U = 0$ in this process, so the only driving force for the expansion is the increase in probability of the system.

If W_1 and W_2 are the numbers of microstates associated with volumes V_1 and V_2, then $S_1 = k \ln W_1$ and $S_2 = k \ln W_2$, so

$$\Delta S = S_2 - S_1 = k \ln \frac{W_2}{W_1} \tag{2.2}$$

The probability that a single molecule will be found in any volume V is proportional to that volume, and the number of microstates accessible to a molecule is proportional to V (Hill 1960, Chapter 4). We therefore can write, for a single molecule, $W_2/W_1 = V_2/V_1$, and for N_A (one mole of) molecules

$$\frac{W_2}{W_1} = \left(\frac{V_2}{V_1}\right)^{N_A} \tag{2.3}$$

Combining Eqs. (2.2) and (2.3) gives as the statistical mechanical result

$$\Delta S = kN_A \ln \frac{V_2}{V_1} \tag{2.4}$$

Entropy in Classical Thermodynamics. Now we are going to treat the isothermal reversible expansion of an ideal gas classically. Our goal is to establish the classical thermodynamic equivalent of the statistical mechanical entropy. We begin with the first law:

$$dU = dq - dw \tag{2.5}$$

On expanding from volume V_1 to volume V_2 against pressure P, the gas is capable of doing work of expansion $dw = P\,dV$. Moreover, we know from our earlier discussion that $dU = 0$ for this process, so we have $dq = P\,dV$. For one mole of an ideal gas $P = RT/V$, giving $dq = RT(dV/V)$, or

$$\frac{dq}{T} = R\frac{dV}{V} \tag{2.6}$$

We will integrate Eq. (2.6) between our expansion limits of V_1 and V_2, giving

$$\int_{\text{state 1}}^{\text{state 2}} \frac{dq}{T} = R \ln \frac{V_2}{V_1} \tag{2.7}$$

Now let us compare Eq. (2.7), derived classically, with Eq. (2.4), derived statistically. These equations describe the same process, and they reveal that consistency between the classical and statistical treatments can be achieved by writing the identities

$$kN_A = R \tag{2.8}$$

$$\int_{\text{state 1}}^{\text{state 2}} \frac{dq}{T} = \Delta S \tag{2.9}$$

and Eq. (2.9) implies

$$\frac{dq}{T} = dS \tag{2.10}$$

These are powerful results. From Eq. (2.8) we achieve a physical interpretation of the proportionality constant k in Eq. (2.1), Boltzmann's definition of entropy, as

$$k = \frac{R}{N_A} \qquad (2.11)$$

where k is the gas constant per molecule; this quantity is known as the *Boltzmann constant*. It has the value $k = 1.38 \times 10^{-23} \, \text{J} \, \text{K}^{-1}$. Any equation containing R is on a per mole basis; replace the R with k and the equation is on a per molecule basis.

According to Eq. (2.10), the differential entropy change is equal to the differential heat change divided by the absolute temperature. Moreover, from Eq. (2.7), since V is a state function, the entropy S is a state function. With a combination of statistical and classical arguments we can make some general statements about entropy changes. From statistical mechanics we had seen that ΔS increases during a spontaneous process, so we infer that $\Delta S = 0$ at equilibrium. Reverting to a differential symbolism, these results give us

$dS > 0$, for a spontaneous (irreversible) process

$dS = 0$, for a system at equilibrium

Recall that in a reversible process the system is always virtually at equilibrium, and the system is then capable of performing the maximum work (because irreversible losses, such as to friction, are minimized). In a spontaneous (irreversible) process, the amount of work that can be done is less than the maximum. From the first law, since dU is a state function and is the same no matter what path is taken, we have

$$dU = dq_{\text{rev}} - dw_{\text{rev}} = dq_{\text{irr}} - dw_{\text{irr}}$$

so

$$dq_{\text{rev}} - dq_{\text{irr}} = dw_{\text{rev}} - dw_{\text{irr}}$$

Since $dw_{\text{rev}} > dw_{\text{irr}}$, it follows that $dq_{\text{rev}} > dq_{\text{irr}}$. We therefore can write

$$\frac{dq_{\text{rev}}}{T} > \frac{dq_{\text{irr}}}{T}$$

The entropy is a state function, independent of path, so the differential dS has a definite value for a given process regardless of whether that process is carried out reversibly. Equation (2.10) for the classical definition of entropy can be more explicitly written

$$dS = \frac{dq_{\text{rev}}}{T}$$

Classically, then, the entropy increase is equal to the heat change in an isothermal reversible process divided by the absolute temperature at which the heat change occurs. All spontaneous (i.e., natural) processes occur with a gain of entropy by the system and the surroundings. Note that it is conceivable for the system to experience an entropy decrease ($dS < 0$), but this will inevitably be accompanied by a more-than-compensating entropy increase in the surroundings.

2.2. THE SECOND LAW OF THERMODYNAMICS

Statement of the Second Law. Entropy plays a critical role in thermodynamic analysis, because it is the missing factor that we were seeking to allow us to predict the direction of change in atomic or molecular systems. The essential result constitutes the *second law* of thermodynamics, which can be stated in several ways, not all of them obviously equivalent, but in fact all of them providing the same message. Here are some of them:

1. Heat does not spontaneously flow from a cold body to a hot body.
2. Spontaneous processes are not thermodynamically reversible.
3. The complete conversion of heat into work is impossible without leaving some effect elsewhere.
4. It is impossible to convert heat into work by means of a constant temperature cycle.
5. All natural processes are accompanied by a net gain in entropy of the system and its surroundings.

This last statement is most useful to us. Let us write

$$dS_{\text{net}} = dS_{\text{system}} + dS_{\text{surroundings}}$$

Then the second law says

$dS_{\text{net}} > 0$ (spontaneous processes)
$dS_{\text{net}} = 0$ (reversible processes)

Interpretations of Entropy. Entropy is an abstract concept of thermodynamics and statistical mechanics that plays a practical role in providing a criterion for equilibrium. Despite its technical and abstract nature, it has passed into popular culture and language, where its use is sometimes casual and inexact. Let us consider some interpretations that have been given to entropy. The statistical mechanical picture is clearest. We found that the entropy increases logarithmically with the number of microstates accessible to the system, and concluded that entropy is correlated with the increase in "mixed- up- ness" of the system [Denbigh (1966, p. 55) attributes this term to Gibbs]. Entropy is widely interpreted as a measure of *randomness* or of *disorder*, an increase in entropy being associated with an increase in these properties. This is because spontaneous processes occur with an increase in entropy and lead to more extensive mixing of the units in a system. This interpretation directly concerns the configurational entropy, which measures the spatial disposition of units; in addition there is the thermal entropy, which measures the distribution of quantum states having different energies. (But note that an increase in configurational entropy might conceivably be accompanied by a decrease in thermal entropy; it is the net entropy change that is decisive.) E. A. Guggenheim [cited by Denbigh (1966, p. 56)] refers to entropy as a measure of *spread*, that is, dispersion over a larger number of quantum states, either configurational or thermal.

A fundamental basis of the second law is closely connected to these interpretive notions. As we have seen, it is possible to convert work completely into heat, but we cannot completely convert heat into work. The reason for this dissymmetry lies in the atomic structure of matter. Doing work means making use of the *directed* motion of an assemblage of particles (as by rubbing a metal block on a surface, or drilling a hole in a solid with a drill bit). This work is converted (through friction) to heat, which raises the temperature of the contacting bodies. The temperature increase reflects the increased kinetic energy of the atoms in the bodies, and (this is the essential point) the motions of these atoms are undirected, as they are largely chaotic. There is no possible way to transform completely this *undirected* motion (heat) back into work, without adding energy from the surroundings. The basis of this irreversibility is the increased randomness on the atomic scale. A modern version describes this phenomenon (increased spread or randomness, therefore increased entropy) as reflecting a loss of information about the system.

It is often said that the entropy of the universe is constantly increasing. This is correct to the extent that we understand the universe, but the statement, if taken as an analogy with chemical systems, implies that the universe is approaching an equilibrium state, when dS will be zero; and this we do not know.

Summary of Fundamental Thermodynamics. Our development of the first and second laws of thermodynamics has provided the entire basis of this subject. Everything else (and there is a great deal more) follows from this by introducing definitions of new quantities or functions and manipulating them mathematically. Before we proceed, we summarize our results[4] in Table 2.1.

Table 2.1. The laws of thermodynamics

Law	State Function	Characteristic
0	T	Determines thermal equilibrium
1	U	Conservation of energy
		(The energy of the universe is constant)
		(You can't get something for nothing)
2	S	Determines direction of spontaneous change
		(The entropy of the universe is increasing)
		(You can't break even)

2.3. APPLICATIONS OF THE ENTROPY CONCEPT

Entropy Relationships. A few simple manipulations will demonstrate the involvement of entropy in thermodynamic relationships. The first law is $dU = dq - dw$. If the only work done in a process is work of expansion, then $dw = P\,dV$. Moreover, we have seen that $dS = dq/T$, so $dq = T\,dS$, and we get

$$dU = T\,dS - P\,dV \tag{2.12}$$

as another statement of the first law. The product $T\,dS$ (or $T\,\Delta S$) is pervasive in thermodynamics, and this is its source; observe that this product is an energy.

Now rearrange Eq. (2.12) to

$$dS = \frac{dU + P\,dV}{T} \tag{2.13}$$

and consider processes at constant pressure. From the definition of enthalpy applied to Eq. (2.12) we find

$$dS = \frac{dH}{T} \tag{2.14}$$

We recall that the heat capacity at constant pressure is defined $C_P = dH/dT$, so $dH = C_P\,dT$. Using this in Eq. (2.14) gives

$$dS = C_P\frac{dT}{T} \tag{2.15}$$

where the constant pressure condition is understood and is not explicitly indicated. We can integrate Eq. (2.15) between the limits T_1 and T_2:

$$\Delta S = S_2 - S_1 = \int_{T_1}^{T_2} C_P\frac{dT}{T} = \int_{T_1}^{T_2} C_P\,d\ln T \tag{2.16}$$

If C_P is substantially independent of temperature over the integration range, Eq. (2.16) becomes

$$\Delta S = C_P \ln \frac{T_2}{T_1} \tag{2.17}$$

at constant pressure [a corresponding equation, $\Delta S = C_v \ln (T_2/T_1)$, applies at constant volume].

An interesting case of Eq. (2.16) arises when we set $T_1 = 0\,\text{K}$, giving

$$S = S_0 + \int_0^T C_P\,d\ln T \tag{2.18}$$

The quantity S_0 is to be interpreted as the value of the entropy at the absolute zero. Planck in 1912 proposed that S_0 may assume the value zero at 0 K for a perfect crystal, which possesses no disorder. This proposal is known as the *third law of thermodynamics*. By means of the third law combined with Eq. (2.18), it is possible to evaluate the entropy S of substances from measurements of C_P as a function of temperature. The procedure is to plot experimental values of C_P against $\ln T$ for the entire range of experimental temperatures. Since $T = 0\,\mathrm{K}$ is unattainable, the curve thus generated is extrapolated to 0 K with the aid of a theoretical function. The area under the curve, from 0 K up to any specified temperature, is then equal to the entropy of the substance at that temperature.

Entropy Changes. Despite the possibility afforded by the third law to evaluate absolute entropies of substances, in nearly all practical applications of the entropy concept we evaluate *changes* in entropy. Here we will see some examples of such determinations. Later in the book we will consider the estimation of entropy changes for additional types of processes.

From the definition $dS = dq/T$ it is evident that the units of entropy are energy per degree kelvin, and it is expressed either in $\mathrm{J\,K^{-1}}$ or $\mathrm{cal\,K^{-1}}$. Since entropy is an extensive property we convert it to an intensive property by expressing it on a per mole basis. Consequently ΔS values will always be encountered in the units $\mathrm{J\,K^{-1}\,mol^{-1}}$ or $\mathrm{cal\,K^{-1}\,mol^{-1}}$ (the combination $\mathrm{cal\,K^{-1}\,mol^{-1}}$ is sometimes referred to as the *entropy unit*, abbreviated e.u.).

We will calculate the entropy changes accompanying phase changes, as when a solid melts (fusion) or a liquid evaporates (vaporization). These processes can be carried out reversibly at constant temperature (the temperature being called the melting point, T_m, for fusion, or the boiling point, T_b, for vaporization.[5] The system is not isolated, because heat must be supplied in order that the process take place. The heat supplied in the fusion process is ΔH_f, the heat of fusion; whereas ΔH_v, the heat of vaporization, is furnished in the vaporization process. These enthalpy changes are expressed on a per mole basis. Many experimental ΔH_f and ΔH_v values are available in the common reference handbooks.

From Eq. (2.14) applied to our present concern we can write

$$\Delta S_\mathrm{f} = \frac{\Delta H_\mathrm{f}}{T_\mathrm{m}} \tag{2.19}$$

$$\Delta S_\mathrm{v} = \frac{\Delta H_\mathrm{v}}{T_\mathrm{b}} \tag{2.20}$$

Table 2.2 shows enthalpy data for a few phase changes.

Example 2.1. Calculate the entropy of fusion of benzoic acid.

$$\Delta S_\mathrm{f} = \frac{\Delta H_\mathrm{f}}{T_\mathrm{m}} = \frac{4320\ \mathrm{cal\,mol^{-1}}}{395.25\ \mathrm{K}} = +10.93\ \mathrm{cal\,K^{-1}\,mol^{-1}}$$

Table 2.3 gives ΔS_f and ΔS_v results for the processes described in Table 2.2.

Table 2.2. Heats of fusion and vaporization for some solids and liquids

Substance	mp[a] (°C)	ΔH_f (kcal mol^{-1})	bp[b] (°C)	ΔH_V (kcal mol^{-1})
Benzoic acid	122.1	4.32	—	—
Phenol	40.9	2.75	—	—
Acetone	—	—	56.2	6.95
Water	0.0	1.436	100.0	9.717

[a]Melting point.
[b]Boiling point.

Table 2.3. Entropies of fusion and vaporization

Substance	ΔS_f (cal K^{-1} mol^{-1})	ΔS_v (cal K^{-1} mol^{-1})
Benzoic acid	+10.93	—
Phenol	+8.76	—
Acetone	—	+21.11
Water	+5.26	+26.04

It has been known since 1884 that for very many nonassociated liquids (i.e., liquids whose molecules do not interact strongly with each other), $\Delta S_v \approx 21\,\mathrm{cal\,K^{-1}\,mol^{-1}}$. This empirical observation is known as *Trouton's rule*, and it provides a simple though approximate estimate of ΔH_v by means of Eq. (2.20), since the boiling point is easily measured. Such a convenient generalization cannot be made for ΔS_f values, although some definite patterns have been observed [see Yalkowski and Valvani (1980); in Chapter 10 we make use of these observations].

Notice that all ΔS_f and ΔS_v values are positive, because the system in each case is proceeding from a state of relative order to a state of relative disorder. Molecules in the liquid state possess a larger number of accessible quantum states (both configurational and thermal) than in the more restricted solid state, and similarly for the vaporization process.

We will subsequently learn how to calculate ΔS for chemical reactions, where we will find that ΔS can be either positive or negative, just as with ΔH values, depending on the direction in which the reaction is written. Very generally we anticipate that if the product state (the right-hand side of the equation) possesses more particles (molecules or ions) than the reactant state, ΔS will be positive, reflecting the availability to the system of more microstates.

PROBLEMS

2.1. Predict the sign of ΔS for these processes.

(a) Crystallization of benzoic acid from its melt.

(b) Evaporation of spilled gasoline.

(c) This chemical reaction:

$$Me_2C{=}CH_2 + Cl_2 \rightarrow Me_2CClCH_2Cl$$

2.2. Look up the boiling point of benzene, and estimate its molar heat of vaporization.

2.3. The heat of fusion of 4-nitroaniline is $5.04\,kcal\,mol^{-1}$. Look up its melting point, and calculate its entropy of fusion.

2.4. Sublimation is the process in which a solid is transformed directly to the vapor state. The heat of sublimation of naphthalene is $17.6\,kcal\,mol^{-1}$ at 25°C. Calculate its entropy of sublimation.

2.5. Calculate the entropy change during the isothermal expansion of 0.5 mol of an ideal gas from 100 ml to 1 L.

2.6. The heat capacity of chloroform in the vicinity of 600 K is $20.4\,cal\,K^{-1}\,mol^{-1}$. Calculate the entropy change per mole when chloroform is brought from 550 to 625 K.

2.7. Derive an equation for the molar entropy change when the pressure on an ideal gas is isothermally changed from P_1 to P_2 atm. [*Hint*: Start with Eq. (2.4).]

NOTES

1. We are making the unstated assumption that the molecules behave independently, so that each has a probability of $\frac{1}{2}$ of being in the left chamber. The probability that both will be in the left chamber is the product of the individual probabilities.

2. Probability theory gives a simple expression for calculating the number of ways N objects can be distributed into n_1 of type 1, n_2 of type 2, and so on; this is the expression:

$$\frac{N!}{n_1!n_2!\ldots}$$

where $N!$ is read N factorial, and is the product $1 \cdot 2 \cdot 3 \cdot 4 \cdots (N-1) \cdot N$. For our system this gives $8!/4!4! = 70$.

3. In making this statement we are neglecting concurrent energy changes; specifically, we are assuming $\Delta U = 0$ (for the present). Note also that we measure *changes* in entropy, ΔS, so the statement says that if ΔS is positive, the process is spontaneous.

4. The concept of entropy was introduced by Clausius in 1854, and he introduced the word *entropy* in 1865. This is how Clausius expressed the first and second laws:

Die Energie der Welt ist constant.
Die Entropie der Welt strebt einem Maximum zu.

5. The boiling point is commonly considered to be the temperature at which the liquid and vapor are in equilibrium at atmospheric pressure. However, Eq. (2.20) can also be applied to data at other pressures, with the appropriate temperature inserted.

3

THE FREE ENERGY

3.1. PROPERTIES OF THE FREE ENERGY

The Gibbs Free Energy. We have seen that for a mechanical system (which consists of relatively few bodies or "particles") the condition for a spontaneous process is that the potential energy change be negative, whereas for a chemical system (which consists of an almost unimaginably large number of particles) we learned that, even when no energy change occurs, spontaneous processes can take place, and we concluded that spontaneous processes occur with an increase in entropy. Now we are going to bring this together, recognizing that there are two factors involved in determining the direction of chemical change: the system seeks to minimize its energy *and* to maximize its entropy, and the position of equilibrium depends upon a combination of (and perhaps a compromise between) these factors. Several thermodynamic functions have been proposed to describe the situation, but we will make use of only one of these, which is particularly useful for our purposes because it invokes the commonly controlled experimental conditions of temperature and pressure. This function, termed *Gibbs free energy G,*[1] is defined as follows:

$$G = H - TS \tag{3.1}$$

This equation is actually a definition. Since H, T, and S are state functions, G is also a state function. As seen from its definition, the Gibbs free energy (which is often referred to simply as the "free energy" for convenience) is an energy quantity. We are, for the present, restricting attention to a closed system, which is one across whose boundaries no matter is exchanged with the surroundings.

Since by definition $H = U + PV$, Eq. (3.1) can be written

$$G = U + PV - TS \tag{3.2}$$

and its complete differential is

$$dG = dU + P\,dV + V\,dP - T\,dS - S\,dT \tag{3.3}$$

We saw earlier [Eq. (2.12)] that if the only work done in a reversible process is work of expansion, the first law can be written

$$dU = T\,dS - P\,dV \tag{3.4}$$

which, combined with Eq. (3.3), gives

$$dG = V\,dP - S\,dT \tag{3.5}$$

Equation (3.5) shows how the free-energy change depends on changes in the pressure and the temperature for a reversible process in a closed system.[2] If the temperature is constant, $dT = 0$, and from Eq. (3.5)

$$\left(\frac{\partial G}{\partial P}\right)_T = V \tag{3.6}$$

If the pressure is constant, $dP = 0$, and from Eq. (3.5), we obtain

$$\left(\frac{\partial G}{\partial T}\right)_P = -S \tag{3.7}$$

From the definition Eq. (3.1), if the temperature is constant, we obtain

$$dG = dH - T\,dS \tag{3.8}$$

or, in incremental form

$$\Delta G = \Delta H - T\,\Delta S \tag{3.9}$$

This last equation is an especially useful relationship because experimentally we measure these incremental quantities. Observe in this equation how ΔG, the change in free energy, is composed of an energy component, ΔH, and an entropic term, $-T\,\Delta S$.

We can obtain some insight into the meaning of free energy from the following development. We can write the work done by or on the system as

$$dw = dw_{\text{expansion}} + dw_{\text{additional}}$$

where $dw_{expansion} = P\,dV$ and $dw_{additional}$ represents work other than $P\,dV$ work (such as electrical work). The first law is $dU = dq - dw$, and for a reversible process $dq = T\,dS$. Combining these relationships gives

$$-dw_{additional} = dU + P\,dV - T\,dS$$

But $dU + P\,dV = dH$, so finally, by comparison with Eq. (3.8), we have $-dG = dw_{additional}$.

It is for this reason that the free energy change is said to be a measure of the maximum work available from a process (exclusive of work of expansion). That is, $-dG = dw - P\,dV$. When the system can do no useful work, $dG = 0$; a spontaneous process has a negative value of dG (or of ΔG). In a chemical reaction the approach to the position of equilibrium may be from either direction, depending on the initial conditions (i.e., the concentration of the reacting species). Figure 3.1 shows this schematically.

The essential characteristic of the Gibbs free-energy function is its combination of both the energy and entropy components in a form that reveals how these two thermodynamic concepts compete to generate a compromise that determines the position of equilibrium in a chemical process.[3] A more negative ΔH favors spontaneous reaction, and a more positive ΔS favors spontaneous reaction, in both instances by making ΔG more negative.

We are now in a position to better understand our earlier calculations of entropies of fusion and vaporization. These systems were at equilibrium, so $\Delta G = 0$, and, from Eq. (3.9), $\Delta S = \Delta H/T$.

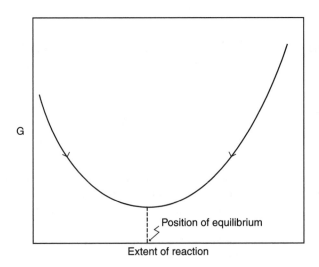

G

Position of equilibrium

Extent of reaction

Figure 3.1. Free energy of a reacting chemical system, showing how the direction of the reaction depends on the initial state of the system.

Pressure Dependence of the Free Energy. From either Eq. (3.5) or Eq. (3.6), at constant temperature,

$$dG = V\,dP \tag{3.10}$$

Now let us consider the special case of one mole of an ideal gas, so $PV = RT$ and $V = RT/P$, giving

$$dG = RT\,\frac{dP}{P} = RT\,d\ln P \tag{3.11}$$

Integrating between the limits of P_1 and P_2, we obtain

$$\Delta G = RT\,\ln\frac{P_2}{P_1} \tag{3.12}$$

which could alternatively have been integrated to the form

$$G = G^* + RT\,\ln P \tag{3.13}$$

where G^* is the constant of integration.

Although Eqs. (3.12) and (3.13) apply only to ideal gases, the mathematical form of these equations turns out to be ubiquitous, and we will subsequently encounter the form of Eq. (3.13) in several contexts.

Temperature Dependence of the Free Energy. If the definition $G = H - TS$ is combined with Eq. (3.7), we obtain

$$G = H + T\left(\frac{\partial G}{\partial T}\right)_P \tag{3.14}$$

Next divide through by T^2 and rearrange to the form of Eq. (3.15):

$$-\frac{G}{T^2} + \frac{1}{T}\left(\frac{\partial G}{\partial T}\right)_P = -\frac{H}{T^2} \tag{3.15}$$

Now we call attention to the nonobvious fact that the left-hand side of Eq. (3.15) is equal to the derivative $d(G/T)/dT$:

$$\frac{d(G/T)}{dT} = -\frac{G}{T^2} + \frac{1}{T}\frac{dG}{dT} \tag{3.16}$$

Combining Eqs. (3.15) and (3.16) therefore yields

$$\left[\frac{\partial(G/T)}{\partial T}\right]_P = -\frac{H}{T^2} \tag{3.17}$$

The incremental form of Eq. (3.17) is

$$\left[\frac{\partial(\Delta G/T)}{\partial T}\right]_P = -\frac{\Delta H}{T^2} \tag{3.18}$$

Equations (3.14), (3.17), and (3.18) are equivalent forms of the *Gibbs–Helmholtz equation*. We will later make use of Eq. (3.18).

3.2. THE CHEMICAL POTENTIAL

Definition of the Chemical Potential. All of the relationships that we have seen to this point deal with closed systems (no matter can enter or leave the system) in complete internal equilibrium (no chemical reactions are occurring in the system). But of course we are very interested in chemical reactions, and we would also like to be able to describe open systems, in which matter may be exchanged between the system and its surroundings. In order to do this we expand our concept of the free energy to include the amounts (numbers of moles) of the chemical constituents of the system, writing

$$G = f(T, P, n_1, n_2, \ldots) \tag{3.19}$$

where n_1 is the number of moles of chemical substance 1, and so on. From Eq. (3.19) we write out the total differential

$$dG = \left(\frac{\partial G}{\partial T}\right)_{P,n_1,n_2,\ldots} dT + \left(\frac{\partial G}{\partial P}\right)_{T,n_1,n_2,\ldots} dP + \left(\frac{\partial G}{\partial n_1}\right)_{T,P,n_2,\ldots} dn_1$$

$$+ \left(\frac{\partial G}{\partial n_2}\right)_{T,P,n_1,\ldots} dn_2 + \cdots \tag{3.20}$$

where the subscripts indicate the quantities that are held constant during the evaluation of the partial derivatives. We have already dealt with the partial derivatives $(\partial G/\partial T)$ and $(\partial G/\partial P)$, and now we turn our attention to the new quantities appearing in Eq. (3.20). These partial derivatives are called *partial molar free energies*. They have this significance: they represent the change in the total free energy of the system when one mole of constituent $i(i = 1, 2, \ldots)$ is added while T, P, and all other constituent amounts are held constant. This quantity is so important that it has been given the special name *chemical potential* and its own symbol μ. Thus we define[4]

$$\left(\frac{\partial G}{\partial n_i}\right)_{T,P,n_j \neq n_i} = \mu_i \tag{3.21}$$

Now let us rewrite eq. (3.20), making use of eqs. (3.6), (3.7), and (3.21):

$$dG = -S\,dT + V\,dP + \mu_1\,dn_1 + \mu_2\,dn_2 + \cdots \qquad (3.22)$$

which can be written more succinctly as

$$dG = -S\,dT + V\,dP + \sum \mu_i\,dn_i \qquad (3.23)$$

The chemical potential μ is an intensive property, its units being energy per mole, as can be seen from its definition, Eq. (3.21).

Now let us consider Eq. (3.22) at constant temperature and pressure:

$$dG_{T,P} = \mu_1\,dn_1 + \mu_2\,dn_2 + \cdots \qquad (3.24)$$

On integration this gives

$$G_{T,P} = n_1\,\mu_1 + n_2\,\mu_2 + \cdots \qquad (3.25)$$

which can be generally differentiated to give

$$dG_{T,P} = (n_1\,d\mu_1 + \mu_1\,dn_1) + (n_2\,d\mu_2 + \mu_2\,dn_2) + \cdots \qquad (3.26)$$

which is rearranged to

$$dG_{T,P} = (n_1\,d\mu_1 + n_2\,d\mu_2 + \cdots) + (\mu_1\,dn_1 + \mu_2\,dn_2 + \cdots) \qquad (3.27)$$

Comparison of Eqs. (3.24) and (3.27) leads to

$$n_1\,d\mu_1 + n_2\,d\mu_2 + \cdots = 0 \qquad (3.28)$$

This last equation is called the *Gibbs–Duhem equation*.

Dependence of Chemical Potential on Pressure. We had earlier applied Eq. (3.6), reproduced here, to establish the dependence of the free energy of a closed system on pressure [Eq. (3.13)]:

$$\left(\frac{\partial G}{\partial P}\right)_T = V \qquad (3.29)$$

We are now interested in mixtures, that is, systems of more than one substance, so we must make use of chemical potentials (partial molar free energies). We state without derivation the analog to Eq. (3.29), which is intuitively evident[4]

$$\left(\frac{\partial \mu_i}{\partial P}\right)_T = \bar{V}_i \tag{3.30}$$

where $\bar{V}_i$ is the *partial molar volume* of substance i. The physical interpretation of this quantity is that it is the volume per mole of i at the composition specified. (In general, $\bar{V}_i$ is not equal to V_i, the molar volume of pure i, because of intermolecular interactions in the mixture.)

Now let us consider a mixture of ideal gases. From Eq. (3.30), the variation in chemical potential for constituent i can be written $d\mu_i = \bar{V}_i \, dP$, where P is the total pressure. Since the total number of moles n in the ideal-gas equation $PV = nRT$ is just the sum $(n_1 + n_2 + \cdots)$, we obtain

$$V = (n_1 + n_2 + \cdots)\frac{RT}{P}$$

so the partial molar volume of i is

$$\bar{V}_i = \left(\frac{\partial V}{\partial n_i}\right)_{T,P,n_j \neq n_i} = \frac{RT}{P} \tag{3.31}$$

which is nicely simple (because we are dealing with ideal gases). Therefore we can write

$$d\mu_i = \bar{V}_i \, dP = RT\frac{dP}{P} = RT \, d \ln P \tag{3.32}$$

For a mixture of ideal gases, we have

$$p_i = x_i P \tag{3.33}$$

where p_i is the partial pressure of gas i and x_i is its mole fraction. At constant x_i, therefore, $d \ln p_i = d \ln P$, giving, from Eq. (3.32)

$$d\mu_i = RT \, d \ln p_i \tag{3.34}$$

which is integrated to

$$\mu_i = \mu_i^* + RT \ln p_i \tag{3.35}$$

where μ_i^* is the constant of integration. According to Eq. (3.35), the chemical potential of i is logarithmically related to its partial pressure. The value of μ_i^*

can be evaluated by setting $p_i = 1$ atm; then we see that μ_i^* is the chemical potential of gas i when $p_i = 1$ atm.

Although these ideas seem rather remote from our main interests, they are leading to an important result. In particular, Eq. (3.35), and its predecessor Eq. (3.13), possess the general form

$$\mu_i = \text{constant} + RT \ln (\text{composition variable})$$

which will recur in important contexts. We will also have to pay some attention to the constant term.

The Fugacity. In the development leading to Eq. (3.35), we supposed that we were dealing with a mixture of ideal gases, and the resulting expression for the chemical potential was very simple. In real circumstances gases are not ideal (although at low pressures their behavior may closely approach ideality). We therefore must accept that Eq. (3.35) will not be an exact description for real-gas mixtures. The simplicity of the equation is so attractive, however, that standard practice is to preserve the form of the equation by replacing the partial pressure p_i with a quantity symbolized f_i and called the *fugacity*. Thus Eq. (3.35) applied to real gases becomes

$$\mu_i = \mu_i^* + RT \ln f_i \tag{3.36}$$

The fugacity may be thought of as a measure of the "escaping tendency" of the gaseous constituent (consider Latin *fugio*, to flee; Italian *fuggire*, to flee; French *fugace*, fleeting; English *fugitive*). Again μ_i^* is the value of μ_i when the logarithmic term vanishes, that is, when $f_i = 1$. Of course, when $f_i = 1$, p_i probably does not equal 1 for a real gas, but as the pressure becomes smaller, p_i and f_i approach each other, and ultimately as $p_i \to 0$, $f_i/p_i \to 1$. Thus the ratio f_i/p_i is a measure of the extent of nonideal behavior of gas i in the mixture.

Experimental methods are available for the measurement of fugacities. We will not pursue this aspect of the problem, except to note that fugacity has the units of pressure.

Activity and Activity Coefficient. We now turn to liquid mixtures, which are of great importance in pharmaceutical, chemical, and biological systems. Equation (3.36) applies to each constituent in a liquid solution because (as we will prove in Chapter 4) at equilibrium the chemical potential of each constituent is equal in the liquid phase and in the vapor phase in contact with it; therefore the fugacity f_i of component i is the same in the liquid and the vapor phases. But it is more convenient to express the chemical potential in a liquid solution in terms of a quantity having units more familiar than those of pressure. We therefore build on the foregoing developments, anticipating that the form of Eq. (3.36) is applicable, to write, for constituent i in a liquid mixture,

$$\mu_i = \mu_i^\circ + RT \ln a_i \tag{3.37}$$

This equation is of great importance to us. The quantity a_i is called the *activity* of constituent i, μ_i is its chemical potential, and μ_i° is the *standard chemical potential* of i. Evidently $\mu_i^\circ = \mu_i$ when $a_i = 1$. Of course, the activity a_i and the chemical potential μ_i depend on the conditions of temperature, pressure, and composition of the system.

At this stage in our treatment the activity is still a concept without a context. Let us relate this concept to an experimental observable by focusing attention on a solution of solute i in a liquid solvent. Let c_i be the concentration (in $\mathrm{mol\,L^{-1}}$) of the solute. Then we write the activity of i as

$$a_i = \gamma_i c_i \tag{3.38}$$

where γ_i, a proportionality constant, is called the *activity coefficient*. Combining Eqs. (3.37) and (3.38), we obtain

$$\mu_i = \mu_i^\circ + RT \ln \gamma_i c_i \tag{3.39}$$

Why do we need the activity and the activity coefficient at all? Why not just write

$$\mu_i = \mu_i^\circ + RT \ln c_i \tag{3.40}$$

The answer to these questions is that real solutions do not behave ideally (just as real gases do not behave ideally). When treating gases we replaced the pressure p_i with the fugacity f_i, and saw that the ratio f_i/p_i is a measure of nonideal behavior. Now in treating liquids we replace the concentration c_i with the activity a_i, and use the ratio $a_i/c_i = \gamma_i$ as a measure of nonideal behavior. The source of the nonideal behavior is the noncovalent forces of interaction between molecules and ions. These interactions perturb the chemical and physical properties of the molecules characteristic of their isolated states, when they are sufficiently far apart that they are not sensibly affected by other particles. We therefore expect that deviations from ideal behavior will become greater as the molecules are forced closer together, which will happen as the pressure increases (for gases) or as the concentration increases (for liquids).

Let us now return to our consideration of Eqs. (3.37) and (3.39). At the moment we cannot use these equations, because the only quantity that we presumably know is the concentration c_i. It is necessary to introduce some definitions and to adopt some conventions. First, here are the definitions:

The *standard state* (with respect to constituent i) is that state of the system in which $a_i = 1$; then $\mu_i = \mu_i^\circ$.

The *reference state* (with respect to constituent i) is that state of the system in which $\gamma_i = 1$; then $a_i = c_i$.

From this point on, the rigor with which applications are made depends on the level of accuracy required in the results. Here are conventions that provide realistic approximations for practical calculations that do not require the highest accuracy.

1. The fugacity of a *gas* may be taken equal to its pressure (or partial pressure) in atm, at low to moderate pressures.
2. The activity of a liquid *solvent* in a solution is equal to its mole fraction. It follows that the activity of a pure liquid is 1.00.
3. The activity of a pure *solid* is 1.00. (This is consistent with convention 2.)
4. The activity of a *solute* in an infinitely dilute liquid solution (concentrations of $\sim \leq 10^{-4}$ M may be considered infinitely dilute for this purpose) may be taken equal to its molar concentration. Thus, $\gamma_i = 1.00$; the solute is in its reference state.
5. The activity coefficient of an uncharged solute may be taken as 1.00 at any concentration (because uncharged molecules experience much weaker forces of interaction than do ions).

The reference state of a solute is usually taken to be the infinitely dilute solution, so that $\gamma_i \to 1$ as $c_i \to 0$. (Activity coefficients of ions are more complex than has been implied by our treatment, as a consequence of the impossibility of experimentally studying an ionic solution of either a cation or an anion by itself.) Table 3.1 (Harned and Owen 1958, pp. 484, 488) lists some experimental values of activity coefficients to give a sense of the extent to which solution behavior may depart from ideality. It is also possible to calculate theoretically the activity coefficients of ions by means of the Debye–Hückel theory. Chapter 8 treats ionic activity coefficients in more detail.

Table 3.1. Activity coefficients of hydrochloric acid and sodium chloride in aqueous solutions at 25°C

	γ	
m^a	HCl	NaCl
0.001	0.965	—
0.002	0.952	—
0.005	0.928	0.928
0.007	—	0.917
0.01	0.905	0.903
0.02	0.875	0.873
0.03	—	0.851
0.04	—	0.835
0.05	0.831	0.822
0.06	—	0.812
0.08	—	0.794
0.10	0.797	0.780

[a] Molality.

Source: Harned and Owen (1958, pp. 484, 488).

Table 3.2. Equations relating chemical potentials to composition variables

System	Equation	Equation Number
Pure ideal gas	$G = G^* + RT \ln P$	(3.13)
Mixture of ideal gases	$\mu_i = \mu_i^* + RT \ln p_i$	(3.35)
Mixture of real gases	$\mu_i = \mu_i^* + RT \ln f_i$	(3.36)
Ideal liquid mixture	$\mu_i = \mu_i^\circ + RT \ln c_i$	(3.40)
Real liquid mixture	$\mu_i = \mu_i^\circ + RT \ln a_i$	(3.37)
Real liquid mixture	$\mu_i = \mu_i^\circ + RT \ln \gamma_i c_i$	(3.39)

In most of the practical situations of interest to us we deal with mixtures, so the proper notation and terminology consists of μ, the chemical potential, and $\Delta\mu$, the change in chemical potential. For pure substances, there is no difference between μ and G, the molar free energy, or between $\Delta\mu$ and ΔG. In common practice we tend to be careless and to use G and ΔG where we really should be using μ and $\Delta\mu$, but this should cause no confusion. Note, however, that when we are talking about the free energy or free-energy change of the *system*, G or ΔG is appropriate even for mixtures. The chemical potential rightly applies to specific constituents of the mixture.

It may be helpful to collect the several equations having the form characteristic of (e.g.) Eq. (3.37). Table 3.2 lists these equations.

PROBLEMS

3.1. Calculate the activity of 0.02 m HCl at 25°C.

3.2. Calculate the free-energy change accompanying the process

$$NaCl(0.005\,m) \rightarrow NaCl(0.05\,m)$$

3.3. Estimate the free-energy difference $\Delta\mu = \mu - \mu^\circ$ for a solution 0.25 M in sucrose.

3.4. On the basis of the results of Problems 3.2 and 3.3, comment on the spontaneity or nonspontaneity of making a solution more concentrated.

NOTES

1. After J. Willard Gibbs, a physicist at Yale University, who provided much of the theoretical development of thermodynamics and statistical mechanics in the second half of the nineteenth century. The *Helmholtz free energy A*, defined $A = U - TS$, is more useful than G under conditions of constant volume. We will not make use of A (but see also note 2).

2. Each of the functions U, H, G, and A can be written in parallel form as a function of two variables, namely (for closed systems)

$$dU = T\,dS - P\,dV$$
$$dH = T\,dS + V\,dP$$
$$dA = -S\,dT - P\,dV$$
$$dG = V\,dP - S\,dT$$

These all contain the same information, but it is because G is expressible as a function of the variables P and T that we find it especially useful. If a system is at equilibrium, any infinitesimal change is reversible. The preceding four relationships, which are called *characteristic functions*, provide equivalent criteria for equilibrium. From the first one, at constant entropy and volume (i.e., $dS = 0, dV = 0$), the condition for equilibrium is $dU = 0$. From the second, at constant entropy and pressure, $dH = 0$ defines equilibrium; from the third, at constant temperature and volume, $dA = 0$ at equilibrium; finally, at constant pressure and temperature, the condition for equilibrium is $dG = 0$.

3. It is not too fanciful to draw an analogy with a political science setting, in which each society must choose its own compromise position between the extremes of maximum security (the energy component) and maximum liberty (the entropy component).

4. Partial molar quantities are sometimes indicated with the conventional letter symbol and a bar above it, so the chemical potential μ_i may also be written $\bar{G}_i$.

4

EQUILIBRIUM

4.1. CONDITIONS FOR EQUILIBRIUM

We have concluded that a spontaneous process, at constant temperature and pressure, possesses a negative value of dG (or of ΔG), and that the condition for equilibrium is that $dG = 0$ (or $\Delta G = 0$). We are now going to examine some specific systems to uncover an important consequence of the preceding statements.

First, suppose that the system consists of a single pure substance at constant temperature and pressure, the substance existing (at this temperature and pressure) in two phases at equilibrium. A solid and its melt at the melting point, or a liquid and its vapor at the boiling point, are the most common examples of such a system. We will use the solid (s)–liquid (l) equilibrium in what follows. Since the system is at equilibrium, we know that $\Delta G = 0$, where ΔG is the free energy change per mole associated with the process. Writing the process as

$$\text{Solid} \rightleftharpoons \text{liquid}$$

we have, from our general definition of incremental change in a process,

$$\Delta G = G_l - G_s$$

where G_l and G_s are the molar free energies of the substance in the liquid and solid phases, respectively. But since $\Delta G = 0$, we conclude

$$G_s = G_l \tag{4.1}$$

at equilibrium. Thus, for a pure substance, whenever two (or three) phases are in equilibrium, at fixed temperature and pressure, the molar free energy of the substance has the same value in each phase.

Now we will extend this argument to a closed system at constant temperature and pressure, where the system is at equilibrium and contains P phases ($P = a, b, c, \ldots$) and C components ($C = 1, 2, 3, \ldots$).[1] Since this is a mixture, we use chemical potentials (partial molar free energies) rather than molar free energies. Imagine infinitesimally small amounts dn of components being transferred from one phase to another. Since the system remains at equilibrium during this reversible process, $dG = 0$, and we write out Eq. (3.24) for the system, obtaining (Glasstone 1947, p. 238)

$$\begin{aligned}
&\mu_{1(a)}dn_{1(a)} + \mu_{1(b)}dn_{1(b)} + \cdots + \mu_{1(P)}dn_{1(P)} \\
&+ \mu_{2(a)}dn_{2(a)} + \mu_{2(b)}dn_{2(b)} + \cdots + \mu_{2(P)}dn_{2(P)} \\
&\qquad\qquad \vdots \\
&+ \mu_{C(a)}dn_{C(a)} + \mu_{C(b)}dn_{C(b)} + \cdots + \mu_{C(P)}dn_{C(P)} = 0
\end{aligned} \tag{4.2}$$

which is succinctly written

$$\sum \mu_{C(P)}dn_{C(P)} = 0 \tag{4.3}$$

Since the system is closed, the total amount of each component is constant, giving

$$\begin{aligned}
dn_{1(a)} + dn_{1(b)} + \cdots + dn_{1(P)} &= 0 \\
dn_{2(a)} + dn_{2(b)} + \cdots + dn_{2(P)} &= 0 \\
\vdots \\
dn_{C(a)} + dn_{C(b)} + \cdots + dn_{C(P)} &= 0
\end{aligned} \tag{4.4}$$

or

$$\sum dn_{C(P)} = 0 \tag{4.5}$$

The only way in which Eqs. (4.2) and (4.4) [or Eqs. (4.3) and (4.5)] can simultaneously be satisfied is if

$$\begin{aligned}
\mu_{1(a)} &= \mu_{1(b)} = \cdots \mu_{1(P)} \\
\mu_{2(a)} &= \mu_{2(b)} = \cdots \mu_{2(P)} \\
\vdots \\
\mu_{C(a)} &= \mu_{C(b)} = \cdots \mu_{C(P)}
\end{aligned} \tag{4.6}$$

Thus, under these conditions (consisting of P phases, C components, where the closed system is at equilibrium at fixed temperature and pressure), *the chemical potential of each individual component has the same value in all phases.* This is an obvious generalization of our earlier result for a pure substance. Since, from Eq. (4.6), we have for component i, $\mu_{i(a)} = \mu_{i(b)} = \cdots \mu_{i(P)}$, it follows that, at equilibrium, $d\mu_i = 0$ for the transfer of an infinitesimal amount of component i from one phase to another.[2]

4.2. PHYSICAL PROCESSES

Phase Transitions (***Single Component***). We now return to a system consisting of a single component in a closed system at fixed temperature and pressure. This substance is capable of existing in three states of matter, the solid, the liquid, and the gas (vapor). The manner in which these states are controlled by the values of temperature and pressure is readily displayed on a pressure–temperature *phase diagram*. Figure 4.1 shows a schematic phase diagram. For each chemical substance the phase diagram must be experimentally determined.

Any selected pair of coordinates P, T determine the state of the system. Of special interest are those coordinates describing the lines in the phase diagram, for along these lines two phases coexist in equilibrium. Thus line OC describes the melting transition; at any point on this line the solid and liquid phases are in equilibrium, and the value of T corresponding to any given value of P is the *melting point* at that pressure. The line is very steep because the melting point is not very sensitive to pressure changes (i.e., the melting point does not change much when the pressure is changed).

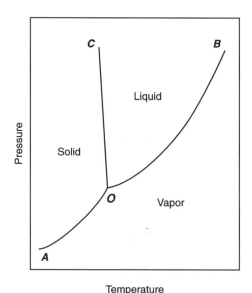

Figure 4.1. Pressure–temperature phase diagram of a pure substance.

Along the line OB the liquid and its vapor are in equilibrium, so the value of T on this line is the *boiling point* corresponding to the selected P value. Observe that the boiling point is quite sensitive to pressure.[3] Along the line OA the solid and the vapor are in equilibrium. The direct conversion of solid to vapor is called *sublimation*.[4] At point O all three phases coexist in equilibrium. This is obviously a unique set of circumstances; it is called the *triple point*. The triple point of water is 273.16 K (i.e., 0.01°C) and 4.58 mm Hg pressure.

Now we treat phase transitions thermodynamically. Consider a pure substance at temperature and pressure such that two phases, 1 and 2 (which may be gas, liquid, or solid), are in equilibrium. Thus $G_1 = G_2$, and so $dG_1 = dG_2$, which means that if the temperature or pressure is changed infinitesimally, the changes in free energy of the two phases will be identical and the phases will remain in equilibrium. From Eq. (3.5) we write $dG = V\,dP - S\,dT$, or

$$V_1\,dP - S_1\,dT = V_2\,dP - S_2\,dT$$

Rearranging, we obtain

$$\Delta S\,dT = \Delta V\,dP$$

where $\Delta S = S_2 - S_1$ and $\Delta V = V_2 - V_1$. Therefore

$$\frac{dP}{dT} = \frac{\Delta S}{\Delta V} \tag{4.7}$$

But the system is at equilibrium, so $\Delta G = \Delta H - T\,\Delta S = 0$, giving $\Delta S = \Delta H/T$, or, from Eq. (4.7)

$$\frac{dP}{dT} = \frac{\Delta H}{T\,\Delta V} \tag{4.8}$$

This is the *Clapeyron equation*. It describes the slope of the line in the phase diagram for a pure substance.

The Clapeyron equation is especially useful when applied to the liquid–vapor transition (boiling), and in this application we usually can employ an approximate version. Writing Eq. (4.8) specifically for this transition, we obtain

$$\frac{dP}{dT} = \frac{\Delta H_{vap}}{T\,\Delta V_{vap}} \tag{4.9}$$

where T is the boiling temperature and $\Delta V_{vap} = V_{vapor} - V_{liquid}$. We neglect the molar volume of the liquid as being very small relative to the molar volume of the vapor. We also will assume that the vapor phase behaves ideally, so $V_{vap} = RT/P$. Combining these approximations with Eq. (4.9) yields

$$\frac{1}{P}\frac{dP}{dT} = \frac{\Delta H_{vap}}{RT^2} \tag{4.10}$$

or

$$\frac{d \ln P}{d T} = \frac{\Delta H_{vap}}{RT^2} \tag{4.11}$$

These two equations are versions of the *Clausius-Clapeyron equation*, which relates the boiling point T to the vapor pressure P.

If ΔH_{vap} should happen to be essentially constant (independent of temperature), we can integrate the Clausius–Clapeyron equation. First integrating generally gives

$$\ln P = -\frac{\Delta H_{vap}}{RT} + \text{constant} \tag{4.12}$$

or

$$\log P = -\frac{\Delta H_{vap}}{2.3\,RT} + C \tag{4.13}$$

where C is a constant. Equations (4.12) or (4.13) provide a means for evaluating the molar heat of vaporization ΔH_{vap} from vapor pressure-temperature data.

Example 4.1. Table 4.1 gives vapor pressure–temperature data for *n*-octane. Calculate ΔH_{vap}.

Figure 4.2 is a plot of the data according to Eq. (4.13). From the plot we evaluate the slope as $-2091\ K$. Equation (4.13) shows this identity:

$$\text{Slope} = -\frac{\Delta H_{vap}}{2.3R}$$

Thus we calculate

$$\Delta H_{vap} = -2.3(1.987\ \text{cal mol}^{-1}\ \text{K}^{-1})(-2091\ \text{K})$$
$$= 9568\ \text{cal mol}^{-1}$$
$$= 9.57\ \text{kcal mol}^{-1}$$
$$= 40.0\ \text{kJ mol}^{-1}$$

Table 4.1   Vapor pressure–temperature data for *n*-octane

t (°C)	T (K)	$1/T$	P (mm Hg)	$\log [P$ (mm Hg)$]$
−14.0	259.15	0.00386	1	0.000
+19.2	292.35	0.00342	10	1.000
45.1	318.25	0.00314	40	1.602
65.7	338.85	0.00295	100	2.000
104.0	377.15	0.00265	400	2.602
125.6	398.75	0.00251	760	2.881

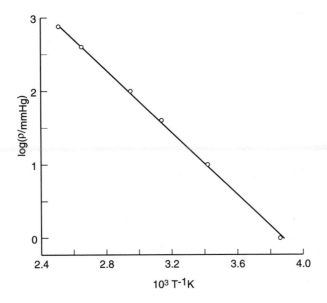

Figure 4.2. Plot of Eq. (4.13) for *n*-octane. Data from Table 4.1.

The heat of vaporization is positive because heat is absorbed by the system during the vaporization process.

We can also integrate the Clausius–Clapeyron equation between the limits T_1 and T_2, presuming that ΔH_{vap} is essentially constant in this temperature range. From Eq. (4.11), we obtain

$$\int_{P_1}^{P_2} d \ln P = \frac{\Delta H_{\text{vap}}}{R} \int_{T_1}^{T_2} \frac{dT}{T^2}$$

which gives

$$\ln \frac{P_2}{P_1} = -\frac{\Delta H_{\text{vap}}}{R} \left(\frac{1}{T_2} - \frac{1}{T_1} \right) = \frac{\Delta H_{\text{vap}}}{R} \left(\frac{T_2 - T_1}{T_1 T_2} \right) \qquad (4.14)$$

or

$$\log \frac{P_2}{P_1} = \frac{\Delta H_{\text{vap}}}{2.3R} \left(\frac{T_2 - T_1}{T_1 T_2} \right) \qquad (4.15)$$

Example 4.2. The vapor pressure of water is 17.535 mm Hg at 20.0°C and 31.824 mm Hg at 30.0°C. Calculate the heat of vaporization of water in this temperature interval.

Using Eq. (4.15), we have

$$\log \frac{31.824}{17.535} \doteq \frac{\Delta H_{vap}}{(2.3)(1.987)} \left(\frac{10}{293.15 \times 303.15} \right)$$
$$\Delta H_{vap} = 10,530 \, cal \, mol^{-1}$$
$$= 10.53 \, kcal \, mol^{-1}$$

In Examples 4.1 and 4.2 we see how heats of transition are determined. With such ΔH values at hand, we can calculate entropies of transition as shown in Example 2.1.

The Phase Rule (Multiple Components). We have already developed the condition for equilibrium in a system at equilibrium containing multiple phases and components; the condition is that the chemical potential of each component be the same in all phases [Eq. (4.6)]. This will lead us to a general rule connecting the number of phases, the number of components, and the number of variables (this last variable is called the *degrees of freedom*) that must be specified in order to define the system completely (in a thermodynamic sense). Let P be the number of phases and C the number of components (see note 1). Here are the steps in the reasoning:

1. The composition of a phase containing C components can be specified by giving $C - 1$ concentrations. This is because the final concentration can be obtained by difference.
2. If there are P phases, in order to completely define the compositions of all phases, $P(C - 1)$ concentrations must be specified. This is the total number of concentration variables in the system.
3. To the $P(C - 1)$ concentration variables must be added the temperature and pressure variables. This gives us

$$\text{Total number of variables} = P(C - 1) + 2$$

4. Since for component 1 we know that $\mu_{1(phase \, a)} = \mu_{1(phase \, b)} = \dots$, and similarly for all C components, this condition gives $C(P - 1)$ independent equations, which fix $C(P - 1)$ variables.[5]
5. The number of variables left undetermined (i.e., the number of degrees of freedom) is equal to the total number of variables minus the number of variables that are determined by the equilibrium condition. Thus

$$\text{Number of degrees of freedom} = P(C - 1) + 2 - C(P - 1)$$

or

$$F = C - P + 2 \tag{4.16}$$

This last equation is the *phase rule* of Gibbs.

We will apply the phase rule to the phase diagram of Fig. 4.1 in order to learn how it works. First consider the liquid–gas equilibrium. There are two phases and one component, so $F = 1 - 2 + 2 = 1$. This means that specifying one degree of freedom suffices to completely define the system. If we choose to specify the temperature (as our one degree of freedom), the condition of equilibrium uniquely guarantees that the pressure will be fixed at the value given by the line OB corresponding to the specified temperature. Alternatively, we might have specified the pressure; then the temperature would be defined by the system. In this system as described we cannot independently choose both the temperature and the pressure.

Next consider the triple point O. Here $P = 3$ and $C = 1$, so $F = 0$. There is no freedom to alter the system variables while maintaining the system at the triple point.

A very practical kind of system is that of a pure solid substance placed in contact with a pure liquid, which we call the *solvent*. To be specific, let us add solid benzoic acid to water. Presuming that sufficient benzoic acid has been added so that at equilibrium some solid is present, how many degrees of freedom does the system possess?

The process that occurs is dissolution of benzoic acid in water. Evidently $P = 2$, for two phases, solid benzoic acid and liquid solution, are present. Moreover, $C = 2$, for the system can be prepared from benzoic acid and water. The phase rule gives us $F = 2 - 2 + 2 = 2$ degrees of freedom. These are the temperature and the pressure, both of which must be fixed in order to completely define the position of equilibrium of the system. (In practice this system is not very sensitive to pressure, which is commonly the ambient atmospheric pressure, but it is very sensitive to the temperature.) An equivalent description of this system is that at fixed temperature and pressure, the concentration of dissolved benzoic acid is invariant; no further degrees of freedom remain. We call this invariant dissolved concentration the *equilibrium solubility* of benzoic acid at the experimental temperature.

4.3. CHEMICAL EQUILIBRIUM

The Equilibrium Constant. We now turn to a treatment of chemical reactions, namely, processes in which chemical bonds (covalent bonds) or noncovalent interactions are formed or broken, or both. Because liquid systems are of special interest to us, suppose that the process occurs in a homogeneous (single phase) liquid system. Let the generalized balanced chemical reaction be written

$$aA + bB \rightleftharpoons mM + nN \tag{4.17}$$

where A and B represent the reactant chemical species; M and N are the product chemical species; and a, b, m, n are stoichiometric coefficients in the balanced reaction.[6] For the moment we do not require that the system be at equilibrium, but the temperature and pressure are fixed.

As is our usual practice, the incremental change in free energy is defined (on a per mole basis) as the difference between the final state and the initial state:

$$\Delta G = \sum G_{\text{products}} - \sum G_{\text{reactants}} \tag{4.18}$$

Recognizing that our reaction system is a mixture, we know that we should express the free energies of reactants and products in terms of chemical potentials; thus Eq. (4.18) becomes

$$\Delta G = m\mu_M + n\mu_N - a\mu_A - b\mu_B \tag{4.19}$$

Notice that each term on the right is the product of an intensity factor (e.g., μ_M, chemical potential per mole) and a capacity factor (m, number of moles).

Next we call on our fundamental relationship for the chemical potential in terms of activity [Eq. (3.37)]:

$$\mu_i = \mu_i^\circ + RT \ln a_i \tag{4.20}$$

We simply substitute from Eq. (4.20) into Eq. (4.19):

$$\Delta G = m\mu_M^\circ + m\,RT \ln a_M + n\mu_N^\circ + n\,RT \ln a_N \\ - a\mu_A^\circ - a\,RT \ln a_A - b\mu_B^\circ - b\,RT \ln a_B$$

Collecting terms and making use of one of the properties of logarithms gives

$$\Delta G = (m\mu_M^\circ + n\mu_N^\circ - a\mu_A^\circ - b\mu_B^\circ) \\ + RT \ln a_M^m + RT \ln a_N^n \\ - RT \ln a_A^a - RT \ln a_B^b$$

which can be written

$$\Delta G = \Delta G^\circ + RT \ln \frac{a_M^m a_N^n}{a_A^a a_B^b} \tag{4.21}$$

where $\Delta G^\circ = m\mu_M^\circ + n\mu_N^\circ - a\mu_A^\circ - b\mu_B^\circ.$[7] Equation (4.21) is called the *reaction isotherm* (the term *isotherm* merely signifies that the equation or phenomenon takes place at, or applies to a constant temperature).

Recall that we have not yet required that the system be at equilibrium. Equation (4.21) gives the free energy change as a function of the activities of reactants and products of the reaction. But it is the equilibrium condition that specifically interests us. Let the activities now be the activities at equilibrium, and define

$$K = \frac{a_M^m a_N^n}{a_A^a a_B^b} \tag{4.22}$$

Moreover, we recall that the condition for equilibrium is that $\Delta G = 0$. Putting this condition and the definition of Eq. (4.22) into Eq. (4.21) gives the simple but very important result

$$\Delta G^\circ = -RT \ln K \qquad (4.23)$$

The quantity K is called the *equilibrium constant* for the reaction; its general form can be inferred from Eq. (4.22). It is conventional to write the products in the numerator and the reactants in the denominator. Notice, therefore, that the reciprocal of K as thus defined is the equilibrium constant for the reaction when written in the reverse direction.

Equilibrium constants can be measured experimentally; in effect, one needs to determine each activity in the definition, and then to calculate K according to Eq. (4.22). Then, with Eq. (4.23), the quantity ΔG° (which is pronounced "delta G naught") is calculated. ΔG° is called the *standard free-energy change* for the reaction, and it is interpreted as the change in free energy, per mole, when the reactants in their standard states are transformed into the products in their standard states. This concept is difficult to visualize in physical terms, and it may be better to note the obvious, namely, that [see Eq. (4.23)] ΔG° and K contain the same information about the system. The logarithmic relationship between ΔG° and K, as well as the form of the equilibrium constant definition, is a direct consequence of the form of Eq. (4.20) for the chemical potential.

In the chemical literature many equilibrium constants are described by adjectives that provide information on the chemical process and on the definition of the constant. For example, a weak acid HA dissociates according to

$$\text{HA} \overset{K_a}{\rightleftharpoons} \text{H}^+ + \text{A}^-$$

Placing the equilibrium constant symbol over the arrows tells the reader how the constant is to be defined; in this case

$$K_a = \frac{a_{\text{H}^+} a_{\text{A}^-}}{a_{\text{HA}}} \qquad (4.24)$$

This particular equilibrium constant is called an *acid dissociation constant* (or *acid ionization constant*). For a reaction, especially a reaction involving noncovalent interactions, having the form

$$\text{A} + \text{B} \overset{K}{\rightleftharpoons} \text{M}$$

the equilibrium constant

$$K = \frac{a_{\text{M}}}{a_{\text{A}} a_{\text{B}}}$$

may be called an *association constant, formation constant, stability constant*, or *binding constant*. Turn the reaction around, and its equilibrium constant (which will be the reciprocal of K) becomes a dissociation constant or instability constant.

Example 4.3. For the acid dissociation of acetic acid in water at 25°C, the experimental value of K_a is 1.75×10^{-5}. Calculate $\Delta G°$ for this process.

We can use Eq. (4.23) directly or in the form

$$
\begin{aligned}
\Delta G° &= -2.303 \, RT \log K_a \\
&= -(2.303)(1.987 \, \text{cal mol}^{-1}\text{K}^{-1})(298.15 \, \text{K})(-4.757) \\
&= +6490 \, \text{cal mol}^{-1} \\
&= +6.49 \, \text{kcal mol}^{-1}
\end{aligned}
\tag{4.25}
$$

From either Eq. (4.23) or (4.25) we obtain these correspondences:

If $K < 1$, $\Delta G° > 0$.
If $K = 1$, $\Delta G° = 0$.
If $K > 1$, $\Delta G° < 0$.

In Example 4.3, $\Delta G°$ has a positive sign because K is smaller than unity. This tells us that, at equilibrium, the reactant state is "favored" in this process.

The units of the equilibrium constant require comment. From its definition in terms of activities, it is clear that we need to know the units of activities. Our earlier conventions concerning standard states and reference states provide guidance. Evidently the activities of solvents and solids, which are taken equal to their mole fractions in practical work, are dimensionless, because the mole fraction is dimensionless. The activities of uncharged molecules are taken equal to the concentrations (usually in mol L^{-1}) of these molecules, so the activities are reasonably given the same units. To maintain consistency, it is advisable to assign the units of concentration to the activities of other solution species.

According to these recommendations, the unit of the acid dissociation constant K_a is [from Eq. (4.24)] M (i.e., mol L^{-1}). However, units are conventionally not stated for K_a values.[8] The standard free-energy change $\Delta G°$ can be related to a standard enthalpy change $\Delta H°$ and a standard entropy change $\Delta S°$ by the usual form:

$$
\Delta G° = \Delta H° - T \, \Delta S°
\tag{4.26}
$$

$\Delta H°$ and $\Delta S°$ are interpreted analogously to $\Delta G°$, that is, in terms of the process in which reactants are transformed into products, and all species are in their standard states.

Temperature Dependence of the Equilibrium Constant. The Gibbs–Helmholtz equation [Eq. (3.18), repeated here as Eq. (4.27)] has a useful form for our present purpose:

$$
\frac{d(\Delta G/T)}{dT} = -\frac{\Delta H}{T^2}
\tag{4.27}
$$

From Eq. (4.23), $\Delta G° = -RT \ln K$, rearrangement gives

$$\frac{\Delta G°}{T} = -R \ln K \tag{4.28}$$

Combination of Eqs. (4.27) and (4.28) yields

$$\frac{d \ln K}{dT} = \frac{\Delta H°}{RT^2} \tag{4.29}$$

Equation (4.29), the *van't Hoff equation*, describes how the equilibrium constant varies with the temperature. The quantity $\Delta H°$ is the standard enthalpy change, sometimes called the *heat of reaction*. If $\Delta H°$ is essentially independent of temperature, general integration of Eq. (4.29) gives

$$\ln K = -\frac{\Delta H°}{RT} + \text{constant} \tag{4.30}$$

or

$$\log K = -\frac{\Delta H°}{2.3RT} + C \tag{4.31}$$

Alternatively, integration between the temperature limits T_1 and T_2 gives

$$\ln \frac{K_2}{K_1} = \frac{\Delta H°}{R} \left(\frac{T_2 - T_1}{T_1 T_2} \right) \tag{4.32}$$

$$\log \frac{K_2}{K_1} = \frac{\Delta H°}{2.3R} \left(\frac{T_2 - T_1}{T_1 T_2} \right) \tag{4.33}$$

These integrated equations may seem familiar; they have the same form as the vapor pressure equations (4.12)–(4.15), and they are used similarly.

Free-Energy, Enthalpy, and Entropy Changes in Chemical Reactions.

We now have at hand all the thermodynamic theory needed to calculate (from the appropriate experimental data) these standard thermodynamic quantities for a chemical reaction: $\Delta G°$, $\Delta H°$, and $\Delta S°$. These are the steps:

1. From measurement of the equilibrium constant K at a given temperature, calculate $\Delta G°$ from

$$\Delta G° = -RT \ln K \tag{4.34}$$

2. From measurements of K at several temperatures, calculate $\Delta H°$ by means of one of Eqs. (4.30)–(4.33).
3. From $\Delta G° = \Delta H° - T \Delta S°$, calculate $\Delta S°$.

Table 4.2   Dependence of equilibrium constant on temperature for the binding of methyl *trans*-cinnamate and 8-chlorotheophylline anion in water

T (°C)	K (M^{-1})	T (K)	$1/T$	$\log K$
15.5	11.6	288.65	0.00346	1.064
25.0	8.7	298.15	0.00335	0.940
40.0	5.9	313.15	0.00319	0.771

Since K in general varies with temperature, evidently $\Delta G°$ does as well. When integrating the van't Hoff equation we assumed that $\Delta H°$ is a constant, independent of temperature, and although this may constitute an acceptable approximation for many reactions, it is not generally true, and it may lead to poor estimates of $\Delta H°$ and $\Delta S°$. The data themselves, if carefully interpreted, will reveal whether $\Delta H°$ is reasonably constant over the temperature range that was investigated experimentally.

Example 4.4. These are data (Table 4.2) for the equilibrium constant (a stability constant) describing the noncovalent association between methyl *trans*-cinnamate and 8-chlorotheophyllinate in aqueous solution. Find $\Delta G°$, $\Delta H°$, and $\Delta S°$ at 25°C.

1. From Eq. (4.34), or its equivalent, we have

$$\Delta G° = -(2.303)(1.987 \, \text{cal mol}^{-1} \, \text{K}^{-1})(298.15 \, \text{K}) \log 8.7$$
$$= -1282 \, \text{cal mol}^{-1}$$
$$= -1.28 \, \text{kcal mol}^{-1}$$

2. $\Delta H°$ will be obtained from a plot according to Eq. (4.31); this is called a *van't Hoff plot*:

$$\log K = -\frac{\Delta H°}{2.3 \, RT} + C$$

$$\text{Slope} = -\frac{\Delta H°}{2.3 \, R}$$

Figure 4.3 shows the plot, which is acceptably straight over the temperature range given in the table; this linearity is consistent with the constancy of $\Delta H°$ over this temperature range. The slope of the line is 1083 K, giving for $\Delta H°$

$$\Delta H° = -(2.3)(1.987 \, \text{cal mol}^{-1} \, \text{K}^{-1})(1083 \, \text{K})$$
$$= -4996 \, \text{cal mol}^{-1}$$
$$= -5.00 \, \text{kcal mol}^{-1}$$

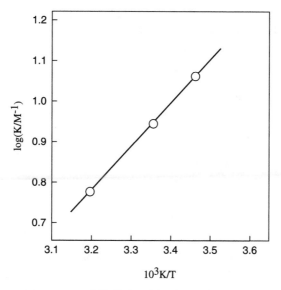

Figure 4.3. van't Hoff plot of the data in Table 4.2.

3.

$$\Delta S° = \frac{-(\Delta G° - \Delta H°)}{T}$$

$$= \frac{-1.28 - (-5.00)\,\text{kcal mol}^{-1}}{-298.15\,\text{K}}$$

$$= -0.0125\,\text{kcal mol}^{-1}\,\text{K}^{-1}$$

$$= -12.5\,\text{cal mol}^{-1}\,\text{K}^{-1}$$

We can interpret these results chemically. The reaction has the form

$$A + B \overset{K}{\rightleftharpoons} C$$

where A is methyl cinnamate and B is 8-chlorotheophyllinate; C is the complex formed from these. Since $K > 1$, $\Delta G° < 0$; the product C is favored over the reactants. But this result is seen to be a consequence of a competition between $\Delta H°$ and $\Delta S°$. $\Delta H°$ is negative, so the enthalpy change makes a favorable contribution to $\Delta G°$ (it makes $\Delta G°$ more negative). The negative value of $\Delta H°$ suggests that fairly strong noncovalent binding is occurring between A and B, because $\Delta H°$ is an energy value. On the other hand, the negative value of $\Delta S°$ opposes product formation by making a positive contribution to $\Delta G°$ (because of the negative sign in $\Delta G° = \Delta H° - T\,\Delta S°$). The negative entropy change may arise because two particles (A and B) are being transformed into a single C particle, with a resultant decrease in number of configurational and thermal microstates of the system. If we were to write this reaction as

$$C \overset{K'}{\rightleftharpoons} A + B$$

we would find that $K' = 1/K$, and that $\Delta G°$, $\Delta H°$, and $\Delta S°$ each possesses the same numerical value as found in this example, but with the opposite sign.

A subtlety of such calculations, often overlooked, is that the numerical values of $\Delta G°$ and $\Delta S°$ (but not of $\Delta H°$) depend on the concentration scale in which the equilibrium constant is expressed. In thermodynamic terms this is stated as follows: The numerical values of $\Delta G°$ and $\Delta S°$ depend on the choice of standard state.

PROBLEMS

4.1. The vapor pressure of heptane, C_7H_{16}, is 100 mm Hg at 41.8°C and 760 mm Hg (i.e., 1 atm) at 98.4°C. Calculate its molar heat of vaporization over this temperature range.

4.2. The equilibrium constant for this reaction in aqueous solution at 25°C is $21.5 \, M^{-1}$:

$$\text{Theophylline} + \text{salicylate anion} \overset{K}{\rightleftharpoons} \text{complex}$$

Calculate the standard free energy change for this reaction.

4.3. These are literature data for the vapor pressure of ethyl acetate, $CH_3COOC_2H_5$, as a function of temperature. Calculate the heat of vaporization.

t (°C)	P (mm Hg)
−43.4	1
−13.5	10
9.1	40
27.0	100
59.3	400
77.1	760

4.4. A quantity pK_a is defined by the relationship

$$pK_a = -\log K_a$$

where K_a is the acid dissociation constant of a weak acid in water. Obtain an equation by which the standard free-energy change can be calculated directly from the pK_a.

4.5. The pK_a value of phenol is 10.0 at 25°C. Write the chemical reaction, define K_a, and calculate $\Delta G°$ for the process.

4.6. The pK_a value of chloroacetic acid, $ClCH_2COOH$, is 2.87 at 25°C, and its heat of ionization ($\Delta H°$) has been measured to be -1.12 kcal mol^{-1}. Calculate its standard entropy of ionization.

4.7. The ionization (acid dissociation) of chloroacetic acid takes place in aqueous solution according to

$$ClCH_2COOH \overset{K_a}{\rightleftharpoons} H^+ + ClCH_2COO^-$$

In view of this, attempt to rationalize the sign of $\Delta S°$ obtained in Problem 4.6.

4.8. The equilibrium constant for the addition of hydrogen cyanide to acetaldehyde is 7100 M^{-1} at 25°C. Calculate $\Delta G°$.

$$CH_3CHO + HCN \overset{K}{\rightleftharpoons} CH_3\underset{\underset{CN}{|}}{\overset{\overset{OH}{|}}{CH}}$$

NOTES

1. A *component* is defined in this way: C, the number of components, is the minimum number of substances needed to make up the equilibrium mixture. For example, pure water contains H_2O, H_3O^+, OH^-, and a mixture of hydrogen-bonded water multimers, but these are all connected by (established by) equilibria, so $C = 1$; you need take only one substance, water, to create this system.

2. The equilibrium condition $d\mu_i = 0$ also applies to the case $P = 1$, as in a liquid solution, and it determines the direction in which solute diffusion takes place. If a nonequilibrium distribution of solute exists, the solute particles will diffuse in the direction so as to achieve the condition $d\mu_i = 0$ throughout the solution. This means that the direction of diffusion is from regions of higher chemical potential to regions of lower chemical potential.

3. Conventionally the boiling point is considered to be the temperature at which the liquid and vapor are in equilibrium at atmospheric pressure. This definition can be assumed when the pressure is not stated.

4. Sublimation is less familiar than melting or boiling, but it can be important. Salicylic acid readily sublimes. An old bottle of aspirin tablets may contain partially hydrolyzed aspirin (acetylsalicylic acid). The products are acetic acid (a liquid, whose vapor smells like vinegar) and salicylic acid, which may sublime and then condense in white crystals on the wall of the bottle.

5. The multiplier is $P - 1$ rather than P because if we know $C(P - 1)$ relationships, we have exhausted the independent equations. for instance, suppose $C = 2$ (components numbered 1,2) and $P = 3$ (phases labeled a,b,c). Then the $C(P - 1) = 2 \times 2 = 4$ independent equations are

$$\mu_{1(a)} = \mu_{1(b)} \qquad \mu_{2(a)} = \mu_{2(b)}$$

$$\mu_{1(b)} = \mu_{1(c)} \qquad \mu_{2(b)} = \mu_{2(c)}$$

The equations $\mu_{1(a)} = \mu_{1(c)}$ and $\mu_{2(a)} = \mu_{2(c)}$ are not independent, but follow from the preceding four equations.

6. Our modern interpretation of a balanced chemical reaction views the species symbols as representing atoms, molecules, or ions, but the balanced reaction does not necessarily imply an atomic viewpoint. The reaction simply describes an experimental observation and is a classical thermodynamic concept.

7. It would be perfectly correct to write $\Delta\mu^\circ$ instead of ΔG°. The latter symbolism is used in order to be consistent with conventional practice.

8. An alternative viewpoint is that activities are dimensionless, thus requiring the activity coefficient to have units. Each point of view is acceptable provided it is consistently applied throughout a calculation. Observe, in this connection, that many thermodynamic equations, exemplified by Eqs. (4.12) and (4.23), direct us to take the logarithm of a physical quantity that may possess units. Of course, we cannot take the logarithm of a unit, and so we proceed (as described in Appendix B) by applying "quantity algebra." For example, we can write $P = 1.5$ atm, from which it follows that $P\,(\text{atm}) = 1.5$, a pure number, whose logarithm can be taken. Similarly, in Example 4.3, $K_a = 1.75 \times 10^{-5}$ M, so $K_a\,(\text{M}) = 1.75 \times 10^{-5}$, and Eq. (4.25) should strictly be written

$$\Delta G^\circ = -2.303RT \log\left[K_a\,(\text{M})\right]$$

Figure 4.3 shows how this convention is properly used to label the axes of a graph.

II

THERMODYNAMICS OF PHYSICAL PROCESSES

5

INTRODUCTION TO PHYSICAL PROCESSES

5.1. SCOPE

The separation of properties or processes into physical and chemical categories is arbitrary but useful, and in most instances it is not notably ambiguous. Here are the criteria adopted in making the present separation:

1. All covalent bond changes (which necessarily result in alterations in primary molecular structure) are *chemical*. This category includes most of the reactions of interest in organic chemistry, inorganic chemistry, and biochemistry. Part III deals with such processes.
2. All changes in physical state or phase that do not involve covalent bond changes are *physical*. Such processes include melting, vaporization, sublimation, dissolution, partitioning, and adsorption. These are of concern in Part II.
3. There is an exception—electrolyte dissociation and behavior is treated generally, in Part II, as a physical phenomenon, but the special case of acid–base equilibrium is discussed as a chemical phenomenon in Part III.
4. An ambiguous area remains, consisting of changes in noncovalent interactions roughly in the $\Delta G°$ range of 0–10 kcal mol^{-1}. These processes include molecular complex formation (binding phenomena of many types) and conformational changes. We classify these as *chemical*, and treat them in Part III.

Some slight repetition of material from Part I will be encountered in Part II, where it is inserted for convenience.

5.2. CONCENTRATION SCALES

Solution composition can be expressed on a physical (empirical) basis in terms of the quantities measured in the laboratory. These are the common concentration scales of this type:

Percent by Weight. The number of grams of solute contained in 100 g of solution. The concentration of the strong mineral acids, as available commercially, are expressed as percent by weight.

Percent Weight/Volume (% w/v). The number of grams of solute contained in 100 mL of solution. This scale is often used to describe the composition of solutions of solids in liquids.

Percent by Volume. The number of mL of solute contained in 100 mL of solution. Solutions of liquids in liquids are commonly specified in this way. It is important to note a possible ambiguity in this designation. Consider these two operations: (1) 80.0 mL of ethanol is dissolved in water to make a final total volume of 100 mL; (2) 80.0 mL of ethanol is mixed with 20.0 mL of water. These solutions have different compositions, because preparation 2 does not yield a final volume of 100 mL. In thermodynamic terms, the partial molar volume of ethanol is not equal to its molar volume. In molecular terms, the spatial and energetic character of the ethanol–water interaction is different from those of ethanol-ethanol or water-water interactions. Solution 1 has a composition of 80.0% by volume of ethanol. The composition of solution 2 is most easily specified in terms of its *volume fraction* φ, where the volume fraction φ_i of component i is defined

$$\varphi_i = \frac{V_i}{\sum_{i=1}^{n} V_i}$$

Thus solution 2 has volume fraction $\Phi_1 = 0.20$ of water and $\Phi_2 = 0.80$ of ethanol. In order to communicate without possible confusion, statements of solution composition should specify clearly, as, for example, by describing the manner of preparing the solution, which concentration scale is meant.

Observe that these physical concentration scales constitute the three combinations of mass/mass, mass/volume, and volume/volume. Other units may, however, often be encountered. For example, milligram percent is the number of milligrams of solute contained in 100 mL of solution. Another common unit is milligrams per milliliter (mg/mL), which is numerically equal to grams per liter (g/L). Very dilute solutions may be expressed in parts per million (ppm), which is the number of grams of solute contained in 10^6 g of solution. (If the solvent is water, this is effectively the number of grams of solute in 10^6 mL of solution.) Similarly, ppb means parts per billion.

The chemical concentration scales are based on the concept of the amount of substance as expressed in number of moles:

Molarity (c)—the number of moles of solute contained in 1000 mL of solution. Molarity has the units mol L^{-1}, which is often designated M; it is expressed as mol dm^{-3} in SI units. Some investigators use the unit millimolar (mM), which denotes the number of millimoles contained in 1000 mL of solution; for example, 0.030 M and 30 mM have the same meaning. Molarity is a very practical concentration scale, but it has the disadvantage that the molarity of a solution depends on the temperature, because the volume is temperature-dependent.

Molality (m)—the number of moles of solute per 1000 g of solvent. The molality is temperature-independent, and for this reason is often preferred in precise physical chemical experimental work.

Mole fraction (x)—the number of moles of solute divided by the total number of moles in the solution. The mole fraction is temperature-independent. A convenient attribute of the mole fraction (as of all fractional quantities) is that the sum of the mole fractions of all constituents in a solution is unity.

In general the molarity, molality, and mole fraction scales are not directly proportional to each other, but in very dilute solutions of a solute i the relationships are

$$x_i = \frac{c_i M_1}{1000\rho_1} \qquad (x_i \ll 1) \tag{5.1}$$

$$x_i = \frac{m_i M_1}{1000} \qquad (x_i \ll 1) \tag{5.2}$$

where subscript 1 refers to the solvent and i to the solute. In these dilute solutions Eqs. (5.1) and (5.2) show that the various concentration scales are proportional to each other; M_1 is the molecular weight of the solvent, and ρ_1 is its density.

5.3. STANDARD STATES

In Chapter 3 we encountered the concept of the standard state, and here we will extend the treatment by explicitly invoking the concentration scales used in laboratory work. We begin with Eq. (3.37), repeated here:

$$\mu_i = \mu_i^{\circ} + RT \ln a_i \tag{5.3}$$

In this equation, μ_i is the chemical potential (partial molar free energy) of constituent i in a liquid mixture, μ_i° is its standard chemical potential, and a_i is its activity. The activity, which can be thought of as an "effective concentration," is related to the actual concentration by

Activity = activity coefficient × concentration

where the activity coefficient is a number that accounts for deviations from ideal behavior. Let us recall these definitions:

The *standard state* (with respect to constituent i) is that state of the system in which the activity of i is unity; then, from Eq. (5.3), $\mu_i = \mu_i^\circ$.

The *reference state* (with respect to constituent i) is that state of the system in which the activity coefficient of i is unity; then its activity equals its concentration.

For the present let us suppose that the system is in its reference state (for constituent i), so the activity coefficient is unity, and the activity is equal to the concentration. But we have seen that concentrations can be expressed in molarity, molality, or mole fraction. For constituent i in a given system, Eq. (5.3) may be written in terms of each of these concentration units:

$$\mu_i = \mu_i^\circ + RT \ln c_i \tag{5.4}$$

$$\mu_i = \mu_m^\circ + RT \ln m_i \tag{5.5}$$

$$\mu_i = \mu_x^\circ + RT \ln x_i \tag{5.6}$$

The situation represented by Eqs. (5.4)–(5.6) is analogous to the specification of mechanical potential energy, say, of a rock on top of a hill. We can only speak numerically of energy *differences*, and we calculate the potential energy of the rock as the product mgh, where m is its mass, g is the gravitational acceleration, and h is its height. But before we can make the calculation we must define a state at which $h = 0$, and this is arbitrary, meaning that we can choose any state we wish. We might, in the case of the rock on the hill, choose to measure h from the valley floor, but we could just as well choose sea level as this state. Equations (5.4)–(5.6) present the same kinds of choices. In each case μ_i is the same definite quantity (corresponding to the potential energy of the rock on the hill). Each equation can be rearranged to the form

$$\mu_i - \mu_c^\circ = RT \ln c_i$$

using Eq. (5.4) as an example. Since, for a given solution, c_i, m_i, and x_i have different numerical values, so, too, do the quantities $(\mu_i - \mu_c^\circ)$, $(\mu_i - \mu_m^\circ)$, and $(u_i - \mu_x^\circ)$. Each of these quantities gives the value of the chemical potential u_i *relative to its standard state value*. Each expression is thermodynamically acceptable; they differ only in the values they assign to the standard potential. We can easily find the relationship between these different standard chemical potentials. Let us compare Eqs. (5.4) and (5.6). Recalling that we have assumed that the system is in its reference state, which usually is the infinitely dilute solution, we can use Eq. (5.1), substituting it into (5.6) to eliminate x_i, and setting Eqs. (5.4) and (5.6) equal to yield

$$\mu_c^\circ = u_x^\circ + RT \ln \frac{M_1}{1000\rho_1}$$

For example, if the solvent is water, then $M_1 = 18$ and $\rho_1 = 1.0$, and we find $\mu_c^\circ = \mu_x^\circ - RT \ln 55.5$. Concluding this exposition, we see that the selection of a standard state is arbitrary, and that we select a standard state when we choose a concentration scale. [Some authors write of "adopting the 1 M standard state," for example, which merely means that the molar scale was used, with Eq. (5.4) showing that when $c_i = 1$, then $\mu_i = \mu_c^\circ$.]

In the more general case where activity coefficients may deviate from unity, Eqs. (5.4)–(5.6) become

$$\mu_i = \mu_c^\circ + RT \ln \gamma_c c_i \tag{5.7}$$

$$\mu_i = \mu_m^\circ + RT \ln \gamma_m m_i \tag{5.8}$$

$$\mu_i = \mu_x^\circ + RT \ln \gamma_x x_i \tag{5.9}$$

where the subscript i has been omitted from the μ° and γ terms to reduce typographical clutter. In general γ_c, γ_m, and γ_x differ for the same system, although in dilute solutions they have nearly the same value (Glasstone 1947, p. 355). Certain conventions allow us to carry out calculations to levels of accuracy appropriate to many practical situations where extreme accuracy is not required. We will adopt these conventions, which are repeated from Chapter 3 for convenience:

1. The fugacity of a *gas* is taken equal to its pressure (or partial pressure) in atm, at low to moderate pressures.
2. The activity of a liquid *solvent* in a solution is equal to its mole fraction. It follows that the activity of a pure liquid is 1.00, and that this is its standard state. (This convention also applies to liquid solutes if desired.)
3. The activity of a pure *solid* is 1.00; this is the same as convention 2.
4. The activity of a *solute* in an infinitely dilute solution will be taken equal to its molar concentration; that is, $\gamma_c = 1.00$; the solute is in its reference state. The standard state is rather peculiar; it approximates to the 1 M solution, but at this concentration the solution probably does not behave ideally, so although its activity is unity by definition, some of its properties are those of the reference state. (We further expand on this in Section 7.2.)
5. The activity of an *uncharged solute* will be taken as 1.00 at any concentration. This is an approximation justified by recognizing that uncharged molecules experience much weaker forces of interaction than do ions. The approximation improves as the solution is made more dilute.
6. The activity coefficient of an *ion* can be drawn from experimentally determined results (Harned and Owen 1958) or calculated from theory, as will be described in Section 8.3.

It is instructive to write Eq. (5.7) in this expanded form:

$$\mu_i = \mu_i^\circ + RT \ln c_i + RT \ln \gamma_i \tag{5.10}$$

This equation shows how the numerical value of the chemical potential μ_i receives a contribution from the arbitrarily assigned standard state (μ_i°), a contribution from $RT \ln c_i$, which describes the composition dependence of the ideally behaved constituent, and a contribution from $RT \ln \gamma_i$, which describes the nonideal behavior of the constituent. Although not explicitly indicated, γ_i is also composition-dependent, and as $c_i \to 0$, $\gamma_i \to 1$.

PROBLEMS

5.1. Calculate the mole fraction x_2 of benzoic acid in an aqueous solution 1.5 mM in benzoic acid. Also calculate the mole fraction x_i of water in this solution.

5.2. Concentrated hydrochloric acid is labeled to contain about 38.0% by weight of HCl, and its density is about 1.19 g mL^{-1}. Calculate the approximate molar concentration of HCl in this solution.

5.3. What is the molar concentration of pure water?

5.4. Calculate the difference between standard chemical potentials in dilute aqueous solution based on the molar and the mole fraction standard states, at 25°C.

5.5. Obtain an equation with which molar and molal concentrations may be interconverted in dilute solution.

5.6. Consider a liquid solution of solvent 1 and solute 2. Let n_1 and n_2 respectively be the numbers of moles of solvent and solute in a given mass of solution, whose density is ρ. Then derive an *exact* equation relating x_2 and c_2. [*Hint:* The correct result must reduce to Eq. (5.1) in very dilute solution.]

6

PHASE
TRANSFORMATIONS

6.1. PURE SUBSTANCES

Phase Diagrams. In this section we treat equilibria in heterogeneous systems, that is, systems consisting of more than one phase. A phase of matter is uniform in chemical composition and physical state. It may be subdivided, but it remains a single phase. For example, a system consisting of ordinary crushed ice dispersed in water possesses two phases: ice and water. These types of systems were treated briefly in Chapter 4. Figure 6.1, which appeared earlier as Fig. 4.1, is a pressure–temperature phase diagram for the simplest case, a pure substance possessing only one form of each of the three phases solid, liquid, and vapor (gas). (A pure substance can have only a single vapor phase, and most pure substances have only a single liquid phase,[1] but many solid phases may exist, as will be described below.)

The line OC in Fig. 6.1 describes all systems in which the solid and liquid phases coexist in equilibrium; that is, any pair of P, T coordinates on this line describe the *melting temperature* of the solid at that pressure. Similarly line OB gives the *boiling temperature* as a function of pressure, and line OA gives the *sublimation temperature*. Point O is called the *triple point*, a unique pair of P, T values at which the solid, liquid, and vapor are in mutual equilibrium. The slopes of these lines are given by Eq. (6.1), the Clapeyron equation, from Chapter 4:

$$\frac{dP}{dT} = \frac{\Delta H}{T\,\Delta V} \tag{6.1}$$

where ΔH is the enthalpy change for the process and ΔV is the volume change. For the special case of the liquid–vapor transition (boiling), this equation is usually used

67

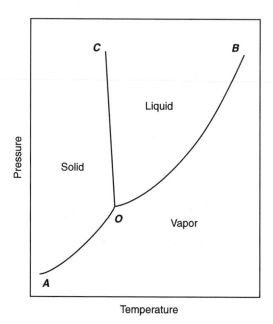

Figure 6.1. Pressure–temperature phase diagram of a pure substance.

in the approximate version called the *Clausius–Clapeyron equation*:

$$\frac{d\ln P}{dT} = \frac{\Delta H_{\text{vap}}}{RT^2} \tag{6.2}$$

In its integrated forms the Clausius–Clapeyron equation becomes

$$\log P = -\frac{\Delta H_{\text{vap}}}{2.3RT} + C \tag{6.3}$$

or

$$\log\frac{P_2}{P_1} = \frac{\Delta H_{\text{vap}}}{2.3R}\left(\frac{T_2 - T_1}{T_1 T_2}\right) \tag{6.4}$$

where C is a constant; ΔH_{vap}, the molar heat of vaporization, is assumed to be a constant throughout the temperature range of interest; and the equations relate boiling temperature to pressure.

The Gibbs phase rule is

$$F = C - P + 2 \tag{6.5}$$

where P is now the number of phases in the system at equilibrium, C is the number of components, and F is the number of degrees of freedom.[2] F is the number of variables that must be fixed in order to completely define the system. For example, along line OC in Fig. 6.1 there are two phases (solid and liquid) and one component (since this is the diagram for a pure substance), so $F = 1 - 2 + 2 = 1$. According to this result, the system along line OC possesses one degree of freedom. This means that we can select *either* the pressure *or* the temperature at will (provided the value lies within the OC range); the other variable is then established by the equilibrium.

At the triple point O, $F = 1 - 3 + 2 = 0$; the system has no degrees of freedom. The three phases solid, liquid, and vapor are all in equilibrium, and if this condition is to be maintained, neither the temperature nor the pressure may be altered.

Figure 6.1 and the Clausius–Clapeyron equation show that the pressure may be a fairly sensitive function of temperature along the vaporization line OB. By definition the *normal boiling point* T_b is the boiling temperature when $P = 1$ atm; this is the boiling temperature usually measured in the laboratory (or the kitchen). The melting point (also called the *freezing point*) is not very sensitive to pressure.

Polymorphism. A pure substance may be capable of existing in more than one crystalline solid form. Each such crystalline solid is a separate phase, and these forms are called *polymorphs*. The phenomenon of polymorphism (also known as *allotropy*) is widespread, and it has pharmaceutical ramifications. Polymorphs have different arrangements of the molecules in their crystal structures, but chemically they are identical. The two or more polymorphs of a substance possess different free energies, and the polymorph that has the lowest free energy is the thermodynamically most stable form. The other forms are thermodynamically unstable relative to the stable form, but it may happen that the rate of transformation from the unstable to the stable forms is so slow as to be negligible or practically unimportant, in which case the unstable polymorph is said to be *metastable*. For example, the element carbon can exist in two polymorphic forms called *graphite* and *diamond*. Graphite is the thermodynamically stable form, and diamond is metastable with respect to it, but although diamond is thermodynamically unstable, the timescale on which it transforms to the more stable form is of no human concern. Some polymorphic transformations may be quite fast, however.

A given substance may possess numerous polymorphs—phenobarbital has at least 8 and may have 11 of them—but according to the phase rule, the maximum number of phases, including solid phases, that can coexist in equilibrium is $P = C + 2$ (i.e., P is maximized when F is set to 0); for a pure substance this is three phases. Figure 6.2 is the phase diagram of water at extremely high pressures (Findlay et al. 1951). This phase diagram (which is based on the experimental work of P. W. Bridgman) shows six ice polymorphs; these are labeled ice I (this is ordinary ice), ice II, ice III, ice V, ice VI, and ice VII (the reported discovery of ice IV was erroneous). Observe that a maximum of three phases may exist at any fixed combination of temperature and pressure.

The pharmaceutical significance of polymorphism lies in two features: (1) the different crystal forms have different physical properties and (2) polymorphs may interconvert on a pharmaceutically pertinent time scale. These features have led to

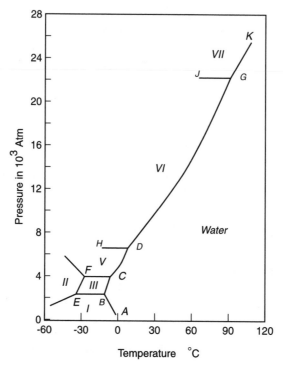

Figure 6.2. Pressure–temperature phase diagram of water at high pressures, showing the six ice polymorphs. [Reproduced by permission from Findlay et al. (1951).]

much pharmaceutical research in this area (Carstensen 1973, pp. 113–124; Haleblian and McCrone 1969; Haleblian 1975; Florence and Attwood 1981, Chapter 2). It has been found that the solubilities of polymorphic forms of a drug are different. If the solubility of the less stable form is greater than that of the more stable form, its solution will be unstable with respect to the more stable solid form because it is supersaturated with respect to this form. Precipitation may occur unexpectedly in such a situation unless some form of stabilization can be devised. The bioavailability of a drug may depend on the drug's polymorphic form. Chemical stability of drugs, and the physical stability of pharmaceutical dosage forms, may be dependent on the polymorphic form of the drug and its propensity for transformation to a more stable polymorph.

Note that the formation of a crystalline hydrate (or other solvate), in which the compound crystallizes with one or more molecules of solvent in its crystal structure, is not true polymorphism; a crystal hydrate is not chemically the same substance as the unhydrated substance.

The Amorphous State. We have seen that a pure substance may assume any one of several crystalline solid forms called *polymorphs*. There exists yet another possibility called the *amorphous* or *glassy* state, in which the substance appears to be solid in its consistency, yet X-ray diffraction data show the absence of the periodic array of molecules characteristic of the crystalline state. The amorphous (i.e., formless) state is really the supercooled liquid, which, although below its normal freezing point, has not adopted the orderly arrangement of molecules characteristic of the crystal. Although it appears to be a solid, it is really a highly viscous liquid. Presumably some kinetic barrier to crystallization permits super-cooling to take place. This pathway to the amorphous state is not the only one, how-ever, and it has been found possible to generate amorphous samples by subjecting crystalline solids to high-energy processes such as grinding, milling, and freeze drying. The amorphous state is best detected by means of X-ray powder spectra.

The amorphous state is unstable with respect to (it is of higher energy than) the crystalline solid, to which it may revert on a generally unpredictable timescale. Its pharmaceutical advantages and disadvantages follow from these properties. Higher solubility and bioavailability may be achieved with amorphous solids, but transfor-mation to the crystalline state is a possibility. Experimental study of each substance is required to establish its characteristic behavior.

The amorphous state is often studied by means of differential scanning calori-metry (DSC), in which the temperature of the sample is raised while the heat absorbed or released by the sample is monitored. Figure 6.3 shows DSC curves for two amorphous samples of the drug indomethacin (Yoshioka et al. 1994). One sample (dashed lines) had been prepared by rapidly cooling the melted drug; the other sample (solid lines) had been more slowly cooled. Besides these amorphous samples, indomethacin also forms two crystalline polymorphs: the α form with melting point 155°C and the γ with melting point 161°C.

As the temperature sweeps through the range 35–65°C, in Fig. 6.3a, both amor-phous samples show endothermic peaks (they are absorbing heat) as they undergo a transition. The onset of this transition, at about 50°C, is called the *glass transition temperature*, T_g. With increased temperatures, the samples undergo crystallization in Fig. 6.3b, with the release of heat (the heat of crystallization, which can be mea-sured from the areas under the crystallization peaks). Finally, in Fig. 6.3c, both samples melt. Observe that the two melting crystalline samples are actually

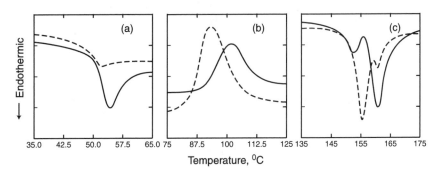

Figure 6.3. DSC traces of two amorphous samples of indomethacin. See text for explanation. Reproduced by permission from Yoshioka et al. (1994).

mixtures of the α and γ polymorphs (each curve has two components), but they differ in terms of which polymorph is present in major fraction.

The properties of the amorphous state are a consequence of its high energy content, which is its dominant characteristic. It is a relatively unstudied state of matter, for which increasing pharmaceutical applications may be expected.

6.2. MULTICOMPONENT SYSTEMS

This is an abbreviated treatment of this topic, limited in these two ways: (1) we consider only binary (i.e., two-component) systems, and (2) we omit certain topics as not particularly pertinent to our interests (fractional distillation is an example). Fuller treatments are available (Rossini 1950, Chapter 32; Atkins 1994, Chapter 8).

Liquid–Liquid Systems. We will omit consideration of the vapor phase, in principle by postulating that it is excluded from the system, in practice by working (usually) under the ambient fixed atmospheric pressure. We begin by considering a system of two liquids. Of course, whether a substance is a liquid or a solid depends (at fixed pressure) on the temperature, but common usage denotes as liquids those substances that exist in this state at or near room temperature. Pairs of liquids often are classified as essentially completely immiscible (such as mercury and water), as completely miscible in all proportions (e.g., ethanol and water), or as partially miscible (e.g., diethyl ether and water). The completely immiscible case need not concern us, since it effectively consists of two separate pure substances. Completely miscible systems are dealt with in Chapter 7. We are left to consider those pairs of liquids that are miscible in some proportions but are immiscible in other proportions.

Inasmuch as we have fixed the pressure, the two experimental variables by means of which the system may be manipulated are the temperature and the composition of the system, and phase diagrams are commonly constructed with these variables as the coordinates. Usually the composition is expressed as mole fraction or as percent by weight. Figure 6.4 shows a schematic temperature–composition phase diagram for a partially miscible pair of liquids, 1 and 2. Any combination of temperature and composition giving a point outside the phase boundary line describes a homogeneous system; in this region 1 and 2 are mutually miscible. Note that small concentrations of 1 will dissolve in 2, and vice versa; moreover, as the temperature increases, the extent of mutual solubility increases. At any temperature above T_c (which is called the upper critical temperature), the two liquids are miscible in all proportions.

But if the temperature–composition combination places the system under (within) the phase boundary line, two phases form. One phase is predominantly 1 saturated with 2, the other is largely 2 saturated with 1. At any given temperature, say, T' in Fig. 6.4, the horizontal *tieline pr* connects the arms of the phase diagram, and the compositions of the two phases are given by x_p and x_r. Moreover, if x_q is the

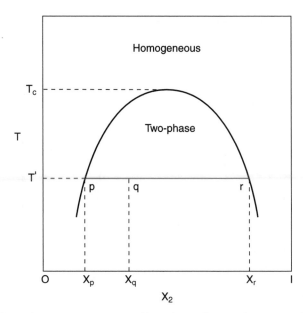

Figure 6.4. Schematic temperature–composition phase diagram for two partially immiscible liquids 1 and 2; x_2 is the mole fraction of 2, and T_c is the upper critical temperature.

overall composition of the system, the amounts of the two phases are in the ratio of the distances pq/qr. Figure 6.5 shows the experimental phase diagram for the phenol–water system [see Findlay et al. (1951, p. 95); the melting point of phenol is ~41°C, and phenol is being treated as a liquid in this context]. This diagram is helpful in determining the ranges of compositions that will yield homogeneous solutions of phenol in water at room temperature (25°C). Liquified Phenol U.S.P. contains 89% by weight of phenol, placing it in the single-phase region of the diagram.

Example 6.1. 50.0 g of Liquified Phenol U.S.P. is diluted with 50.0 mL of water at room temperature. Analyze the outcome of this procedure.

Since Liquified Phenol contains 89% w/w of phenol, and the density of water is 1.0 g mL^{-1}, the system as prepared contains 44.5% w/w phenol with a total weight of 100 g. Figure 6.5 shows the 25°C tieline with point q given by the 44.5% system composition. This point lies within the two-phase boundary, so the system will separate into two layers. Reading the compositions of the layers at points p and r tells us that one phase will contain 8% phenol and the other phase will contain 71% phenol. The ratio $pq/qr = (44.5 - 8)/(71 - 44.5) = 1.38$.

We can go further than this. Since 100 g of total system contains 44.5 g of phenol, we can write

Weight of phenol in aqueous layer + weight of phenol in phenolic layer = 44.5 g

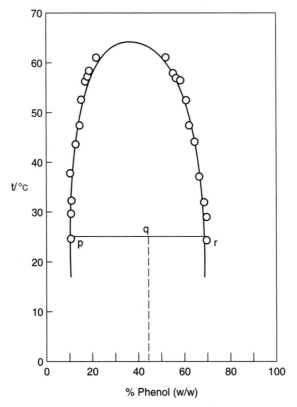

Figure 6.5. Phase diagram for the phenol–water system. See discussion in Example 6.1.

Letting x be the weight of the aqueous layer in 100 g of sample gives

$$0.08x + 0.71(100 - x) = 44.5$$

resulting in $x = 42.1$ g as the weight of the aqueous layer and therefore 57.9 g as the weight of the phenolic layer. The aqueous layer contains $(0.08)(42.1) = 3.4$ g of phenol, and the phenolic layer contains $(0.71)(57.9) = 41.1$ g of phenol. Note, incidentally, that $pq/qr = 1.38 = 57.9/42.1$.

In these two-component systems each phase is a solution, which can be defined as a phase of variable composition. Notice that we have not identified one of the components as the solute and the other as the solvent; such a designation has no thermodynamic significance, and is done solely for our convenience.

Liquid–Solid Systems. Imagine a two-component system consisting of two solids A and B brought to a temperature above the melting points of both. Then in the simplest instance a one-phase system will form consisting of a liquid solution

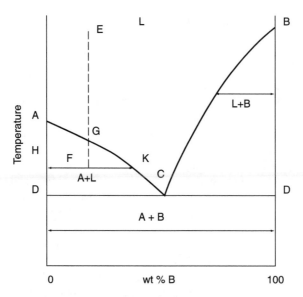

Figure 6.6. The simplest solid–liquid phase diagram for a two-component system of A and B, where L represents the liquid (solution) phase; C is the eutectic point. [Reproduced by permission from Findlay et al. (1951).]

of A and B (Findlay et al. 1951, p. 135). Referring to Fig. 6.6, the area labeled L (for liquid phase) will include the system as described, its precise location in the diagram depending on the temperature and the composition.

The points A and B in Fig. 6.6 represent the melting points of solids A and B. Now let the temperature be lowered (always allowing the system to remain at equilibrium). Suppose the system initially is represented by point E. When the temperature reaches point G, pure solid A will begin to form, and as the temperature continues to fall (as heat is withdrawn from the system), more solid is formed. Throughout the area ADC the system consists of pure solid A dispersed in a solution of A and B. Its composition is given by tielines, such as HK in the figure.

When the system temperature reaches level C, the temperature ceases to fall, even though heat continues to be withdrawn from the system; point C has no degrees of freedom. (Recall that we have fixed the pressure.) At point C, solid A, solid B, and solution phase are in mutual equilibrium. The solid phase at this point is a finely divided two-phase dispersion of crystalline A and B called a *eutectic*, and C is the *eutectic point*. Microscopic examination reveals that the eutectic is a mixture and not a single phase. The composition of the eutectic mixture is fixed for a given pair of substances. Observe that the eutectic melts at a lower temperature than either of its pure components. Eutectic formation is observed widely in geologic deposits and metal alloys, and the phenomenon is of pharmaceutical importance. Numerous drugs form eutectic mixtures, with the consequence that they may liquify at ambient temperature owing to the melting point decrease characteristic at the eutectic point. Acetaminophen, aspirin, menthol, phenacetin, phenol, and thymol are some of these substances that are prone to eutectic formation. Special care in formulating or compounding these compounds is necessary (Thompson 1998, p. 34.5).

We tend to think of curves such as AC and BC in Fig. 6.1 as freezing point (or melting point) curves, but from the thermodynamic point of view they can just as well be viewed as solubility curves. Suppose, for example, that A is a liquid at room temperature but that B is a solid. Then the curve BC can be interpreted as the solubility of B in A. We will not pursue this line of interpretation because Chapter 10 is entirely concerned with solubility.

A traditional laboratory technique for the confirmation of identity of a solid substance is to mix some of the sample with an authentic specimen, and to measure the melting point. If this *mixed melting point* is the same as that of the melting point of the authentic specimen, the sample is very likely the same compound. If, on the other hand, the melting point of the mixture is decreased, the two substances are different. This is a consequence of the mutual depression of melting points seen in Fig. 6.6 when two components are mixed.[3]

The region in Fig. 6.6 labeled $A + B$ and lying entirely below point C may consist merely of the two crystalline phases of A and B (leaving aside the phenomenon of polymorphism). But another possibility is that A and B may form a *solid solution*, which is a homogeneous single-phase state of matter, no different in principle from a liquid solution. Some drugs are known to form solid solutions (Carstensen 1977, pp. 23–26).

PROBLEMS

6.1. Suppose that a solution is prepared at 70°C to contain 65% by weight of phenol in water. The solution is slowly cooled. At what temperature will it separate into two phases?

6.2. Calculate the degrees of freedom at the eutectic point C in Fig. 6.6.

NOTES

1. Some substances reveal the existence of a second liquid phase called the *liquid crystalline phase*. It is recognized by its optical properties.

2. The number of components may differ from the number of constituents. Here is a simple way to determine C, the number of components: C is equal to the minimum number of bottles of pure substances required to prepare the system in the laboratory.

3. The melting of ice on winter roads by spreading salt is another manifestation of the phenomenon. NaCl and H_2O from a eutectic of composition 23.3% NaCl at a eutectic temperature of -21.1°C.

7

SOLUTIONS OF
NONELECTROLYTES

7.1. IDEAL SOLUTIONS

A nonelectrolyte is a substance that is uncharged and that does not sensibly give rise to ions. Our analysis will be sufficiently general if we consider solutions of two nonelectrolytes, labeled 1 and 2; the results can be extended to more components if necessary. For the present we limit discussion to single-phase systems.

A convenient starting place is with the experimental observation known as *Raoult's law*, which describes a particularly simple type of solution behavior in the form of

$$p_i = x_i P_i^* \tag{7.1}$$

Raoult's law states that the partial pressure p_i of constituent i over its solution is directly proportional to its mole fraction in the solution, where the proportionality constant P_i^* is the vapor pressure of the pure liquid (i.e., when $x_i = 1$). An ideal liquid solution is then one in which Raoult's law is obeyed over the entire range of composition, at all temperatures and pressures. As may be imagined, Raoult's law represents a limit of simple behavior toward which certain systems tend, rather than an exact description, but if the solution components are chemically very similar, and are nonpolar molecules, behavior very close to the ideal may be observed. A solution of benzene and toluene illustrates such behavior.

It can be proved (Glasstone 1947, p. 320) that if Raoult's law applies to one of the constituents of a solution, then it must also apply to the other. Figure 7.1 shows Raoult's law behavior for an ideal solution. Since the total pressure is the sum of the partial pressures, then

$$P = x_1 P_1^* + x_2 P_2^* \tag{7.2}$$

This is the equation of the topmost line in Fig. 7.1.

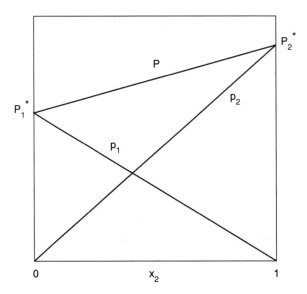

Figure 7.1. Raoult's law behavior of both components of an ideal solution; p_1 and p_2 are the partial pressures; P is the total pressure.

We know from Chapter 4 that at equilibrium the chemical potentials of constituent i are equal in the vapor and liquid phases, or $\mu_i(g) = \mu_i(l)$. We also can write [see Eq. (3.35)], for a mixture of ideal gases, that

$$\mu_i(g) = \mu_i^*(g) + RT \ln p_i$$

If we combine this relationship with the foregoing equality and with Raoult's law, we obtain

$$\mu_i(l) = \mu_i^\circ(l) + RT \ln x_i \qquad (7.3)$$

where $\mu_i^\circ(l) = \mu_i^*(g) + RT \ln P_i^*$. Equation (7.3) may be taken as an alternative description of an ideal-liquid solution (Smith 1977, p. 78). The standard chemical potential $u_i^\circ(l)$ is the chemical potential of pure component i (i.e., when $x_i = 1$).

We can develop the thermodynamic properties of the ideal solution as follows. The total free energy of the solution is given by

$$G = \mu_1 x_1 + \mu_2 x_2 \qquad (7.4)$$

where x_1 and x_2 are mole fractions. The free-energy change on mixing 1 and 2 is equal to the free energy of the solution after mixing minus the free energy of the pure components before mixing, or

$$\Delta G_{\text{mix}} = \sum \mu_i x_i - \sum \mu_i^\circ x_i \qquad (7.5)$$

Substituting from Eq. (7.3) into Eq. (7.5) leads to

$$\Delta G_{\text{mix}}^{\text{ideal}} = RTx_1 \ln x_1 + RTx_2 \ln x_2 \tag{7.6}$$

as the ideal free energy of mixing. Since the mole fractions are less than one, the free energy of mixing is negative and the process is spontaneous.

The entropy of mixing is easily obtained by applying the relationship [Eq. (3.7)]

$$\left(\frac{\partial \Delta G}{\partial T}\right)_P = -\Delta S \tag{7.7}$$

to Eq. (7.6). The result is

$$\Delta S_{\text{mix}}^{\text{ideal}} = -Rx_1 \ln x_1 - Rx_2 \ln x_2 \tag{7.8}$$

Therefore the entropy of mixing is positive, as we would expect. From the identity $\Delta G = \Delta H - T \Delta S$ we obtain, making use of Eqs. (7.6) and (7.8):

$$\Delta H_{\text{mix}}^{\text{ideal}} = 0 \tag{7.9}$$

Finally, from Eq. (3.6), we obtain

$$\left(\frac{\partial \Delta G}{\partial P}\right)_T = \Delta V \tag{7.10}$$

applying this to Eq. (7.6), we get

$$\Delta V_{\text{mix}}^{\text{ideal}} = 0 \tag{7.11}$$

Equations (7.6), (7.8), (7.9), and (7.11) give the essential thermodynamic properties of the ideal solution. We can make some molecular interpretations of these results. In an ideal solution, the three pairwise interactions between 1–1 molecules, 2–2 molecules, and 1–2 molecules are all energetically and spatially identical, so replacement of a 1 molecule by a 2 molecule anywhere in the solution leads to no energy or volume changes; hence $\Delta H_{\text{mix}}^{\text{ideal}} = 0$ and $\Delta V_{\text{mix}}^{\text{ideal}} = 0$. (It is these stringent constraints that account for the rarity of experimental examples of ideal solutions, because if two real molecules have different identities, their energies and space-filling requirements will differ to at least some degree.) The ideal entropy of mixing is positive because the mixed system is more disordered than is the initial system of separated species and the number of configurational microstates is greater. Since $\Delta H_{\text{mix}}^{\text{ideal}} = 0$ and $\Delta S_{\text{mix}}^{\text{ideal}} > 0$, the negative value of $\Delta G_{\text{mix}}^{\text{ideal}}$ is entirely entropy-driven.

7.2. NONIDEAL SOLUTIONS

It will be no surprise to learn that few real solutions behave ideally. Nevertheless, fairly simple behavior is widely observed in solutions that are very dilute with respect to one component. It will now be convenient to designate the component (to be labeled component 1) that is present in great excess as the *solvent*, and component 2, present in low concentration, as the *solute*. The solvent is obviously a liquid, but the solute may be either a liquid or a solid.

First consider Fig. 7.2, which shows vapor pressure–composition curves for both solution components when derivations from ideality occur. In this figure the dashed lines show ideal Raoult's law behavior (compare with Fig. 7.1), whereas the solid lines show positive deviations from Raoult's law (Fig. 7.2a) and negative deviations (Fig. 7.2b).[1] The two components may exchange roles as solvent and solute depending on which is in excess.

Now, in a dilute solution (i.e., dilute with respect to component 2, the solute), the solvent, component 1, approaches a mole fraction of unity, and its vapor pressure approaches that expected from Raoult's law; this behavior can be seen in Fig. 7.2, where the dashed and solid lines approach asymptotically as x appoaches unity. This is reasonable behavior, since in this circumstance (the very dilute solution), the solvent molecules are surrounded essentially only by other solvent molecules, and hence are practically unperturbed by solute molecules. But it is otherwise for the solute molecules in dilute solution, for then each solute molecule finds itself in an environment of essentially only solvent molecules, which is clearly not typical of the purely solute environment. Consequently the solute does not follow Raoult's law in dilute solution.

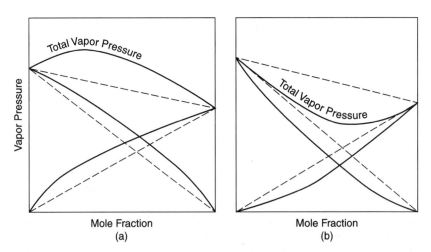

Figure 7.2. Nonideal solution behavior showing positive deviations (a) and negative deviations (b) from Raoult's law. The mole fraction scale runs from 0 to 1 for one of the components and from 1 to 0 for the other.

Despite this result, a certain simplicity of behavior by the solute can be discerned. Experiment shows that, in the very dilute solution, the vapor pressure of the solute is, in the limit of zero concentration, a linear function of its mole fraction, as in

$$p_2 = x_2 k_2^x \tag{7.12}$$

which should be compared with Raoult's law, Eq. (7.1). Equation (7.12) is called *Henry's law*, and the constant of proportionality k_2^x is the Henry's law constant. The distinction between Raoult's law and Henry's law is easily seen graphically in Fig. 7.3.

The thermodynamic description of solute behavior in very dilute solutions is based on Henry's law, and it leads, by the same kind of argument used for ideal solutions, to Eq. (7.13), which is very similar to Eq. (7.3) for the ideal solution, except that the standard chemical potential incorporates the Henry's law constant:

$$\mu_2 = \mu_2^* + RT \ln x_2 \tag{7.13}$$

We saw in Chapter 5 that we may base our standard state definitions on either the mole fraction, the molal, or the molar concentration scales. Equations (7.12) and (7.13) make use of the mole fraction convention, and this is shown in Fig. 7.3 and again in Fig. 7.4a. Figure 7.4b shows the significance of the standard

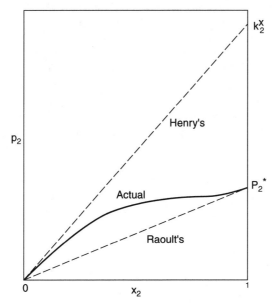

Figure 7.3. P_2^* is the vapor pressure of the pure solute ($x_2 = 1$), and the actual vapor pressure curve tends to this value. The Henry's law constant k_2^x is a hypothetical value obtained by linear extrapolation to $x_2 = 1$ of the tangent to the actual curve at $x_2 = 0$.

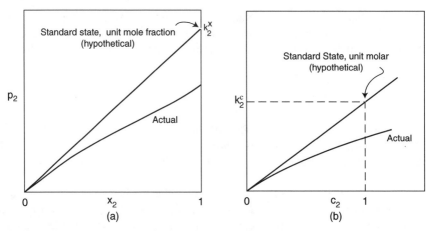

Figure 7.4. Henry's law constant k_2^x on the (a) mole fraction scale and (b) on the molar scale. These standard states are different. They are both hypothetical, because real behavior (solid curves) deviates from these linear extrapolations based on very dilute behavior.

state convention on the molar scale. Note how the superscript x or c is used with the Henry's law constant to clarify the definition. Of course k_2^x and k_2^c are different; their relationship can be worked out as we did in Chapter 5 [see also Grant and Higuchi (1990, p. 93)].

Finally we must consider nonideal solution behavior outside the very dilute solution range. We have seen how to cope with this behavior (Section 5.3) by defining activity coefficients, so that the actual behavior is quantitatively expressed by an activity coefficient that measures the deviation between real and ideal behavior. Now we can see that the adoption of a criterion of ideal behavior is critical to expressing the extent of deviation from this ideal. We are here approaching from a different direction an issue already faced in Section 5.3. At that point we had defined the activity of the solvent to be equal to its mole fraction. We now see that this is equivalent to assuming that Raoult's law is obeyed by the solvent, which is a reasonable assumption in the dilute solution range. The activity of the solute, on the other hand, we took as equal to its molar concentration in the very dilute range. This is a Henry's law reference state; the standard state is as shown in Fig. 7.4b. In Chapter 8 we will learn how to estimate activity coefficients for ionic species, which are notorious for their nonideal behavior; except in very concentrated solutions, however, the activity coefficients of nonelectrolytes can be taken as unity for most practical work.

The thermodynamic properties of real solutions are sometimes expressed in terms of *excess functions*, which are defined as the difference between the actual value of the function and the ideal value. For example, the excess entropy of mixing is

$$S^E = \Delta S_{\text{mix}}^{\text{real}} - \Delta S_{\text{mix}}^{\text{ideal}}$$

The excess functions can be positive or negative.[2]

7.3. PARTITIONING BETWEEN LIQUID PHASES

The Partition Coefficient. Suppose that we bring two immiscible liquids in contact, and then incorporate a nonelectrolyte solute such that its concentration is in the dilute solution range. The solute will distribute itself between the two phases, each of which constitutes a solution.[3] Since the phases will arrange themselves according to their densities, let us identify them as the upper (U) and lower (L) phases. The distribution of solute between the phases is called *partitioning*. The typical separatory funnel operation exemplifies this system. We take the pressure and temperature as fixed.

At equilibrium the chemical potentials of the solute in the upper and lower phases are equal:

$$\mu_2^U = \mu_2^L \tag{7.14}$$

These chemical potentials will be written out for the Henry's law molar standard state definition, giving

$$\mu_U^* + RT \ln c_U = \mu_L^* + RT \ln c_L \tag{7.15}$$

where for convenience the subscript 2 is omitted, assuming that the solute is meant.

Rearrangement of Eq. (7.15) gives

$$\Delta\mu^\circ = -RT \ln \frac{c_U}{c_L} \tag{7.16}$$

where $\Delta\mu^\circ = \mu_U^* - \mu_L^*$. Comparison of Eq. (7.16) with the important equation [Eq. (4.23)]

$$\Delta G^\circ = -RT \ln K \tag{7.17}$$

shows that the ratio c_U/c_L has the character of an equilibrium constant. In fact, it is the equilibrium constant of this "reaction":

Solute in phase L $\rightleftharpoons$ solute in phase U

This quantity is labeled P and is called the *partition coefficient*:

$$P = \frac{c_U}{c_L} \tag{7.18}$$

Partition coefficients are usually expressed in terms of their base 10 logarithms, log P. This makes the numerical values directly proportional to the standard free-energy change, according to Eq. (7.17), and it provides convenient magnitudes, since P itself can be much smaller or larger than unity.

Log P values have great utility in drug discovery and drug delivery research programs. For these purposes the solvent of the upper phase is usually selected to be 1-octanol, with water serving as the lower phase solvent. The partition coefficient is then defined as

$$P = \frac{c_{\text{octanol}}}{c_{\text{water}}} \tag{7.19}$$

Since water is more polar than is octanol, very polar solutes tend to have greater affinity for the aqueous phase and therefore to have P values smaller than unity, whereas nonpolar solutes have P values greater than unity. Consequently log P is often used as a quantitative measure of a compound's polarity.[4]

Log P values can be measured experimentally by the separatory funnel technique, or modifications of it. Sometimes it is useful to be able to predict a log P value, as for example if a compound of interest is not available or has not yet been synthesized. Empirical methods, making use of a large body of experimental log P values, have been developed that allow log P to be estimated solely on the basis of knowledge of the solute's molecular structure (Leo et al. 1971; Nys and Rekker 1974).

Table 7.1 lists a few log P values. Notice, for the series of normal alcohols, how the trend of log P values appears to accord with our qualitative notions of the polarities in this series. The log P of the aromatics is also consistent with expectations.

Example 7.1. 170.0 mg of benzylpenicillin (MW 334.4) was shaken with 10.0 mL of 1-octanol and 25.0 mL of water. After the phases separated, the aqueous phase was analyzed and found to contain 7.20×10^{-4} M benzylpenicillin. Calculate the partition coefficient of benzylpenicillin in this system.

The total number of moles of benzylpenicillin is $n_{\text{total}} = w/M$, where w is the weight in grams and M is the molecular weight. Obviously n_{total} is the sum of the amounts in the octanol and aqueous phases, or

$$n_{\text{oct}} + n_{\text{aq}} = n_{\text{total}}$$

We also have the partition coefficient definition,

$$P = \frac{c_{\text{oct}}}{c_{\text{aq}}}$$

Table 7.1. Log P (octanol/water) for some solutes

Solute	Log P	Solute	Log P
Methanol	−0.74	Benzene	2.13
Acetic acid	−0.24	Phenol	1.46
Ethanol	−0.32	Aniline	0.94
1-Propanol	0.34	Toluene	2.69
1-Butanol	0.88	Naphthalene	3.37
1-Pentanol	1.40	Aspirin	1.21

and the concentrations (in mol L^{-1}) are given by

$$c_{oct} = \frac{n_{oct}}{V_{oct}} \qquad c_{aq} = \frac{n_{aq}}{V_{aq}}$$

where the volumes are in liters. These equations suffice to solve the problem. We find $n_{total} = 0.170/334.4 = 5.08 \times 10^{-4}$ mol. Then, from the definition of c_{aq}, we obtain

$$n_{aq} = c_{aq}V_{aq}$$
$$= (7.20 \times 10^{-4} \text{mol L}^{-1})(0.025 \text{ L})$$
$$= 0.18 \times 10^{-4} \text{mol}$$

It follows that $n_{oct} = n_{total} - n_{aq}$, or $n_{oct} = 5.08 \times 10^{-4} - 0.18 \times 10^{-4} = 4.90 \times 10^{-4}$ mol, and therefore that

$$c_{oct} = \frac{4.90 \times 10^{-4} \text{ mol}}{0.01 \text{ L}}$$
$$= 4.90 \times 10^{-2} \text{ mol L}^{-1}$$

Finally

$$P = \frac{c_{oct}}{c_{aq}} = \frac{4.90 \times 10^{-2}}{7.20 \times 10^{-4}}$$
$$= 68.1$$

or $\log P = 1.83$.

Example 7.2. Log P (octanol/water) of caffeine is -0.07 at 25°C. Calculate the standard free-energy change for the partitioning process.
From Eq. (7.17), we have

$$\Delta\mu° = -2.303RT \log P$$
$$= (-2.303)(1.987 \text{ cal mol}^{-1} \text{ K}^{-1})(298.15 \text{ K})(-0.07)$$
$$= 96 \text{ cal mol}^{-1} = 400 \text{ J mol}^{-1}$$

The interpretation of $\Delta\mu°$ is that it is the free-energy change when one mole of caffeine in its standard state in water is transferred to its standard state in octanol. (This quantity is sometimes called the *transfer free energy*.)
From the log P value we find $P = 0.85$. Caffeine partitions nearly equally between the octanol and water phases, with a very slight preference for the water.

Solvent Extraction. Partitioning of a solute between immiscible phases is a valuable analytical technique, and it forms the basis of some chromatographic separation methods. In the simplest case we have the type of system described in the preceding discussion. Let p be the fraction of solute present in the upper phase and q the fraction in the lower phase, so $p + q = 1$. This quantity p is defined as

$$p = \frac{\text{amount of solute in upper phase}}{\text{total amount of solute}} \tag{7.20}$$

If c_U and c_L are the concentrations and V_U and V_L are the volumes of the upper and lower phases, then

$$p = \frac{c_U V_U}{c_U V_U + c_L V_L} \tag{7.21}$$

Let us define the ratio of phase volumes as

$$R = \frac{V_U}{V_L} \tag{7.22}$$

and of course $P = c_U/c_L$ from Eq. (7.18). Combining these relationships gives

$$p = \frac{PR}{PR + 1} \tag{7.23}$$

and so

$$q = \frac{1}{PR + 1} \tag{7.24}$$

Note that the product PR is equal to the ratio (amount in upper phase)/(amount in lower phase); this quantity is called the *capacity factor*. Equation (7.23) gives the fraction of solute extracted into the upper phase, and $100p$ is the percent extracted.

Example 7.3. Log P (octanol/water) $= 0.70$ for ethyl acetate. If 10.0 mL of an aqueous solution of ethyl acetate is extracted with one-25.0 mL portion of octanol, what percentage of the ethyl acetate will be extracted into the octanol layer?
    Since log $P = 0.70, P = 5.0$. We also have $R = 2.50$. Applying Eq. (7.23) gives $p = 0.926$, so 92.6% will be found in the octanol.

    Unless P is very large, a significant fraction of solute will be found in both phases after a single extraction, as seen in Example 7.3. If the experimental goal is to remove essentially all the solute from one phase into the other, common practice is to reextract with fresh portions of the extracting solvent, pooling the extracts, until the solute has been quantitatively removed. We can calculate the number of extractions required to extract any specified fraction of solute.

Table 7.2. Calculation of the progress of extraction

n	Fraction of Total Extracted in nth Extraction	Total Fraction Extracted	Fraction Remaining
1	p	p	$1 - p = q$
2	pq	$p + pq$	$1 - (p + pq) = q^2$
3	pq^2	$p + pq + pq^2$	$1 - (p + pq + pq^2) = q^3$
.	.	.	.
.	.	.	.
.	.	.	.
n	$pq^{(n-1)}$	$\sum_{n=1}^{n} pq^{(n-1)}$	q^n

As earlier, p is the fraction of solute extracted into the upper phase in a single extraction, and q is the fraction in the lower phase. The first line in Table 7.2 shows the state of the extraction after the first extraction.

If we accept the assumption that P is a true equilibrium constant, so that P has the same value irrespective of the absolute concentrations,[5] then the same fraction p of solute remaining in the lower phase will be extracted into the upper phase each time. (We assume that identical volumes of fresh upper phase are used in each extraction.) Then the fraction of *total* solute removed in the nth extraction is equal to the product of the fraction remaining and the fraction extracted in a single extraction:

Fraction of total extracted in nth extraction = fraction of total left after

$$(n - 1)\text{th extraction} \times p \quad (7.25)$$

Applying this equation to the second extraction gives

Fraction of total extracted in 2nd extraction $= pq$

This is entered on the second line of Table 7.2. The total fraction extracted is now equal to the sum of the fractions extracted in the first and second extractions, which is $p + pq$, and the fraction remaining is $1 -$ total fraction extracted, which is equal to q^2 as seen in Table 7.2. In this way Table 7.2 is completed.

A final convenient expression is obtained by noting that

Total fraction extracted $= 1 -$ fraction remaining

or, from the final entry in Table 7.2, after n extractions

$$\text{Total fraction extracted} = 1 - q^n \quad (7.26)$$

Table 7.3. Multiple extractions of a solute with
$P = 5$ and $R = 1$

Number of Extractions, n	Total Extracted (%)
1	83.33
2	97.21
3	99.53
4	99.92
5	99.99

Example 7.4. For the system described in Example 7.3, calculate the total fraction extracted after 1, 2, 3, 4, and 5 extractions, if $R = 1.0$.

Since $P = 5.0$ and $R = 1.0$, we find with Eq. (7.24) that $q = \frac{1}{6} = 0.167$. Applying Eq. (7.26) gives the results in Table 7.3.

Observe the asymptotic approach to complete extraction, which in principle can never be achieved because, in the terms of classical thermodynamics, at equilibrium (which is reached at each stage of the extraction process) the chemical potential of the solute must be identical in both phases, so the solute cannot be absent from one phase and present in the other. In practice, of course, we can often carry out the extraction to an extent that is practically indistinguishable from completion.

Example 7.5. Using the same system of Examples 7.3 and 7.4, for which $P = 5.0$, compare the efficiency of extraction of a 15-mL aqueous solution of ethyl acetate with (a) one 60-mL portion of octanol; (b) four 15-mL portions of octanol.

(a) With Eq. (7.23) and the quantities $P = 5.0, R = 4.0$, we find $p = 0.952$, or 95.2% extracted in this experiment.

(b) With Eq. (7.26) and the quantities $p = 5.0, R = 1.0$, $n = 4$ we find $q = 0.0476$ and total fraction extracted $= 0.9992$, or 99.92% extracted in this experimental design.

Example 7.5 demonstrates an important result of extraction theory. A more efficient extraction is achieved with several extractions than with a single extraction, even when the same volume of extracting solvent is employed in the different operations.

Countercurrent Distribution. Although a single solute can be exhaustively extracted from solution by means of multiple extractions, it is not possible to separate two solutes (leaving one in each phase) by this technique unless the partition coefficient of one of them is effectively zero or infinite. An alternative experimental design, called *countercurrent distribution* (CCD), has been invented to allow solutes having similar (yet quantitatively different) partition coefficients to be separated. The term "countercurrent" means that the two phases move in opposite directions, although actually one phase is held motionless and the other moves, so the phases are in relative motion. Although CCD as a separation technique has been superseded by chromatography, a description is worthwhile for two reasons: (1) since thermodynamic equilibrium can be achieved at each stage of the process, an exact mathematical analysis is possible, and the mathematics turn out to be of a much wider applicability; and (2) CCD constitutes an excellent introduction to the technique of partition chromatography, which in fact was initially developed as a modification of CCD [the present treatment of CCD draws heavily on earlier work (Connors 1982, pp. 357–364)].

The countercurrent distribution experiment uses a train of tubes within which the individual equilibrations occur. At the beginning of the experiment each tube is charged with an identical volume of the lower phase (e.g., water or an aqueous buffer). These tubes are numbered $0, 1, 2, \ldots, r$. Into tube 0 a suitable volume of the upper-phase solvent (e.g., ether) is introduced. The solute is added to tube 0; it is immaterial whether the solute is added in the upper or the lower phase. Figure 7.5 is a schematic rendering of a countercurrent distribution of a single solute; it is assumed, in this case, that $p = q = 0.5$. Figure 7.5a represents the train of tubes as it has been described above, with 16 parts of solute added to the lower phase of tube 0. Now the tube is shaken to allow distribution to occur; in Fig. 7.5b the resulting partitioning of the solute is shown as 8 parts in each phase, since $p = q$ for this particular solute.

Next the upper phase of tube 0 is transferred to tube 1 (this is called the *first transfer*) and fresh solvent is added to tube 0 (Fig. 7.5c). The tubes are equilibrated to give the distribution shown in Fig. 7.5d. This sequence is repeated until three transfers have been effected ($n = 3$), as shown in Fig. 7.5h.

The result of these operations has been to transfer the solute in the direction of motion of the upper phase. This process may be repeated many times. Since only the upper phase is transferred, clearly the solute can progress along the train of tubes only by being extracted into the upper phase. Therefore the greater the value of p, the further along the tube train the solute will progress in a given number of transfers. Actually the solute is distributed over many tubes, as can be seen by the sample shown in Fig. 7.5. If the original sample contains two solutes with different partition coefficients, they will progress along the tubes at different "rates," the substance with the larger partition coefficient traveling faster. In order to separate the solutes it is necessary only to perform enough transfers.

It is possible to predict quantitatively the countercurrent distribution behavior of a solute if its partition coefficient is known for the liquid–liquid system. Since P and R are known quantities, p and q may be calculated.

Suppose that one unit of a single solute is placed in the lower phase of tube 0; the situation may be represented as in the first row of Table 7.4, where, as in the earlier discussion, the tubes are numbered $0, 1, 2, \ldots, r$, and transfers $0, 1, 2, \ldots, n$. Before equilibration all the solute is in the lower phase, and after equilibration a fraction p of the solute is in the upper phase and q is in the lower phase.

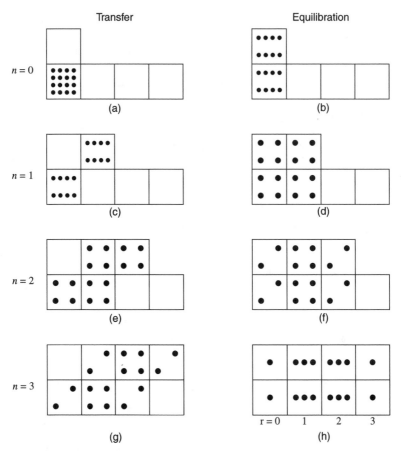

Figure 7.5. Schematic representation of countercurrent distribution with three transfers of a solute with $p = 0.5$. [Reproduced by permission from Connors (1987).]

Next the upper phase of tube 0 is transferred to tube 1 (which contains fresh lower phase) and fresh upper phase is placed in tube 0. The phases are equilibrated. The fraction of total solute extracted into the upper phase of tube 0 will be p times the fraction of solute in the tube, or pq. Similarly, the fraction of solute in the lower phase is q times the fraction of solute in the tube, or q^2. In this way the distribution has been calculated through four transfers, as seen in Table 7.4.

In the last row of the table the total fraction of original solute in each tube is listed. The distribution exhibits a marked symmetry in p and q. Obviously the calculation of such a distribution for many transfers would be extremely laborious, but it is fortunately not necessary to proceed as in the previous example. It has been observed that the total fraction of original solute in each tube is given by the corresponding term in the binomial expansion, $(q + p)^n$. Two implications of this result are (1) for n transfers there are $n + 1$ terms, and therefore $n + 1$ tubes; and (2) the sum of all the terms is 1, since $p + q = 1$, and 1 to any power is 1.

Table 7.4. Calculation of the distribution through four transfers[a]

Transfer Number, n		Tube Number, r				
		0	1	2	3	4
0	B[a]	$0/1$				
	A[b]	p/q				
1	B	$0/q$	$p/0$			
	A	pq/q^2	p^2/pq			
2	B	$0/q^2$	pq/pq	$p^2/0$		
	A	pq^2/q^3	$2p^2q/2pq^2$	p^3/p^2q		
3	B	$0/q^3$	$pq^2/2pq^2$	$2p^2q/p^2q$	$p^3/0$	
	A	pq^3/q^4	$3p^2q^2/3pq^3$	$3p^3q/3p^2q^2$	p^4/p^3q	
4	B	$0/q^4$	$pq^3/3pq^3$	$3p^2q^2/3p^2q^2$	$3p^3q/p^3q$	$p^4/0$
Totals after four transfers		q^4	$4pq^3$	$6p^2q^2$	$4p^3q$	p^4

[a] Before equilibration.
[b] After equilibration.
Source: Reproduced by permission from Connors (1987).

The expansion of the function $(q+p)^n$ is laborious for large n, and an easier calculation is available. The binomial expansion may be written

$$(q+p)^n = q^n + nq^{n-1}p + \frac{n(n-1)}{2}q^{n-2}p^2 + \cdots + p^n$$

which can be expressed

$$(q+p)^n = \sum_{r=0}^{n} \frac{n!}{r!(n-r)!}p^r q^{(n-r)}$$

where r is the number of the corresponding term in the expansion (the quantity $n!$ is called "n factorial" and means $n! = 1 \cdot 2 \cdot 3 \cdot 4 \cdots n$; the relationship $0! = 1$ is a definition). Interpreting this in the context of CCD, we write Eq. (7.27) for the rth term in the binomial expansion

$$T_{nr} = \frac{n!}{r!(n-r)!}p^r q^{(n-r)} \tag{7.27}$$

where the quantity T_{nr} is read "the fraction of total solute contained in both layers of the rth tube after n transfers." A calculated countercurrent distribution is usually exhibited as a plot of T_{nr} versus r. Equation (7.27) is called the *binomial distribution*.

Calculation of the CCD curve may be further simplified. According to statistical theory, the mean of the binomial distribution is equal to np. The mean corresponds to the maximum; therefore the tube number of the maximum in the curve, $r_{\max}$, is given by

$$r_{\max} = np \tag{7.28}$$

This simple expression permits one to calculate the maximum in the CCD curve if p is known. Although n must be an integral number, $r_{\max}$ need not be. Note that $r_{\max}$ is directly proportional to p. If Eq. (7.27) is written for T_{nr} and for $T_{n(r-1)}$, these expressions can be combined to give

$$\frac{T_{nr}}{T_{n(r-1)}} = \frac{p(n-r+1)}{qr} \tag{7.29}$$

with which the fraction of solute in any tube can be calculated if the fraction in an adjacent tube is known.

The easiest way to calculate an entire distribution curve with these equations (assuming that p is known) is to first find $r_{\max}$ with Eq. (7.28). Next calculate T_{nr} with Eq. (7.27) for one tube in the vicinity of $r_{\max}$. Finally calculate the fractions of solute in all surrounding tubes by means of Eq. (7.29). Figure 7.6 shows the results of such a calculation for a typical separation of two solutes; it was assumed that $P_1 = 0.5$, $P_2 = 2.0$, and $R = 1.00$ for this system. In Fig. 7.6a the distribution of each solute is shown after four transfers. In an actual experiment the tube contents would be analyzed for total solutes present, and the experimental curve would therefore represent the sum of the fractions of the individual solutes; this curve is shown as the solid line in Fig. 7.6a. Separation is not yet apparent in this curve. The individual distribution curves, however, show that a partial resolution has occurred, with tubes 0 and 1 enriched in solute 1, tubes 3 and 4 enriched in solute 2, and tube 2 containing equal fractions of solutes 1 and 2.

Figure 7.6b shows the same system after 24 transfers. Separation of the solutes is now apparent. Tubes 0–9 contain essentially only solute 1, whereas tubes 15–24 contain only solute 2. Portions of both solutes will be found in tubes 10–14. If the experiment were extended to a larger number of transfers, a complete separation could eventually be achieved. Note, however, that the width of the "zones," or distribution curves, increases as the number of transfers increases.

In a real experimental situation, the quantity plotted on the vertical axis would usually be an analytic quantity, such as weight of solute per tube, rather than the fraction T_{nr}. It may be noted that from such an experimental distribution curve the quantity $r_{\max}$ may be read and, by utilizing Eqs. (7.28) and (7.23), the partition coefficient may be estimated.

The countercurrent distribution curve is not symmetric (unless $p = q$), but as n becomes larger, the curve approaches very closely a symmetric distribution.

The binomial distribution is a mathematical function that yields the probability of "success" in what are known as *Bernoulli trials*. These are events, such a coin tosses, in which there are only two possible outcomes (heads or tails). The analogy

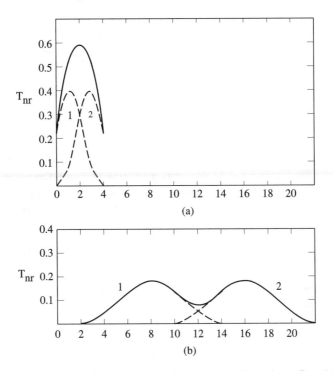

Figure 7.6. Countercurrent distribution of two solutes in a system where $P_1 = 0.5, P_2 = 2.0$, $R = 1.0$: (a) distribution after 4 transfers; (b) distribution after 24 transfers. The calculated points are connected by smooth curves, although in fact the distribution is discontinuous. [Reproduced by permission from Connors (1987).]

to CCD is that a molecule of solute has only two possible choices—it must take up residence in either the upper phase or the lower phase. As the number of transfers becomes very large, the discontinuous (i.e., stepwise) binomial distribution approaches closely a continuous function, the normal distribution, which provides for a faster means of calculating the CCD curve (Connors 1982, pp. 357–364).

PROBLEMS

7.1. Calculate the ideal entropy of mixing and free energy of mixing when 10.0 g of benzene and 15.0 g of toluene are mixed at 25°C.

7.2. For alanine, log P (octanol/water) $= -2.94$. For phenothiazine, log $P = 4.15$. Calculate the standard free energy changes for these phase transfer processes at 25°C.

7.3. These are experimental partial pressures of benzene (B) and toluene (T) over their solutions at 20°C:

X_B	P_B	P_T (mm)
0.00	0	22
0.27	18	17
0.44	34	12
0.55	41	11
0.67	49	8
1.00	75	0

Confirm the validity of Raoult's law for this system by plotting the data. By calculation determine the solution composition at which the partial pressures of benzene and toluene are equal, and check your result on the graph you have plotted. What is the total vapor pressure over the solution at this composition?

7.4. These are partial pressures of chloroform over chloroform-acetone solutions at 35°C:

$x(CHCl_3)$	p (mm)
0.0	0
0.2	34
0.4	82
0.6	148
0.8	225
1.0	293

Plot the data, confirming the asymptotic approach to Raoult's law in the nearly pure chloroform, and the nonideal behavior in dilute solutions of chloroform. Estimate the Henry's law constant.

7.5. How many extractions are necessary to remove 99.9% of a drug from 30 mL of an aqueous solution if it is extracted with 20 mL portions of ether and log P (ether/water) $= 0.54$?

7.6. (a) Consider the distribution of neutral weak acid HA between an organic phase and an aqueous phase. Define the true partition coefficient as $P = [HA]_{org}/[HA]_{aq}$. Presuming that the anion does not detectably partition into the organic phase, derive this relationship between the true partition coefficient P and the apparent partition coefficient P_{app}

$$P_{app} = \frac{P[H^+]}{[H^+] + K_a}$$

where K_a is the acid dissociation constant of HA, $[H^+]$ is the aqueous phase concentration of hydrogen ion, and P_{app} is the ratio of total concentrations of solute in the organic and aqueous phases.

(**b**) Show how P_{app} is related to P at the limits of very low and very high hydrogen ion concentration. How are P and P_{app} related when pH $=$ pK_a?

(**c**) Calculate P_{app} as a function of pH for an acid having p$K_a = 4.0$ and for which $\log P = 1.00$. Plot P_{app} against pH.

7.7. Consider a system consisting of a single solute partitioned among three mutually immiscible phases A, B, and C, the system being at equilibrium.

(**a**) Define the three partiton coefficients.

(**b**) Derive an equation relating one of the partition coefficients to the other two.

(**c**) Derive an equation relating the fraction of solute in phase A to the partition coefficients and the volumes of the two phases.

7.8. A mixture of three compounds was subjected to countercurrent distribution. After 150 transfers, with each tube containing 5 mL of water and 5mL of ether, the maxima in the CCD curve appeared at tubes 30, 75, and 120. Calculate the partition coefficients of the three compounds.

NOTES

1. A solution having the compositon corresponding to either a maximum (Fig. 7.2a) or a minimum (Fig. 7.2b) in the vapor pressure curve will distill as a constant boiling mixture of constant composition, called an *azeotrope*. For instance, 95% alcohol is an azeotrope containing 95.57% by weight (94.9% by volume) of C_2H_5OH.

2. A class of solutions called *regular solutions* is defined to have $S^E = 0$ and $H^E \neq 0$, so that entropically such solutions behave ideally, but they undergo nonideal energy changes. Regular solutions are commonly formed from nonpolar components [see Hildebrandt et al. (1970); see also Chapter 10 (below)].

3. Besides the phenomenon in which the solute distributes between the two phases, the upper phase will be saturated with respect to the lower phase solvent, and vice versa. This mutual saturation alters the solvent properties of the two phases, but it does not affect the thermodynamic argument.

4. P (and therefore also $\log P$) is a perfectly well-defined thermodynamic quantity. The concept that $\log P$ is a measure of polarity is not a part of thermodynamics, however, and since this concept, and othes like it, lie outside of thermodynamics, it is said to be *extrathermodynamic*.

5. From Eq. (7.18), $c_U = Pc_L$, which states that a plot of c_U versus c_L should be linear if P is a constant independent of concentration. This plot is called a *partition* or *distribution isotherm*. A linear partition isotherm shows that P is independent of concentration.

8

SOLUTIONS OF ELECTROLYTES

8.1. COULOMBIC INTERACTION AND IONIC DISSOCIATION

An electrolyte is a substance that produces ions. Since the ions are charged species, the force of interaction between them is a convenient starting point for our discussion. The force of interaction between two particles having charges Q_1 and Q_2, separated by distance r, is given by *Coulomb's law*

$$F = \frac{Q_1 Q_2}{4\pi\epsilon r^2} \qquad (8.1)$$

where ϵ is a property of the medium, to be dealt with shortly. The potential energy of interaction, V, is equal to the product of force and distance. The Coulombic potential energy is therefore

$$V = \frac{Q_1 Q_2}{4\pi\epsilon r} \qquad (8.2)$$

Since the charge on an ion can be written as the product of its valence z (including its sign) and the electronic charge e ($e = 1.602 \times 10^{-19}$ C), Eq. (8.2), for our purposes, is equivalent to

$$V = \frac{z_1 z_2 e^2}{4\pi\epsilon r} \qquad (8.3)$$

For two ions of like charge, V and F are both positive and the force is repulsive, whereas if the ions are of unlike charge, V and F are negative and are attractive.

96

Table 8.1. Dielectric constants of some solvents

Solvent	ϵ_r	Solvent	ϵ_r
n-Hexane	1.89	Methanol	32.6
Cyclohexane	2.02	Nitrobenzene	35
1,4-Dioxane	2.21	Acetonitrile	36.2
Benzene	2.28	N,N-Dimethylformamide	36.7
Diethyl ether	4.34	Ethylene glycol	37.7
Ethyl acetate	6.02	N,N-Dimethylacetamide	37.8
Acetic acid	6.19	Glycerol	42.5
n-Butyl alcohol	17.1	Dimethyl sulfoxide	49
i-Propyl alcohol	17.7	Formic acid	58
Acetone	20.7	Water	78.5
Ethanol	24.3	Formamide	110

The zero of potential energy is taken to be when the ions are separated to infinity $(r = \infty)$.

The quantity ϵ is called the permittivity, and it is best introduced through the expression

$$\epsilon_r = \frac{\epsilon}{\epsilon_0} \tag{8.4}$$

where ϵ_0 is the *permittivity of the vacuum* and ϵ_r is called the *relative permittivity*. Chemists, however, have traditionally referred to ϵ_r as the *dielectric constant*. The relative permittivity or dielectric constant is measured as the electrical capacitance of the medium (solvent) relative to the capacitance of the vacuum. It follows that ϵ_r is a dimensionless number greater than one. Equation (8.3) is often written in the form

$$V = \frac{z_1 z_2 e^2}{4\pi\epsilon_0\epsilon_r r} \tag{8.5}$$

The permittivity of the vacuum ϵ_0 has the value $8.854 \times 10^{-12}\,\mathrm{C^2\,J^{-1}\,m^{-1}}$. Table 8.1 gives some dielectric constant values.

Example 8.1. Calculate the energy of the Coulombic interaction between a sodium ion and a chloride ion, at contact distance, in vacuum and in water.

The ionic radii of Na^+ and of Cl^- (available in reference handbooks) are 0.95 and 1.81 Å, respectively, equivalent to an internuclear distance of $r = 2.76 \times 10^{-10}\,\mathrm{m}$. In vacuum

$$V\,(\text{vacuum}) = -\frac{(1.602 \times 10^{-19}\,\mathrm{C})^2}{4\pi(8.854 \times 10^{-12}\,\mathrm{C^2\,J^{-1}\,m^{-1}})(1)(2.76 \times 10^{-10}\,\mathrm{m})}$$
$$= -8.36 \times 10^{-19}\,\mathrm{J}$$

This is the energy of interaction between one Na^+ and one Cl^-. If we multiply by Avogadro's number to find the energy per mole of sodium chloride, we get

$$V \text{ (vacuum)} = -504 \, \text{kJ mol}^{-1}$$
$$= -120 \, \text{kcal mol}^{-1}$$

a very strong interaction. In water $\epsilon_r = 78.5$, and the calculation gives

$$V \text{ (water)} = -0.106 \times 10^{-19} \, \text{J per ion pair}$$
$$= -6.42 \, \text{kJ mol}^{-1}$$
$$= -1.53 \, \text{kcal mol}^{-1}$$

Example 8.1 shows that the dielectric constant of the medium markedly influences the strength of the interionic interaction energy. The dielectric constant is a measure of the ability of the medium to separate charges of unlike sign. (Not coincidentally, the dielectric constant roughly parallels our chemical notion of solvent polarity, and is often taken as a quantitative measure of polarity.) The larger the dielectric constant, the easier two unlike charges can be separated. The high dielectric constant of water is a manifestation of the very unusual nature of water as a solvent. In fact, the classification of electrolytes into the categories of strong electrolytes (i.e., essentially completely dissociated into ions in solution) and weak electrolytes (incompletely dissociated) is based on the use of water as the solvent. Substances that are strong electrolytes in water act as weak electrolytes in low dielectric constant solvents.[1] Let us pursue this issue by writing Eq. (8.6) for an electrolyte, schematically denoted AB, when dissolved in a solvent:

$$AB \xrightarrow{\text{ionization}} A^+B^- \xrightarrow{\text{dissociation}} A^+ + B^- \qquad (8.6)$$

Ionization is the production of ions,[2] and dissociation is the separation of species (whether ionic or uncharged). The extent of ionic dissociation is reasonably described by Coulomb's law. This is why we do not distinguish between ionization and dissociation for aqueous solutions; because water's dielectric constant is quite large, the force between ions is relatively small, and as soon as ions form, they dissociate. Ion pairs (the species $A^+ B^-$) are seldom detectable in water. But in solvents of low dielectric constant (typically with ϵ_r values less than ~25), the extent of dissociation is reduced, as may be demonstrated by repeating Example 8.1 with some different ϵ_r values. Glacial acetic acid (the term "glacial" simply means essentially pure in this context) is an important analytical solvent that has been carefully studied. Because of its low dielectric constant, ion-pairs can be detected in acetic acid solutions. Letting HOAc represent acetic acid (since acetic acid is CH_3COOH, the symbol Ac represents the acetyl group CH_3CO), a solute acid HX reacts according to

$$HX + HOAc \rightleftharpoons H_2OAc^+X^- \rightleftharpoons H_2OAc^+ + X^-$$

In this scheme HOAc is acting to solvate the hydrogen ion, and H_2OAc^+ in acetic acid is analogous to H_3O^+ in water. For convenience we usually omit the solvent, writing simply

$$HX \rightleftharpoons H^+ X^- \rightleftharpoons H^+ + X^- \tag{8.7}$$

Now, in the conventional manner we define an ionization constant K_i and a dissociation constant K_d as follows, using Eq. (8.7) as the defining reaction.

$$K_i = \frac{[H^+X^-]}{[HX]} \tag{8.8}$$

$$K_d = \frac{[H^+][X^-]}{[H^+X^-]} \tag{8.9}$$

Next we define an overall dissociation constant K_{HX}; we place all dissociated species in the numerator and all undissociated species in the denominator:

$$K_{HX} = \frac{[H^+][X^-]}{c_{HX}} \tag{8.10}$$

where $c_{HX} = [HX] + [H^+X^-]$. In these equations brackets signify molar concentrations. Combining Eqs. (8.8)–(8.10) gives

$$K_{HX} = \frac{K_i K_d}{1 + K_i} \tag{8.11}$$

Similar equations can be written for bases and for salts. One of the consequences is that the pH, which in water is the controlling factor in acid–base equilibria, does not play a comparable role in glacial acetic acid. This is because very little of the acidic species is present as dissociated H^+; most of the acid is in the undissociated form c_{HX}.

8.2. MEAN IONIC ACTIVITY AND ACTIVITY COEFFICIENT

Let us now consider a strong electrolyte, such as a salt in aqueous solution. The solute is completely dissociated into its constituent ions according to

$$M_pX_q \rightleftharpoons pM^{q+} + qX^{p-} \tag{8.12}$$

where p and q denote the number of positive and negative ions, respectively, generated by one molecule of the salt. The following development is motivated by the impossibility of separately varying and studying the cations and the anions; electroneutrality dictates that only their combination in the ratio p/q can be manipulated.

We will adopt the infinite dilution Henry's law reference state in the molar concentration scale for all species. Then we can write for the cation and the anion

$$\mu_+ = \mu_+^\circ + RT \ln a_+ \tag{8.13a}$$

$$\mu_- = \mu_-^\circ + RT \ln a_- \tag{8.13b}$$

and for the solute as a whole

$$\mu_2 = \mu_2^\circ + RT \ln a_2 \tag{8.14}$$

Now we postulate (assuming complete dissociation)

$$\mu_2 = p\mu_+ + q\mu_- \tag{8.15}$$

and analogously

$$\mu_2^\circ = p\mu_+^\circ + q\mu_-^\circ \tag{8.16}$$

Simple algebraic combination of Eqs. (8.13)–(8.16) yields

$$a_2 = a_+^p a_-^q \tag{8.17}$$

We define v as the number of ions generated by one molecule of solute, so

$$v = p + q \tag{8.18}$$

It is now conventional to define the *mean ionic activity* $a_\pm$ by $a_\pm^v = a_2$, giving the following, from Eq. (8.17):

$$a_\pm^v = a_+^p a_-^q \tag{8.19}$$

A self-consistent set of relations is obtained by making these further definitions; the *mean ionic activity coefficient* is

$$\gamma_\pm^v = \gamma_+^p \gamma_-^q \tag{8.20}$$

and the *mean ionic molarity* is

$$c_\pm^v = c_+^p c_-^q \tag{8.21}$$

so that we can write

$$a_\pm = \gamma_\pm c_\pm \tag{8.22}$$

The significance of these relationships is easiest to comprehend for the simplest case of a $1:1$ electrolyte such as NaCl. For this case $p = 1$, $q = 1$, $v = 2$, and we write from the foregoing

$$a_{\pm}^2 = a_+ a_- \tag{8.23a}$$
$$\gamma_{\pm}^2 = \gamma_+ \gamma_- \tag{8.23b}$$
$$c_{\pm}^2 = c_+ c_- \tag{8.23c}$$

Although we separately know c_+ and c_- from c_2, the solute concentration, we cannot separately determine γ_+, γ_-, a_+, and a_-. The effect of the definitions given above is to assign the extent of nonideality equally (when $p = q$) to the cation and the anion.

Example 8.2

(a) What is the mean ionic molarity of an aqueous solution 0.15 M in sodium chloride? Since sodium chloride is completely dissociated, $c_+ = 0.15\,\text{M}$ and $c_- = 0.15\,\text{M}$, giving, from Eq. (8.23c), $c_{\pm} = 0.15\,\text{M}$.
(b) What is the mean ionic molarity of an aqueous solution 0.25 M in K_2SO_4? For this system $p = 2$, $q = 1$, $v = 3$. The concentration of potassium ions, c_+, is 0.50 M and c_-, the concentration of sulfate ions, is 0.25 M. From Eq. (8.21), we have

$$c_{\pm}^3 = (0.50)^2 (0.25)$$
$$c_{\pm} = 0.397\,\text{M}$$

8.3. THE DEBYE–HÜCKEL THEORY

In an infinitely dilute solution each solute ion is resident in an environment that consists effectively only of the solvent (which we continue to treat as a continuum). In such a situation the ion is free to exert whatever effects are characteristic of its identity, unperturbed by other solute species; it is in its Henry's law reference state, and it behaves ideally.

If the ionic concentration of the solution is raised, either by increasing the concentration of the solute of interest or by adding ions of a different electrolyte solute, the environment of our ion changes. As the ionic concentrations increase, the distance between ions decreases, and the Coulombic interaction energies come into play. Ions of like charge tend to repel each other, and ions of unlike charge attract each other. The consequence of these interactions is that instead of a random distribution of ions throughout the solution, an *ionic atmosphere* develops such that the volume centered on a cation possesses a net negative charge, whereas the volume centered on an anion possesses a net positive charge (of course, the solution as a whole is electrically neutral). These charge distributions, constituting perturbations of the infinite dilution environment, are manifested in solute behavior that we interpret as nonideal, and that we measure in terms of a mean ionic activity coefficient.

In 1923 Debye and Hückel developed a quantitative theory of this ionic atmosphere effect. Although the Debye–Hückel theory is not itself part of thermodynamics, its final result has been absorbed into thermodynamics, and it is routinely used to interpret and to predict nonideal behavior in electrolyte solutions. The *Debye–Hückel equation* is written

$$\text{Log}\,\gamma_\pm = -\frac{A|z_+z_-|\sqrt{I}}{1 + aB\sqrt{I}} \tag{8.24}$$

where A and B are constants whose values depend on the dielectric constant and the temperature, and a is closely related to an ionic radius. The quantity I is the *ionic strength* and is defined by Eq. (8.25), where c_i is the molar concentration of ion i and z_i is its charge.

$$I = \tfrac{1}{2}\sum c_i z_i^2 \tag{8.25}$$

In Eq. (8.24), z_+ and z_- are the (absolute values of the) charges on the electrolyte of interest; in Eq. (8.25), the c_i and z_i include *all* the ions in the solution.

For aqueous solutions at 25°C, Eq. (8.24) takes the specific form

$$\text{Log}\,\gamma_\pm = -\frac{0.509|z_+z_-|\sqrt{I}}{1 + \sqrt{I}} \tag{8.26}$$

and at very low ionic strengths Eq. (8.26) approaches Eq. (8.27), which is known as the *Debye–Hückel limiting law*:

$$\text{Log}\,\gamma_\pm = -0.509|z_+z_-|\sqrt{I} \tag{8.27}$$

Example 8.3. What is the ionic strength of (a) a solution 0.10 M in NaCl and 0.05 M in HCl; (b) a solution 0.25 M in K_2SO_4?

(a) $c_{NA^+} = 0.10\,M$, $c_{H^+} = 0.05\,M$, $c_{Cl^-} = 0.15\,M$; $z_i^2 = 1$ for all ions. From Eq. (8.25), we have

$$I = \tfrac{1}{2}(0.10 + 0.05 + 0.15) = 0.15\,M$$

The ionic strength of a solution of 1 : 1 electrolytes is equal to the total solute concentration.

(b) $c_{K^+} = 0.50\,M$, $z_{K^+} = +1$, $c_{SO_4^{2-}} = 0.25\,M$, $z_{SO_4^{2-}} = -2$

$$I = \tfrac{1}{2}(0.50 \times 1 + 0.25 \times 4) = 0.75\,M$$

The ionic strength of a solution containing polyvalent ions reflects the dominant effect of the square of the charge on the ionic atmosphere. Notice that the concentrations of H^+ and OH^- arising from the dissociation of water are not included in the calculation because they make a negligible contribution to the ionic strength.

Example 8.4. Calculate the mean ionic activity coefficient of a $1:1$ electrolyte at concentrations of 0.001, 0.010, and 0.10 mol L^{-1}, in water at 25°C. Use the Debye–Hückel equation in the form of Eq. (8.26), and also the limiting law, Eq. (8.27).

From the given data, $z_+ = +1$, $z_- = -1$, so $|z_+z_-| = 1$, and $I = c$, the molar concentration. These results are found:

	$\gamma_\pm$	
c (M)	Eq. (8.26)	Eq. (8.27)
0.001	0.965	0.964
0.010	0.899	0.889
0.100	0.756	0.690

The results in Example 8.4 show that the limiting law and the full Debye–Hückel equation agree closely in extremely dilute solution, but they begin to differ significantly in the concentration region of ~0.01 M (i.e., when $\sqrt{I} = 0.1$). Above this ionic strength Eq. (8.26) is necessary, but even this equation fails to agree closely with experimental results at ionic strengths above about 0.05 M, where effects specific to each electrolyte are observed. Table 8.2 lists some experimentally determined mean ionic activity coefficients.[3] We expect, from the appearance of the product $|z_+z_-|$ in the Debye–Hückel equation, that different charge types of

Table 8.2. Mean ionic activity coefficients in water at 25°C

	$\gamma_\pm$			
m	HCl	NaCl	CaCl$_2$	ZnSO$_4$
0.001	0.966	0.966	0.888	0.734
0.005	0.928	0.929	0.789	0.477
0.01	0.905	0.904	0.732	0.387
0.02	0.875	0.875	0.669	0.298
0.05	0.830	0.823	0.584	0.202
0.1	0.796	0.778	0.531	0.148
0.2	0.767	0.732	0.482	0.104
0.5	0.757	0.679	0.457	0.063
1.0	0.809	0.656	0.509	0.044
2.0	1.009	0.670	0.807	0.035
3.0	1.316	0.719	1.55	0.041

Source: Data from Glasstone (1947, p. 402).

electrolytes will behave differently, and this is seen. However, it is also observed that electrolytes of the same charge type display behavior characteristic of the individual electrolyte; compare HCl and NaCl in Table 8.2. Empirical extensions of the Debye–Hückel equation have been proposed of the form (at 25°C in water)

$$\text{Log}\,\gamma_{\pm} = -\frac{0.509|z_+z_-|\sqrt{I}}{1 + aB\sqrt{I}} + CI \tag{8.28}$$

where the parameters aB and C are chosen to best fit the experimental data.

Figure 8.1 is a plot of the data from Table 8.2 in a format consistent with the manner in which the Debye–Hückel equation is written, that is, as a plot of $\log\gamma_{\pm}$ against $\sqrt{I}$. Figure 8.1 shows several interesting features. The individual character of the nonideal behavior is clearly evident in the curves for HCl and NaCl. The minima observed in these curves is not predicted by the Debye–Hückel equation, and in some instances the mean ionic activity coefficients rise to values greater than unity. From the limiting law, Eq. (8.27), we can predict the slope of the plot for each charge type of electrolyte at infinite dilution, and these slopes are drawn in Fig. 8.1. The Debye–Hückel limiting law gives a satisfactory account of nonideal electrolyte behavior in very dilute solutions.

The Debye–Hückel theory finds very practical application in obtaining thermodynamic acid dissociation constants for weak acids and bases. An apparent constant is measured experimentally at, necessarily, finite ionic strength, and the theory is used to correct the value to zero ionic strength. This calculation is described in Chapter 13. One powerful consequence of the Debye–Hückel theory is that it provides a firm theoretical basis for the extrapolation of electrolyte experimental

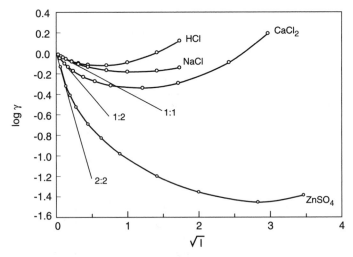

Figure 8.1. Plot of data in Table 8.2. Limiting law slopes are drawn for 1:1, 1:2, and 2:2 electrolytes.

data to infinite dilution; the appropriate independent variable is the square root of the ionic strength.

PROBLEMS

8.1. Write the reactions for ionization and dissociation of a base B in glacial acetic acid.

8.2. Calculate the ionic strengths of these three solutions (from Table 8.2): $3.0\,m$ NaCl; $3.0\,m$ $CaCl_2$; $3.0\,m$ $ZnSO_4$.

8.3. Calculate the mean ionic activity coefficient of $0.05\,m$ NaCl in water at 25°C, and compare your result with the experimental value in Table 8.2.

8.4. Estimate the mean ionic activity of 0.001 M HCl in an aqueous solution containing 0.025 M KCl at 25°C.

8.5. Calculate the ionic strength of a solution containing 0.10 M Na_3PO_4 and 0.05 M KBr.

8.6. Obtain an estimate of the parameter C in Eq. (8.28) for $CaCl_2$ by use of the data in Fig. 8.1. [*Hint:* find the derivative $d\log\gamma_\pm/d\sqrt{I}$ of Eq. (8.28), set equal to zero (at the minimum), and solve for C.]

NOTES

1. The dielectric constant is a bulk property of matter, and its incorporation into Coulomb's law means that we are treating the solvent as a continuum; that is, the molecular (particulate) nature of the solvent is ignored in this treatment.

2. The molecular interpretation of the ionization process may be complex, and will depend on the molecular identity. One possibility is that two kinds of ion pairs may form. One of these, represented A^+B^-, is an *intimate ion pair*; the other, shown as A^+SB^-, where S is a molecule of solvent, is a *solvent-separated ion pair*.

3. See Glasstone (1947, p. 402). These activity coefficients can be measured in various ways. One approach is to measure the derivation from ideality of the *solvent*, and to relate this to the nonideality of the solute.

9

COLLIGATIVE PROPERTIES

Several properties of solutions depend (mainly) only on the *number* of solute particles (molecules or ions) and not on their identity. These are called the *colligative properties*. They are pharmaceutically relevant.

9.1. BOILING POINT ELEVATION

The boiling point of a solution of a nonvolatile solute is higher than is the boiling point of the pure solvent. This observation is readily explicable on the following basis. The normal boiling point T_b of the solvent is the temperature at which its vapor pressure is equal to 1 atm. When a solute is incorporated into the solvent, according to Raoult's law the vapor pressure over the solution is $p_1 = x_1 P_1^*$ [Eq. (7.1)]. (We will use subscript 1 to designate the solvent and 2 for the solute.) Since $x_1 + x_2 = 1$, an increase in x_2 results in a decrease in x_1 and therefore a decrease in p_1, at a given temperature. In order to cause the solvent to boil, it is now necessary to raise the temperature until p_1 becomes 1 atm. This phenomenon is known as the *boiling point elevation*, and it is seen to be a consequence of the vapor pressure lowering by the presence of solute particles. As ordinarily discussed, the boiling point elevation is treated as a phenomenon of nonelectrolyte solutions, but solutions of electrolytes show the same effect. It is necessary to keep in mind that the number of solute particles (i.e., their concentration) is the controlling factor, and if the solute is an electrolyte, the number of particles depends on the charge type and the extent of dissociation. For example, in a 0.10 M aqueous solution of NaCl the effective concentration, as concerns the colligative properties, is 0.20 M.

A thermodynamic description of the boiling point elevation effect can be achieved by the application of concepts that we have already developed. At equilibrium (i.e., at the boiling point), the chemical potential of the solvent is equal in the vapor and liquid phases:

$$\mu_1(g) = \mu_1(l) \tag{9.1}$$

By restricting attention to dilute solutions we can treat the solution as an ideal solution, writing

$$\mu_1(l) = \mu_1^\circ(l) + RT \ln x_1 \tag{9.2}$$
$$\mu_1(g) = \mu_1^\circ(g) + RT \ln p_1 \tag{9.3}$$

Setting these equal, noting that $p_1 = 1$ atm at the boiling point, and writing $\Delta G_{vap}^\circ = \mu_1^\circ(g) - \mu_1^\circ(l)$ gives

$$\Delta G_{vap}^\circ = RT \ln x_1 \tag{9.4}$$

Putting Eq. (9.4) into the form $\Delta G_{vap}^\circ/T = R \ln x_1$ and applying the Gibbs–Helmboltz equation [Eq. (3.18)] leads to

$$\frac{d \ln x_1}{dT} = -\frac{\Delta H_{vap}^\circ}{RT^2} \tag{9.5}$$

where constant pressure is understood.[1]

When $x_1 = 1$, $T = T_b$ (the normal boiling point). Equation (9.5) is integrated between the limits shown:

$$\int_1^{x_1} d \ln x_1 = -\frac{\Delta H_{vap}^\circ}{R} \int_{T_b}^{T} \frac{dT}{T^2}$$

The result is

$$\ln x_1 = -\frac{\Delta H_{vap}^\circ}{R} \left(\frac{1}{T_b} - \frac{1}{T} \right)$$

which can be written

$$\ln x_1 = -\frac{\Delta H_{vap}^\circ}{R} \left(\frac{T - T_b}{TT_b} \right) \tag{9.6}$$

Now define the boiling point elevation as $\Delta T_b = T - T_b$, and, since T and T_b are quite close together, approximate TT_b by T_b^2. Making these substitutions in Eq. (9.6) gives

$$\ln x_1 = -\frac{\Delta H_{vap}^\circ \Delta T_b}{RT_b^2}$$

Since x_2 is small (the solution is dilute), we write[2] $\ln x_1 = \ln(1 - x_2) \approx -x_2$. We also convert x_2, the mole fraction of solute, to m_2, the molality of solute, with $x_2 = m_2 M_1/1000$, where M_1 is the molecular weight of solvent [Eq. (5.2)]. The final result of these substitutions is

$$\Delta T_b = \frac{RT_b^2 M_1 m_2}{1000 \,\Delta H_{vap}^\circ} \qquad (9.7)$$

which can be written $\Delta T_b = K_b m_2$, where

$$K_b = \frac{RT_b^2 M_1}{1000 \,\Delta H_{vap}^\circ} \qquad (9.8)$$

The proportionality constant K_b is called the *boiling point elevation constant* or the *ebullioscopic constant*. Note that K_b can be calculated solely from properties of the solvent, and that ΔT_b depends only on the identity of the solvent and the concentration (not the identity) of the solute.

Example 9.1. The heat of vaporization of water is 9.717 kcal mol^{-1} at its boiling point. Calculate the ebullioscopic constant of water:

$$K_b = \frac{(1.987 \text{ cal mol}^{-1}\text{K}^{-1})(373.15 \text{ K})^2 (18.02 \text{ g mol}^{-1})}{(1000)(9717 \text{ cal mol}^{-1})}$$
$$= 0.513 \text{ K g mol}^{-1}$$

The result in Example 9.1 may appear to say that the boiling point of a 1 *m* solution will be raised 0.513 K, but of course a 1 *m* solution lies outside the dilute solution range where this equation is valid.[3]

9.2. FREEZING POINT DEPRESSION

We have seen in Chapter 6 that the freezing point (melting point) of a two-component system is lowered (relative to a pure substance). A simple quantitative treatment can be based on the assumption that the solute does not dissolve in solid solvent; then the solid that forms is pure solvent. The method is identical in form with that used for the analysis of the boiling point elevation; we replace the chemical potential of the gaseous solvent with that of the solid solvent. The result can be written

$$\Delta T_f = K_f m_2 \qquad (9.9)$$

where $\Delta T_f = T_f - T$ and

$$K_f = \frac{RT_f^2 M_1}{1000 \,\Delta H_f^\circ} \qquad (9.10)$$

where ΔH_f° is the heat of fusion and K_f is the *cryoscopic constant* or *freezing point depression constant*.

Example 9.2. The heat of fusion of water is 6.01 kJ mol^{-1}. Calculate the freezing point depression constant of water:

$$K_f = \frac{(8.314\,\text{J mol}^{-1}\,\text{K}^{-1})(273.15\,\text{K})^2(18.02\ \text{g mol}^{-1})}{(1000)(6010\,\text{J mol}^{-1})}$$

$$= 1.86\,\text{K g mol}^{-1}$$

9.3. OSMOTIC PRESSURE

Consider the experimental arrangement in Fig. 9.1, which shows a solvent compartment (left) and a compartment containing a dilute solution of the same solvent (right), the two compartments separated by a *semipermeable membrane*, which permits the passage of solvent molecules but prevents the passage of solute molecules. The presence of solute in the right-hand compartment reduces the mole fraction of solvent in that compartment, and thereby reduces its activity and chemical potential below their values in the pure solvent in the left-hand compartment.

In order to achieve equilibrium, the chemical potential of the solvent must be equal on both sides of the membrane. There is thus a driving force for the passage of solvent molecules from left to right. (Although it is actually the chemical potential difference that is responsible for this effect, as it can also be rationalized as a simple concentration effect, as the solvent concentration is higher on the left.) The flow of solvent from left to right continues until it is opposed by the backpressure generated by the increased height of solution in the right-hand column. (Or

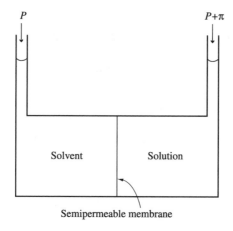

Figure 9.1. Principle of osmosis and the osmotic pressure π.

alternatively, the experiment can be arranged so as to apply an excess pressure to the right until the flow of solvent is exactly balanced.) This phenomenon of the passage of solvent through a semipermeable membrane under the influence of a difference in chemical potentials is called *osmosis*, and the excess pressure (π in Fig. 9.1) that equalizes the chemical potentials is the *osmotic pressure*.

Our thermodynamic analysis of osmosis begins with the statement of osmotic equilibrium

$$\mu_1^\circ(P, T) = \mu_1(P + \pi, T, x_1) \qquad (9.11)$$

where the left side of the equation refers to pure solvent (the left-hand compartment in Fig. 9.1) and the right side, to the solution. The parentheses contain the variables controlling the particular quantities, in order to make explicit how the two sides differ. We assume that the solution is dilute and behaves ideally. Then, on expanding μ_1 in the usual manner, Eq. (9.11) becomes

$$\mu_1^\circ(P, T) = \mu_1^\circ(P + \pi, T) + RT \ln x_1 \qquad (9.12)$$

where now $\mu_1^\circ(P + \pi, T)$ designates the chemical potential of pure solvent at pressure $P + \pi$. We now develop this quantity as in

$$\mu_1^\circ(P + \pi, T) = \mu_1^\circ(P, T) + \int_P^{P+\pi} V_1 \, dP \qquad (9.13)$$

where V_1 is the molar volume of solvent [Eq. (3.6)]. Putting Eq. (9.13) into Eq. (9.12) results in

$$\int_P^{P+\pi} V_1 \, dP = -RT \ln x_1 \qquad (9.14)$$

Treating V_1 as independent of pressure and integrating yields

$$\pi V_1 = -RT \ln x_1 \qquad (9.15)$$

Using once again (see note 2) the approximation (for dilute solution) that $\ln x_1 = -x_2$, Eq. (9.15) becomes $\pi V_1 = x_2 RT$. Now, $x_2 = n_2/(n_1 + n_2)$, which in dilute solution is nearly equal to the mole ratio n_2/n_1. This gives

$$\pi n_1 V_1 = n_2 RT \qquad (9.16)$$

The product $n_1 V_1 = V$, the total volume of the solution, or

$$\pi V = n_2 RT \qquad (9.17)$$

The formal resemblance of Eq. (9.17) to the ideal-gas law is obvious. We can take one further step by noting that the ratio n_2/V is the molar concentration c_2 of the solute:

$$\pi = c_2 RT \tag{9.18}$$

Example 9.3. Calculate the osmotic pressure of an 0.01 M solution at 25°C. Since we find it convenient to express pressure in atmospheres, we use R as 0.08206 L atm mol$^{-}1$ K^{-1}. From Eq. (9.18), we have

$$\pi = (0.01\,\mathrm{mol\,L^{-1}})(0.08206\,\mathrm{L\,atm\,mol^{-1}\,K^{-1}})(298.15\,\mathrm{K})$$
$$= 0.245\,\mathrm{atm}$$

Example 9.3 shows that osmosis is a very sensitive effect, much more so than are the other colligative properties. This same solution would exhibit a boiling point elevation of 0.0051 K (Example 9.1) and a freezing point depression of 0.0186 K (Example 9.2). This sensitivity forms the basis of an experimental method, called *osmometry*, for measuring molecular weights of solutes. Solutions are prepared with known concentrations in grams per liter (g L^{-1}) and their osmotic pressures are measured. From Eq. (9.18) the corresponding molar concentration c_2 is calculated. Since c_2 has the units mol L^{-1} and mol $= g/M_2$ (where M_2 is the molecular weight of the solute), the quantity M_2 can be obtained. In practice deviations from ideality must be taken into account (Atkins 1994, p. 229).

9.4. ISOTONICITY CALCULATIONS

Body membranes, including cell membranes, are semipermeable membranes to some degree. They are generally permeable to water and are impermeable, or nearly so, to many (but obviously not all) solutes. Thus we anticipate the existence of osmotic pressure differences across these membranes. It is known that irritation caused by foreign solutions is in part related to their osmotic pressure; the closer the osmotic pressure of an administered solution is to that of the physiological solution on the other side of the membrane, the less the discomfort that is experienced.

Two solutions are said to be *isoosmotic* if they have the same osmotic pressure. Isoosmoticity is therefore a physical property, based on the thermodynamic concept of Section 9.3. A solution is said to be *isotonic* if it has the same osmotic pressure as a reference body fluid, measured with respect to the appropriate body membrane. Isotonicity is therefore a physiological concept. It is possible for a pair of solutions to be both isoosmotic and isotonic, but they need not be, as when the biological membrane is not perfectly impermeable to the solute. For example, 1.9% boric acid solution (in water, the solvent for all solutions in this section) is both isoosmotic and isotonic with respect to the eye, because the corneal membrane is impermeable to boric acid. On the other hand, 1.9% boric acid is isoosmotic with the red blood cell contents, but it is not isotonic toward this biological medium, because the red blood cell membrane is permeable to boric acid. (Boric acid is often used to render ophthalmic solutions isotonic.)

A solution having an osmotic pressure greater than that of physiological fluids is *hypertonic*; if its osmotic pressure is less than that of physiological fluids, it is *hypotonic*. Consider a red blood cell surrounded by a hypertonic solution. Since the osmotic pressure of the surrounding solution is greater than that inside the cell (i.e., the water activity is less outside than inside the cell), water will flow out of the cell, which shrinks and shrivels. If the red blood cell should be immersed in a hypotonic solution, water will flow into the cell, which swells and may burst. The goal of rendering pharmaceutical solutions isotonic is directed toward preventing or minimizing such physiological consequences.

Experimental work has shown that the freezing point of human blood is $-0.52°C$. We consider that all other physiological fluids are effectively in equilibrium with blood, and so they are isotonic with blood. Although we saw that osmotic pressure is the most sensitive of the colligative properties, the freezing point depression is much the easiest to measure, and so it forms the basis of all isotonicity calculations. Here we will describe the simplest of these, called straightforwardly the *freezing point depression method*. For other methods the literature may be consulted (Thompson 1998, Chapter 10; Windholz 1983, pp. MISC-47–MISC-69; Reich et al. 2000). The basis of the method is the assumption that contributions to the freezing point depression from multiple solutes are additive, and so the goal of the calculation is to achieve a freezing point depression of $-0.52°C$.

Example 9.4. Estimate the concentration of sodium chloride required to produce an isotonic aqueous solution.

The calculation is based on Eq. (9.9), $\Delta T_f = K_f m_2$, with $K_f = 1.86°C$ (see Example 9.2). We seek $\Delta T_f = 0.52°C$ hence we need $m_2 = 0.52/1.86 = 0.28$. But NaCl is a $1:1$ strong electrolyte, so each molecule yields two particles on dissociation; therefore we actually need prepare a solution $0.28/2 = 0.14\,m$. Commonly this molal concentration is expressed as a molar concentration, neglecting the difference; to obtain 0.14 M NaCl, whose molecular weight is 58.5, we take $(0.14)\,(58.5) = 8.19\,g\,L^{-1}$, or 0.82 g/100 mL, which is 0.82%.

Experimentally it is observed that a solution 0.5% in NaCl exhibits a freezing point depression of 0.289°C. Setting up the proportion

$$\frac{0.289°C}{0.5\%} = \frac{0.52°C}{x}$$

we find $x = 0.9\%$ NaCl. The slight discrepancy with the result in Example 9.4 probably is a consequence of nonideal solution behavior. An aqueous solution containing 0.9% (w/v) sodium chloride is isotonic. This solution is called *normal saline* or *physiological saline*.

Because of nonideal solution behavior or incomplete electrolyte dissociation, it is preferable to make use of published freezing point depression data. However, if such data are not available, a very reasonable calculation can be based on the known K_f value of 1.86 together with chemical knowledge of the nature of the solute.

Example 9.5. Give directions for the preparation of 100 mL of isotonic 1% hexamethonium tartrate. The following data are available (Windholz 1983, pp. MISC-47–MISC-69; Reich et al. 2000):

Concentration	ΔT_f
0.5	0.045
1	0.089
2	0.181
3	0.271
5	0.456

We set up the problem in tabular form:

Desired ΔT_f value	0.52°C
ΔT_f of 1% of drug	0.089°C
Difference to be made up	0.431°C

We will use NaCl to make the solution isotonic. From the proportion

$$\frac{0.9\%}{0.52°C} = \frac{x}{0.431°C}$$

we find $x = 0.75\%$. Therefore we proceed by dissolving 1.0 g of hexamethonium tartrate and 0.75 g of NaCl in enough water to make 100 mL.

If data are not available for the concentration we require, interpolation or extrapolation may give the information.

Example 9.6. Prepare 2 oz of 2% isotonic imipramine hydrochloride.

Sources give $\Delta T_f = 0.058°C$ at 0.5% and 0.110°C at 1%. We can plot these data as in Fig. 9.2 and obtain the estimate $\Delta T_f = 0.225°C$ at 2%. (Extrapolation is risky, but it may be our best recourse.) We proceed as before:

Desired ΔT_f value	0.52°C
ΔT_f of 2% of drug	0.225°C
Difference to be made up	0.295°C

Again using NaCl, we obtain

$$\frac{0.9\%}{0.52°C} = \frac{x}{0.295°C}$$
$$x = 0.51\%$$

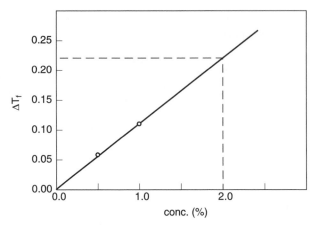

Figure 9.2. Freezing point depression of hexamethonium tartrate. See Example 9.5.

If we needed to prepare 100 mL of the solution we would take 2.0 g of drug and 0.51 g of NaCl. However, only 2 oz (60 mL) of solution is required, so we take $(\frac{60}{100})$ (2) $= 1.2$ g of drug and $(\frac{60}{100})$ (0.51) $= 0.31$ g of NaCl in enough water to make 60 mL.

If the prescription calls for more than one drug, the ΔT_f contributions of the several drugs are summed. In ophthalmic solutions boric acid may be used to make the solution isotonic; 1.9% boric acid solution is isotonic.

Although the several alternative methods of isotonicity calculation are all derived from the freezing point depression method, one of these approaches merits comment because of its simplicity and utility. The principle is as follows. If two isotonic solutions are mixed, the resulting solution is isotonic. For example, if the prescribed amount of drug is dissolved in just enough water to make an isotonic solution, this solution could be diluted to the desired volume with normal saline and the result will be isotonic. The *United States Pharmacopeia* gives formulas for isotonic phosphate buffer solutions that can be used in this way, particularly for ophthalmic solutions.

PROBLEMS

9.1. Starting with Raoult's law, show that the extent of vapor pressure lowering is directly proportional to solute concentration.

9.2. Calculate the boiling point elevation constant of ethanol, whose heat of vaporization is 38.6 kJ mol^{-1}.

9.3. Calculate the freezing point depression constant of glacial acetic acid, whose heat of fusion is 11.7 kJ mol^{-1}.

9.4. Give directions for the preparation of this ophthalmic solution; ΔT_f for 2% pilocarpine nitrate is 0.247:

Pilocarpine nitrate 2%

Make isotonic with boric acid

Qs ad 1 oz

9.5. Estimate ΔT_f of 5% dextrose solution. Dextrose (glucose) is available as the monohydrate, MW 198.2. What concentration of dextrose will yield an isotonic solution?

NOTES

1. $\Delta G_{vap} = \mu_1(g) - \mu_1(l) = 0$, since the system is at equilibrium, but $\Delta G^\circ_{vap} = \mu_1^\circ(g) - \mu_1^\circ(l)$ is not zero; it is the standard free-energy change. It is therefore correct to label the enthalpy change ΔH°_{vap}. However, ΔH°_{vap} is numerically identical to ΔH_{vap}, which appears in the Clausius–Clapeyron equation [Eq. (4.11)]. The reason for this equality is that we have postulated ideal solution behavior, and for the ideal solution, the enthalpy of mixing is zero (Section 7.1). Consequently there is no enthalpy change on bringing the solution from $x_1 = 1$ to $x_1 < 1$.

2. We are using the series expansion $\ln(1-x) = -x + x^2/2 - x^3/3 + \cdots$.

3. Some discrepancies in the form of Eq. (9.8) for k_b will be noted in the literature. some authors (Williamson 1967, p. 102; Atkins 1994, p. 229) omit the factor 1000 in the denominator. Others (Smith 1977, p. 90; Gupta 2000) include the 1000, and assign K_b the unit K. The distinction lies in the units given to the molality m_2, that is, whether molality has the units mol kg^{-1} or mol (1000) g^{-1}, or is considered to be a dimensionless number.

10

SOLUBILITY

10.1. SOLUBILITY AS AN EQUILIBRIUM CONSTANT

The topic of solubility merits special attention because of its great importance in pharmaceutical systems. We can generally anticipate that a drug must be in solution if it is to exert its effect. Typically the type of system we encounter is a pure solid substance (the solute) in contact with a pure liquid (the solvent). We allow equilibrium to be achieved at fixed temperature and pressure, such that at equilibrium the system consists of (excess) pure solid phase and liquid solution of solute dissolved in solvent. According to Gibbs' phase rule, $P = 2$ and $C = 2$, so $F = C - P + 2 = 2$ degrees of freedom. These are the temperature and pressure, which we have specified as fixed. Thus there remain no degrees of freedom; the system is invariant. This means that at fixed temperature and pressure, the concentration of dissolved solute is fixed. We call this invariant dissolved concentration the *equilibrium solubility* of the solute at this pressure and temperature. (We say that the solution is *saturated*.) Our present concern is with how the equilibrium solubility depends on the temperature and on the chemical natures of the solute and the solvent.

Expressed as a reaction, the dissolution process is

$$\text{Pure solute} \rightleftharpoons \text{solute in solution}$$

At equilibrium the chemical potentials of the solute in the two phases are equal, or, letting component 1 be the solvent and component 2 the solute

$$\mu_2 \,(\text{solid}) = \mu_2 \,(\text{soln})$$

Writing out the chemical potentials gives

$$\mu_2^\circ \,(\text{solid}) + RT \ln a_2 \,(\text{solid}) = \mu_2^\circ \,(\text{soln}) + RT \ln a_2 \,(\text{soln}) \qquad (10.1)$$

where the standard state of the solid is the pure solid, and we will adopt as the standard state of the solute in solution the Henry's law definition on the molar concentration scale. Rearranging Eq. (10.1) leads to

$$\Delta\mu^\circ = -RT \ln \frac{a_2 \,(\text{soln})}{a_2(\text{solid})} \qquad (10.2)$$

where $\Delta\mu^\circ = \mu_2^\circ \,(\text{soln}) - \mu_2^\circ \,(\text{solid})$. But the solid is in its standard state, so $a_2 \,(\text{solid}) = 1.0$ by definition, and we obtain

$$\Delta\mu^\circ = -RT \ln a_2 \,(\text{soln}) \qquad (10.3)$$

We have seen that $a_2 \,(\text{soln})$ is invariant—it is the activity corresponding to the equilibrium solubility—so comparison of Eq. (10.3) with the fundamental thermodynamic result

$$\Delta G^\circ = -RT \ln K \qquad (10.4)$$

leads to the conclusion that $a_2 \,(\text{soln})$, the activity of the solute in a saturated solution, must have the character of an equilibrium constant. As a consequence, we can evaluate standard free energy, enthalpy, and entropy changes for the solution process in the usual manner (Chapter 4). These quantities are respectively called the *free energy*, *heat*, and *entropy of solution*.

For nonelectrolyte solutes, particularly those of limited solubility, so that the saturated solution is fairly dilute, it will be acceptable to approximate the activity $a_2 \,(\text{soln})$ by the equilibrium solubility concentration. This is usually in molar concentration units, and is often symbolized s.

10.2. THE IDEAL SOLUBILITY

A thermodynamic argument can predict the equilibrium solubility of a nonelectrolyte, provided it dissolves to form an ideal solution. Ideal behavior does not mean that intermolecular interactions are absent. On the contrary, solids and liquids would not exist without the intermolecular forces of interaction. In the present context, ideal behavior means that the energy of interaction between two solvent molecules is identical to that between one solvent and one solute molecule, so that a solvent molecule may be replaced with a solute molecule without altering the intermolecular energies. (This requires that the solvent and solute molecules have the same size, shape, and chemical nature, a demanding set of limitations.)

Quantitatively, an ideal solution can be defined as one having the following properties (Chapter 7):

$$\Delta H_{\text{mix}} = 0 \tag{10.5}$$

$$\Delta V_{\text{mix}} = 0 \tag{10.6}$$

$$\Delta S_{\text{mix}} = -R(x_1 \ln x_1 + x_2 \ln x_2) \tag{10.7}$$

According to Eqs. (10.5) and (10.6), there is no heat or volume change on mixing the solute and solvent in an ideal solution, and the entropy change is given by Eq. (10.7). Since $x_1 + x_2 = 1$, the logarithmic terms are necessarily negative, so ΔS_{mix} is positive, and this constitutes the "driving force" for dissolution, because of the relationship $\Delta G = \Delta H - T \Delta S$.

If the entropy of mixing is the driving force for dissolution, what is the "resistance"? It is the solute–solute interaction forces, which, for solids, lead to the "crystal lattice energy." These must be overcome for the solute to dissolve. Now, the free-energy change for the dissolution process is the same no matter what reversible mechanism (path) is taken to pass from the initial state (pure solute) to the final state (saturated solution), so we can divide the process as follows (for a solid solute):

Crystalline solute $\rightleftharpoons$ supercooled liquid solute

Pure liquid solvent $\rightleftharpoons$ solvent containing cavity

Supercooled liquid solute $\rightleftharpoons$ saturated solution
+ solvent-containing cavity

Crystalline solute + pure liquid solvent $\rightleftharpoons$ saturated solution

Since in an ideal solution the solvent–solvent interactions match the solvent–solute interactions, the energy required to create molecule-sized cavities in the solvent is offset by the energy recovered when the solute molecules are inserted into these cavities. The energetic cost of the dissolution process then appears in the first step, the melting of the solid. An equivalent viewpoint (Grant and Higuchi 1990, p. 16) is that the enthalpy of solution is given by

$$\Delta H_{\text{soln}} = \Delta H_{\text{fusion}} + \Delta H_{\text{mix}}$$

But $\Delta H_{\text{mix}} = 0$ for an ideal solution, so $\Delta H_{\text{soln}} = \Delta H_{\text{fusion}}$.

The saturation solubility, we have seen, is an equilibrium constant, so the van't Hoff equation [Eq. (4.29)] is applicable

$$\frac{d \ln x_2}{dT} = \frac{\Delta H_f}{RT^2} \tag{10.8}$$

where the solubility is expressed as the mole fraction simply to maintain consistency with Eq. (10.7), and where ΔH_f is the heat of fusion and T is the absolute temperature. We have seen above why the heat of fusion appears in a solubility expression. (Incidentally, a dissolved solid should be viewed as possessing some of the properties of the liquid state, consistent with the above view that fusion is the first step in the dissolution process.) Now suppose that ΔH_f is independent of temperature, which is equivalent to writing, for the solute from Eq. (1.23):

$$\Delta C_p = C_p^{\text{liq}} - C_p^{\text{solid}} = 0 \qquad (10.9)$$

Then integrating Eq. (10.8) from T_m to T gives

$$\ln x_2 = -\frac{\Delta H_f}{R}\left(\frac{T_m - T}{T\,T_m}\right) \qquad (10.10)$$

where T_m is the melting temperature and T is the experimental temperature. Equation (10.10) allows us to calculate the ideal solubility.

Example 10.1. The melting point of naphthalene is 80.2°C, and its heat of fusion at the melting point is 4.54 kcal mol^{-1}. What is the ideal solubility of naphthalene at 20°C?

$$\text{Log}\,x_2 = \frac{-4540\,\text{cal mol}^{-1}}{(2.303)(1.987\,\text{cal mol}^{-1}\text{K}^{-1})}\left(\frac{60.2\,\text{K}}{353.35\,\text{K} \times 293.15\,\text{K}}\right)$$
$$= -0.577$$
$$x_2 = 0.265$$

Deviations from ideality will be manifested by discrepancies from the ideal solubility as calculated with Eq. (10.10). Table 10.1 lists equilibrium solubilities for

Table 10.1. Naphthalene solubility at 20°C

Solvent	x_2
(Ideal)	0.265
Chlorobenzene	0.256
Benzene	0.241
Toluene	0.224
Carbon tetrachloride	0.205
Hexane	0.090
Aniline	0.130
Nitrobenzene	0.243
Acetone	0.183
n-Butanol	0.0495
Methanol	0.0180
Acetic acid	0.0456
Water (25°C)	0.0000039

naphthalene in many solvents. Observe that those solvents most chemically like naphthalene, that is, aromatic and nonpolar solvents, show behavior most closely approximating ideal behavior.

At the melting temperature T_m the solid and liquid forms of the solute are in equilibrium, so $\Delta G_f = 0$ and we get $\Delta H_f = T_m \Delta S_f$, giving Eq. (10.11) as an alternative form of Eq. (10.10):

$$\ln x_2 = -\frac{\Delta S_f(T_m - T)}{RT} \tag{10.11}$$

10.3. TEMPERATURE DEPENDENCE OF THE SOLUBILITY

Since ΔH_f is always a positive quantity, Eq. (10.10) predicts that the solubility of a solid will increase with temperature. Moreover, Eq. (10.10) shows that if two solid substances have the same heat of fusion, the one with the higher melting point will have the lower solubility. Conversely, if they have the same melting point, the one with the lower heat of fusion will have the higher solubility. All of these inferences from Eq. (10.10) refer to systems forming ideal solutions, so deviations from the predictions can occur for real systems. Nevertheless, the increase of solubility with temperature is very widely observed for solids. Even the relationship of solubility to melting point can be a useful guide, though confounding phenomena can introduce complications; for example, hydrogen-bonding or other polar interactions may raise both the melting point and the aqueous solubility. The comparison of the temperature dependence of solubility of solids and gases is instructive; see Table 10.2.

Equation (10.10) can be rearranged to Eq. (10.12):

$$\ln x_2 = -\frac{\Delta H_f}{RT} + \frac{\Delta H_f}{RT_m} \tag{10.12}$$

Table 10.2. The contrary effects of temperature on the solubilities of solids and gases

$$\text{Solid} \underset{}{\overset{\Delta H_f}{\rightleftharpoons}} \text{liquid} \underset{\Delta H_c}{\overset{\Delta H_v}{\rightleftharpoons}} \text{gas}$$

Solids	Gases
Solution is the process of passing from solid to liquid (fusion, ΔH_f)	Solution is the process of passing from gas to liquid (condensation, ΔH_c), which is the reverse of vaporization (ΔH_v)
ΔH_f is *positive*, so x_2 *increases* as T increases	ΔH_v is positive, so ΔH_c is *negative*; thus x_2 *decreases* as T increases

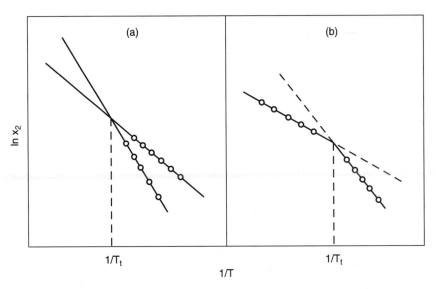

Figure 10.1. Hypothetical solubility van't Hoff plots for polymorphs.

If ΔH_f is essentially constant over the experimental temperature range, Eq. (10.12) predicts that a plot of $\ln x_2$ against $1/T$ will be linear with a slope equal to $-\Delta H_f/R$. The line should terminate at the melting point, where $1/T = 1/T_m$. Often such lines are straight, probably because the usual range of temperatures is small. The slope gives ΔH_f in principle, but in actuality the quantity evaluated from the slope is not precisely ΔH_f because the solution is seldom ideal, and instead the quantity found in this way is termed the *heat of solution*.

Throughout this discussion we have been assuming that the solid phase consists of the pure solid and not a solid solution. Another possible complication arises if the solid substance can exist in two crystalline forms (polymorphs; Chapter 6), which interconvert at transition temperature T_t. The van't Hoff plot can resemble Fig. 10.1a or Fig. 10.1b depending primarily on the kinetics of the transformation. In Fig. 10.1a, the two forms are sufficiently stable that their solubilities can be separately measured at the same temperatures, which are below the transition temperature. Nevertheless, the crystal form having the higher solubility (at a given temperature) is thermodynamically unstable (it is said to be metastable, since its kinetics of transformation permit it to exist for some period during which it acts as if it were stable), and will ultimately be converted to the stable form. Extrapolation of the lines to the transition temperature may be possible. Sulfathiazole in 95% ethanol shows the Fig. 10.1a behavior (Milosovich 1964; Carstensen 1977, p. 7).

In Fig. 10.1b, one form exists in one temperature range, the other form in a temperature range on the other side of T_t. The melting point observed will be that of the higher-melting polymorph. Carbon tetrabromide exemplifies this behavior (Hildebrand et al. 1970, p. 23).

Let us return to the assumption that the change in heat capacities, ΔC_p, is zero, for all the subsequent discussion was based on this assumption. If ΔH_f in fact is a function of temperature, then ΔC_p is not zero. Suppose we make the more reasonable assumption that ΔC_p is a nonzero constant, and write ΔH_f as

$$\Delta H_f = \Delta H_f^m - \Delta C_p(T_m - T) \tag{10.13}$$

where ΔH_f^m is the heat of fusion at T_m. Equation (10.13) is inserted into Eq. (10.8), which can be rearranged and integrated to give Eq. (10.14):

$$\ln x_2^s = \frac{-\Delta H_f^m}{R}\left(\frac{T_m - T}{T T_m}\right) + \frac{\Delta C_p}{R}\left(\frac{T_m - T}{T}\right) - \frac{\Delta C_p}{R}\ln\frac{T_m}{T} \tag{10.14}$$

This equation is useful for assessing the error that may be introduced by making the simple assumption $\Delta C_p = 0$. Suppose, for example, that the experimental temperature is 25°C and the melting point is 100°C. Then the last two terms in Eq. (10.14) become equal to $0.25\Delta C_p/R - 0.22\,\Delta C_p/R = 0.03\Delta C_p/R$. Thus considerable compensation can take place, making the approximation $\Delta C_p = 0$ more acceptable than it might have seemed.

Example 10.2. These are solubility data for nitrofurantoin in water (Chen et al. 1976). Analyze the data to obtain the heat of solution.

$t\,(°C)$	$10^6 x_2$
24	6.01
30	8.57
37	13.16
45	18.99

The data are manipulated as required to make the van't Hoff plot according to Eq. (10.12):

$T\,(10^3\mathrm{K})$	$\log x_2$
3.37	−5.22
3.30	−5.06
3.23	−4.88
3.14	−4.72

The plot is shown in Fig. 10.2. It is possible that the points describe a curve, but this is uncertain with the data as given, for conceivably the scatter is a consequence of experimental random error. A straight line has therefore been drawn. Its slope is

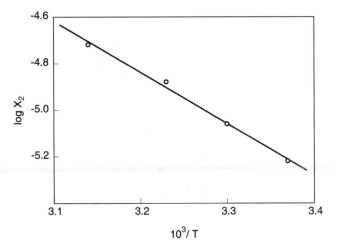

Figure 10.2. van't Hoff plot for nitrofurantoin solubility.

$-2300\,\mathrm{K}$, so we calculate

$$\Delta H_{\text{soln}} = (2300\,\text{K})(1.987\,\text{cal mol}^{-1}\,\text{K}^{-1})$$
$$= 4570\,\text{cal mol}^{-1}$$
$$= 4.57\,\text{kcal mol}^{-1}$$
$$= 19.1\,\text{kJ mol}^{-1}$$

Note that the enthalpy change is labeled ΔH_{soln} to indicate explicitly that this is a heat of solution.

10.4. SOLUBILITY OF SLIGHTLY SOLUBLE SALTS

Many salts exhibit very low solubilities in water. Silver chloride is an example; if aqueous solutions of silver nitrate and sodium chloride are mixed, solid silver chloride precipitates. It is conventional to describe this process as the reverse of the precipitation reaction, namely, as the dissolution of the salt. Let us begin with the simplest case of a $1:1$ sparingly soluble salt MX. The solid crystalline form is ionic. When it dissolves in water the ions dissociate, and no ion pairs are detectable. We therefore write the equilibrium as

$$MX(s) \rightleftharpoons M^+ + X^- \tag{10.15}$$

Proceeding as we have done for several earlier processes, we equate the chemical potentials of the solid and the dissolved solute at equilibrium:

$$\mu(s) = \mu(\text{soln})$$

Expanding these gives

$$\mu°(s) + RT \ln a(s) = \mu_+° + RT \ln a_+$$
$$+ \mu_-° + RT \ln a_-$$

and collecting terms (and noting that $a(s) = 1$ by our standard state definition),

$$\Delta\mu° = -RT \ln a_+ a_- \tag{10.16}$$

where $\Delta\mu° = \mu_+° + \mu_-° - \mu°(s)$. Evidently then [compare with Eq. (10.4)], the product $a_+ a_-$ is an equilibrium constant. By Eq. (8.23a) we see that $a_+ a_- = a_\pm^2$, where $a_\pm$ is the mean ionic activity, and since $a_\pm^2 = \gamma_\pm^2 c_\pm^2$, Eq. (10.16) can be written

$$\Delta\mu° = -RT \ln \gamma_\pm^2 c_\pm^2 \tag{10.17}$$

If no extraneous ions are present, so that the ionic strength is due solely to the ions from the sparingly soluble salt (and hence is very low), the activity coefficient term is essentially unity. Moreover, the molar concentrations of the cation M^+ and the anion X^- are equal, and each is numerically equal to the equilibrium molar solubility of the salt, which is commonly denoted s. Thus Eq. (10.17) becomes

$$\Delta\mu° = -RT \ln s^2 \tag{10.18}$$

Equation (10.17) is exact; Eq. (10.18) is usually a reasonable approximation, and both implicitly define the equilibrium constant for Eq. (10.15). This constant is symbolized K_{sp} and is called the *solubility product*. Since solubility products are very small numbers, it is common to state them as pK_{sp}, where $pK_{sp} = -\log K_{sp}$. Table 10.3 lists some pK_{sp} values.

Table 10.3. Solubility products for slightly soluble salts[a]

Salt	pK_{sp}	Salt	pK_{sp}
BaSO$_4$	9.96	PbCO$_3$	13.13
CaCO$_3$	8.54	PbS	27.9
Ca(OH)$_2$	5.26	MgCO$_3$	7.46
Ca$_3$(PO$_4$)$_2$	28.7	Hg$_2$S	47.0
CuI	11.96	HgS (red)	52.4
AuCl	12.7	HgS (black)	51.8
AuCl$_3$	24.5	AgBr	12.30
Fe(OH)$_2$	15.1	AgCl	9.75
Fe(OH)$_3$	37.4	AgI	16.08

[a] In the temperature range 18–25°C; water is the solvent.

Example 10.3. What is the solubility of silver chloride in water? From Table 10.3, $pK_{sp} = 9.75$ for AgCl, so $K_{sp} = 1.78 \times 10^{-10}$. From Eq. (10.18), $K_{sp} = s^2$, so $s = \sqrt{K_{sp}} = 1.33 \times 10^{-5}$ M.

In the general case of the salt whose formula is $M_p X_q$ the solubility product is defined, in accordance with the usual formulation of equilibrium constants:

$$K_{sp} = c_M^p c_X^q \tag{10.19}$$

The quantity that we label s then depends on the stoichiometry.

Example 10.4. What is the molar solubility of ferrous hydroxide?
From Table 10.3, $pK_{sp} = 15.1$, or $K_{sp} = 7.9 \times 10^{-16}$. The dissolution reaction is

$$Fe(OH)_2 \rightleftharpoons Fe^{2+} + 2OH^-$$

so $K_{sp} = c_{Fe} c_{OH}^2$. (The charges on the subscripts are omitted for clarity.) Since each molecule of Fe (OH)$_2$ that dissolves yields one Fe^{2+} ion, we define the solubility as the concentration of ferrous ion, or $c_{Fe} = s$. The stoichiometry yields $c_{OH} = 2 c_{Fe}$, so the result is[1]

$$K_{sp} = s \times (2s)^2 = 4s^3$$

Therefore $s = 5.8 \times 10^{-6}$ M.

Example 10.5. What is the solubility of silver chloride in 0.02 M KCl? Assume activity coefficients are unity.
Again we set $c_{Ag} = s$, the solubility. The solubility product is defined $K_{sp} = c_{Ag} c_{Cl}$; however, the chloride concentration has been augmented by the addition of potassium chloride, so we write $c_{Cl} = 0.02 + s$; that is, the chloride concentration is the sum from two sources, the KCl and the AgCl. We therefore have $K_{sp} = s(0.02 + s)$, which is a quadratic equation that can be solved for s. Before doing that, however, it is worth trying the approximation $c_{Cl} = 0.02$, which involves neglecting the relatively small contribution from dissolution of the AgCl. Thus

$$K_{sp} = 0.02s = 1.78 \times 10^{-10}$$
$$s = 8.9 \times 10^{-9} \, M$$

First note that the approximation seems well justified. More interestingly, observe that the solubility of silver chloride has been reduced from about 1×10^{-5} M in water (Example 10.3) to about 1×10^{-8} M in 0.02 M KCl. This is an example of the *common ion effect*. The solubility of any slightly soluble salt can be reduced by adding an excess of one of its constituent ions.

The accuracy of such calculations can be improved by making use of the Debye–Hückel equation to estimate the values of mean ionic activity coefficients.

10.5. SOLUBILITIES OF NONELECTROLYTES: FURTHER ISSUES

Salt Effects. In Example 10.5 we encountered one type of salt effect. There is another type of salt effect that is observed when the solubility of a nonelectrolyte is studied as a function of ionic strength (or of the concentration of an added electrolyte). Compare the nonelectrolyte solubility in the absence and presence of added salt. Since the solid solute is present in both cases

$$\mu(\text{solid}) = \mu(c_s = 0) = \mu(c_s)$$

where c_s is the concentration of added salt. Therefore $a(c_s = 0) = a(c_s)$, or

$$s_0 \gamma_0 = s \gamma \tag{10.20}$$

where s_0 and s are the solubilities in the two cases. Thus $\gamma/\gamma_0 = s_0/s$; and since $\gamma_0 = 1$ is a reasonable assumption, $\gamma = s_0/s$, and we have a method for measuring nonelectrolyte activity coefficients. Moreover, it is found experimentally that the quantity log (s_0/s) often varies linearly with c_s, or

$$\text{Log}\frac{s_0}{s} = k_s c_s \tag{10.21}$$

If $s_0/s > 1$, then k_s is positive, and the nonelectrolyte is said to be "salted out"; if $s_0/s < 1$, then k_s is negative, and the solute is "salted in." These are called the "salting-out and salting-in effects," and the constant k_s is known as the Setschenow constant.

Regular Solution Theory. We have seen that an ideal solution has thermodynamic mixing quantities $\Delta H_{\text{mix}} = 0$ and $\Delta S_{\text{mix}} = -R(x_1 \ln x_1 + x_2 \ln x_2)$. A *regular solution* is defined to be one having an ideal entropy of mixing but a nonideal enthalpy of mixing. Recall also that the ideal solubility of a nonelectrolyte (i.e., the solubility when a nonelectrolyte forms an ideal solution) is given by

$$\ln x_2 = \frac{-\Delta H_f}{R}\left(\frac{T_m - T}{T T_m}\right) \tag{10.22}$$

where ΔC_p is assumed to be zero or negligible. The molecular interpretation of an ideal solution is that the energy of interaction of a solute molecule with a solvent molecule is identical with the energy of interaction of two solvent molecules.

The molecular interpretation of regular solution theory is quite different; in regular solution theory the energy of 1–2 interactions (where 1 is the solvent, 2 is the solute) is approximated as the geometric mean of 1–1 and 2–2 interaction energies, or[2]

$$U_{12} = (U_{11}U_{22})^{1/2} \tag{10.23}$$

This approximation results in regular solution theory being applicable mainly to fairly nonpolar systems, that is, nonpolar nonelectrolytes dissolved in nonpolar solvents. For our present interest, the essential result (Hildebrand and Scott 1964, p. 271) of regular solution theory is embodied in Eq. (10.24), which may be compared with Eq. (10.22):

$$\ln x_2 = -\frac{\Delta H_f}{R}\left(\frac{T_m - T}{T T_m}\right) - \frac{V_2 \varphi_1^2}{RT}(\delta_1 - \delta_2)^2 \qquad (10.24)$$

where V_2 is the molar volume of solute and φ_1 is the volume fraction concentration of solvent in the solution. The quantities δ_1 and δ_2 are the *solubility parameters* of the solvent and solute. These are physical properties with the following significance.

The term ΔH_{vap}, the molar heat of vaporization, is the enthalpy required to effect the transformation of one mole of liquid to its vapor state. During this process all the solvent–solvent interactions (which are responsible for the existence of the liquid phase) are overcome. A quantity called the *cohesive energy density* (CED) is defined

$$CED = \frac{\Delta H_{vap} - RT}{V} \qquad (10.25)$$

where V is the molar volume of the liquid. We anticipate, and we find, that liquids with strong intermolecular interactions (especially polar "associated" liquids having the potential for strong dipole–dipole and hydrogen-bonding interactions) have larger ced values than do nonpolar liquids. Table 10.4 lists some CED values.

Because of the manner in which CED appears in regular solution theory equations, Hildebrand (Hildebrand et al. 1970; Hildebrand and Scott 1964, p. 271) defined the solubility parameter δ by Eq. (10.26). Table 10.4 also gives δ values.

$$\delta = (CED)^{1/2} \qquad (10.26)$$

Referring now to Eq. (10.24), note that if $\delta_1 = \delta_2$, we recover Eq. (10.22) for the ideal solution; in other words, the condition $\delta_1 = \delta_2$ is equivalent to the condition $\Delta H_{mix} = 0$. The greater the difference $\delta_1 - \delta_2$ (or of $\delta_2 - \delta_1$, because the difference is squared), the greater the deviation from ideality, and, as Eq. (10.24) shows, the lower the solubility that is predicted. This provides a guide for experimental design; to achieve maximal solubility according to regular solution theory, strive to equate the solubility parameters of solvent and solute. Since the solute identity is usually established by the nature of the problem, the experimental variable is the solvent identity. Sometimes mixed solvent systems function better than do pure solvents for this reason. For example, a mixture of ether ($\delta = 7.4$) and ethanol ($\delta = 12.7$) dissolves nitrocellulose ($\delta = 11.2$), although neither pure liquid serves as a good solvent for this solute.[3]

Although the cohesive energy density, and therefore the solubility parameter, is a well-defined physical property for any solvent, regular solution theory is limited

Table 10.4. Cohesive energy densities and solubility parameters

Solvent	CED (cal cm^{-3})	$\delta(\text{cal}^{1/2}\,\text{cm}^{-3/2})$
n-Pentane	50.2	7.0
Cyclohexane	67.2	8.2
1,4-Dioxane	96	10.0
Benzene	84.6	9.2
Diethyl ether	59.9	7.4
Ethyl acetate	83.0	9.1
Acetic acid	102	10.1
n-Butyl alcohol	130.0	11.4
n Propyl alcohol	141.6	11.9
Acetone	95	9.9
Ethanol	168	12.7
Methanol	212	14.5
Acetonitrile	141.6	11.9
Dimethylformamide	146.4	12.1
Ethylene glycol	212	14.6
Glycerol	272	16.5
Dimethylsulfoxide	144	12.0
Water	547.6	23.4

(e.g., by the geometric mean approximation) to solutions of nonpolar substances. It should therefore not be expected to apply quantitatively to polar systems such as aqueous solutions.

Example 10.6. Predict the solubility of naphthalene in n-hexane at 20°C. The solubility parameters are $\delta_1 = 7.3$ and $\delta_2 = 9.9$ (both in $\text{cal}^{1/2}\,\text{cm}^{-3/2}$), and the molar volumes are $V_1 = 132\,\text{cm}^3\,\text{mol}^{-1}$ and $V_2 = 123\,\text{cm}^3\,\text{mol}^{-1}$. See Example 10.1 for additional data.

We use Eq. (10.24), which in Example 10.1 was expressed in terms of log x_2. In that form the first term on the right had the value -0.577, which we need not recalculate. Now we consider the second term. We lack only the quantity φ_1, the volume fraction of solvent. This appears to be a dilemma, because we cannot estimate φ_1 until we know x_2, which is what we want to calculate.

If we anticipate that the solute has a low solubility, it may be acceptable to make the approximation $\varphi_1 = 1$. An alternative is to take the result for an ideal solution (Example 10.1, which gave $x_2 = 0.265$) as a basis for estimating φ_1. We will do the problem in both ways.

(a) Let $\varphi_1 = 1$. Then from eq. (10.24),

$$\text{Log } x_2 = -0.577 - \frac{(123\,\text{cm}^3)(1)^2(7.3 - 9.9\,\text{cal}^{1/2}\,\text{cm}^{-3/2})^2}{(2.303)(1.987\,\text{cal mol}^{-1}\,\text{K}^{-1})(293.15\,\text{K})}$$

$$= -0.577 - 0.620 = -1.197$$

$$x_2 = 0.064$$

(b) The volume fraction is defined as follows:

$$\varphi_1 = \frac{n_1 V_1}{n_1 V_1 + n_2 V_2} \tag{10.27}$$

Suppose $n_1 + n_2 = 1$; from Example 10.1, $x_2 = 0.265$, or $n_2 = 0.265$ and $n_1 = 0.735$. Using these numbers in Eq. (10.27) gives $\varphi_1 = 0.748$. (Note how close φ_1 is to x_1, because V_1 and V_2 are similar.) Repeating the calculation gives

$$\text{Log } x_2 = -0.577 - 0.335 = -0.912$$
$$x_2 = 0.122$$

We therefore predict that x_2 is between 0.064 and 0.122, and we might take the average as our best estimate. The experimental result (Table 10.1) is $x_2 = 0.090$.

Prediction of Aqueous Solubilities. Water is the preferred solvent for liquid dosage forms because of its biological compatibility, but unfortunately many drugs are poorly soluble in water. To be able to predict the aqueous solubility of compounds, even if only approximately, is a valuable capability because it can guide or reduce experimental effort. Water is a highly polar and structured medium in which nonideal behavior is commonly observed, so we must abandon hope that the ideal solubility prediction of Eq. (10.10) will be useful, and even the regular solution theory [Eq. (10.24)] is ineffectual in solving this problem. Effective approaches may be guided by thermodynamic concepts, but they incorporate much empirical (i.e., experimental) content.

Although the ideal solubility equation will not suffice to predict nonelectrolyte solubility in water, the solute–solute interactions responsible for maintaining the crystal lattice must nevertheless be overcome, so Eq. (10.10) will still be applicable as a means of estimating the solute–solute interaction. What must be done in addition is to take account of the solvent–solvent and solvent–solute interactions, for these will in general not offset each other. In a paper that includes a valuable collection of solubility data, Yalkowsky and Valvani (1980) have developed a very useful method based on this approach. They start with Eq. (10.10), which they transform to Eq. (10.11), repeated here:

$$\ln x_2 = -\frac{\Delta S_f (T_m - T)}{RT} \tag{10.28}$$

They then carry out an analysis of experimental entropies of fusion, reaching these conclusions:

For spherical (or nearly so) molecules: $\Delta S_f = 3.5 \text{ cal mol}^{-1} \text{K}^{-1}$
For rigid molecules: $\Delta S_f = 13.5 \text{ cal mol}^{-1} \text{K}^{-1}$

For molecules having $n > 5$ flexible chain atoms: $\Delta S_f = 13.5 + 2.5$
$(n - 5) \, \text{cal mol}^{-1} \, \text{K}^{-1}$

In the following we will use only the result for rigid molecules.

Yalkowsky and Valvani then take the log P value of the solute (where P is the 1-octanol/water partition coefficient) as an empirical measure of the solution phase nonidealities. They combine this with Eq. (10.28), convert to molar concentration, and apply a small statistical adjustment, finally getting Eq. (10.29) for the calculation of rigid nonelectrolyte molar solubility in water at 25°C:

$$\text{Log } c_2 = -0.011(t_m - 25) - \log P + 0.54 \qquad (10.29)$$

where t_m is the solute melting point in centigrade degrees. For liquid nonelectrolytes t_m is set to 25, so the first term vanishes. Log P may be available from experimental studies, but it may have to be estimated by methods cited in Chapter 7.

Yalkowsky and Valvani applied Eq. (10.29) to solubility data on 167 compounds whose solubilities ranged over nine orders of magnitude, finding that the estimated solubilities agreed with the observed solubilities to within 0.5 log unit for all but eight compounds, and in no case was the error greater than a factor of 10. Equation (10.29) is a very practical solution to the problem of predicting aqueous solubilities.

Amidon and Williams (1982) refined the approach of Yalkowsky and Valvani, achieving better accuracy but at the cost of increased complexity in the equation. Grant and Higuchi (1990) describe alternative methods of calculation that are based on different pathways from the initial to the final state.

Equation (10.10) and equations derived from it, such as Eqs. (10.28) and (10.29), contain the difference $(T_m - T)$, showing that a higher melting temperature is reflecting stronger solute–solute interactions in the solid state. As a general but not precise rule, we may anticipate that very polar molecules (or functional groups) will conduce to strong intermolecular interactions by means of electrostatic forces, which for certain groups may include hydrogen bonding. Thus high molecular polarity tends to be associated with high melting temperature, and higher melting temperatures lead to lower solubilities, at least as they are described by Eq. (10.10).

Now consider the special case of water as a solvent. Water is a very polar solvent and is capable of functioning as a hydrogen bond donor and acceptor. Very polar solute molecules will tend to interact strongly with the solvent water; these are the solvent–solute or solvation interactions that increase solubility. But we have seen that highly polar substances tend to have high melting temperatures, so we are led to the tentative conclusion that melting temperature may be an approximate indicator of the extent of solvent–solute interaction. It follows (still arguing in this approximate mode) that the opposing factors of solute–solute (crystal lattice) and solvent–solute (solvation) interactions are both measured by, or at least indicated by, the same quantity, namely, the melting temperature.[4] Thus in some degree we may anticipate that these two factors will compensate each other, with the consequence that the solubility will become essentially independent of the melting temperature. But then the first term in Eq. (10.29) will (approximately) vanish, leading to a dependence solely on log P.

Correlations of log c with log P are well known (Yalkowsky and Valvani 1980; Grant and Higuchi 1990, Chapter 8). Equations (10.30a) and (10.30b) are such correlations, based on solubility data for compounds having a considerable range of structural features. These equations are to be judged solely by their success in reproducing or predicting solubilities; they are purely empirical.

$$\text{Log } c_2 = -\log P - 1.00 \quad \text{(for solids)} \tag{10.30a}$$

$$\text{Log } c_2 = -\log P + 0.27 \quad \text{(for liquids)} \tag{10.30b}$$

A comparison of the performance of Eq. (10.29) with Eqs. (10.30) indicates that Eq. (10.29) is slightly superior, but there are some reversals. If the solute melting point is not available, Eq. (10.30a) offers an alternative method of estimation.

Example 10.7. Estimate the aqueous solubility at 25°C of isophthalic acid, for which log $P = 1.73$ and whose melting temperature is 346°C.

With Eq. (10.29), $\log c_2 = -4.72$; with Eq. (10.30a), $\log c_2 = -2.73$. The experimental result is $\log c_2 = -3.40$. Evidently neither Eq. (10.29) nor Eq. (10.30a) yields a fully satisfactory answer in this case. (Although interestingly their average is 3.73, in error by only about a factor of 2 in the solubility c_2.) Obviously there is scope for improved methods of estimation.

Solubility in Mixed Solvents. If the equilibrium solubility of a solute in water is too low to achieve the desired "target" concentration, a preferred approach in many instances is to incorporate an organic solvent in the aqueous solution, in this way increasing the solubility of the solute. This organic solvent (often called the *cosolvent*) must be miscible with water, at least in the proportions used, and if the solution is to be a dosage form, the cosolvent must be physiologically acceptable. These requirements severely limit the cosolvent selection. But beyond this issue is the matter of the optimal cosolvent concentration in the mixed solvent system of water and cosolvent. As in our treatment of aqueous solubility, we seek methods that are rapid and easy to apply, even though approximate in their accuracy, because the calculation will always be followed by laboratory studies to confirm or refine the numerical estimate.

If the solute and solvent molecules in a solution differ greatly in size, plots of various experimental quantities against solvent composition tend to be more symmetrical when solvent composition is given in volume fraction than in mole fraction (Williamson 1967, p. 44). This observation forms the basis of a model proposed by Yalkowsky and Rubino (1985). For these three-component systems, let water be component 1, the cosolvent component 2, and the solute component 3. The molar solubility of solute in water is written $(c_3)_1$ and its molar solubility in pure cosolvent as $(c_3)_2$. In solvent of any composition the solute solubility is written c_3. Then the Yalkowsky–Rubino model becomes

$$\text{Log } c_3 = \varphi_1 \log (c_3)_1 + \varphi_2 \log (c_3)_2 \tag{10.31}$$

where φ_1 and φ_2 are the volume fractions of water and cosolvent, respectively. Since $\varphi_1 + \varphi_2 = 1$, an equivalent form of Eq. (10.31) is

$$\text{Log } c_3 = \varphi_2[\log (c_3)_2 - \log (c_3)_1] + \log (c_3)_1 \tag{10.32}$$

This equation predicts that $\log c_3$ will be a linear function of φ_2.

Equation (10.31) is a postulate. It can be described as a linear combination model, or as a weighted average; that is, $\log c_3$ is postulated to be an average of $\log (c_3)_1$ and $\log (c_3)_2$, each of these making a contribution according to (weighted by) its volume fraction.

The procedure for testing and using this model is simple. On a graphical scale of φ_2 one plots $\log (c_3)_1$ at $\varphi_2 = 0.0$ and $\log (c_3)_2$ at $\varphi_2 = 1.0$. These points are connected by a straight line, which is the graphical representation of Eq. (10.32). A test of the model consists of plotting experimental solubilities at intermediate values of φ_2 to learn how well they agree with the straight-line prediction. Alternatively, if (as is usually the case) such data are not available, the model is assumed to be (approximately) valid, and that value of φ_2 is read off the line that will achieve a desired target solubility. It is not necessary to carry this operation out graphically, for by rearrangement of Eq. (10.32) we obtain

$$\varphi_2 = \frac{\log c_3 - \log (c_3)_1}{\log (c_3)_2 - \log (c_3)_1} \tag{10.33}$$

With this equation the required volume fraction of cosolvent can be calculated, according to this model.

Figure 10.3 shows solubility data for the system water (1)-ethanol (2)-naphthalene (LePree et al. 1994). The straight line connecting the extreme points constitutes the linear combination model, Eq. (10.32); the points are experimental. Obviously the points do not describe a straight line, so in this sense, and for this system, the model does not appear to be valid. On the other hand, as an approximate guide to the dependence of solubility on solvent composition it may be helpful to the experimentalist, and it is in this sense that the model should be judged. It is not a precise description of physicochemical behavior, but rather is a useful tool in formulation development.

Example 10.8. Propose a water/ethanol mixed solvent composition that will dissolve 2.5 mg mL^{-1} of naphthalene. The solubility of naphthalene in water is 2.14×10^{-4} M, and in ethanol it is 0.675 M.

The target concentration of 2.5 mg mL^{-1} is equivalent to 2.5 g L^{-1}. The molecular weight of naphthalene is 128.2, so the molar target concentration c_3 is 0.0195 M, or $\log c_3 = -1.71$. From the given data we have $\log (c_3)_1 = -3.67$ and $\log (c_3)_2 = -0.17$. Applying Eq. (10.33), we obtain

$$\varphi_2 = \frac{-1.71 - (-3.67)}{-0.17 - (-3.67)}$$

$$= 0.56$$

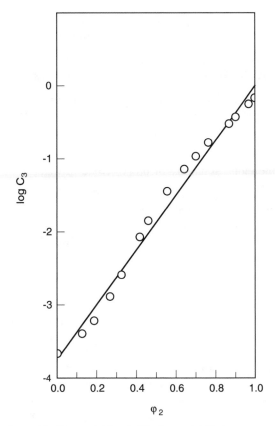

Figure 10.3. The linear combination model for naphthalene solubility in aqueous ethanol solutions.

Thus we predict that a volume fraction of 0.56 ethanol will dissolve the target concentration. This result could also have been obtained by reading from the straight line of Fig. 10.3. It is interesting to note, from the experimental points in Fig. 10.3, that a volume fraction $\varphi_2 = 0.51$ will actually dissolve the target concentration.

More accurate models of solvent effects are available, but these require much experimental effort and are computationally more elaborate.

PROBLEMS

10.1. The melting point of benzoic acid is 122.4°C, and its heat of fusion is 4.44 kcal mol^{-1}. Calculate its ideal solubility at 25°C.

10.2. From the data in Example 10.2, convert the mole fraction solubilities to molar solubilities, construct the van't Hoff plot, and evaluate the heat of solution.

10.3. Derive an equation relating the molar solubility of calcium phosphate to its solubility product, and calculate its molar solubility.

10.4. A solution containing NaBr, NaCl, and NaI is titrated with silver nitrate solution. Predict the order in which the silver halides will precipitate.

10.5. Predict the solubility of iodine in carbon tetrachloride at 25°C. The melting point of iodine is 113.6°C, its heat of fusion is 3.71 kcal mol^{-1}, its molar volume is 59 cm^3, and its solubility parameter is 14.1. The solubility parameter of carbon tetrachloride is 8.6.

10.6. Predict the molar solubility of progesterone in water at 25°C. The melting point of progesterone is 131°C and its log P value is 3.87.

10.7. The solubility of naphthalene in water at 25°C is 2.14×10^{-4} M, and its solubility in dimethylsulfoxide (DMSO) is 1.920 M. Estimate the mixed solvent composition required to dissolve 4 mg mL^{-1} of the solute.

NOTES

1. Equations like this one in Example 10.4 are easily solved by a logarithmic technique. We have $7.9 \times 10^{-16} = 4s^3$, or $1.975 \times 10^{-16} = s^3$. Take logarithms of both sides, obtaining $-15.70 = 3 \log s$, or $-5.235 = \log s$. The antilogarithm gives s.
2. The arithmetic mean of two numbers is $(a+b)/2$; their geometric mean is $(ab)^{1/2}$.
3. As a strategy for optimizing solvent selection, evidently this approach requires an estimate of the solubility parameter of the solute. There are several ways to obtain this. One method is suggested by the example; presumably the solubility parameter of the solvent mixture that maximizes solubility is also the solubility parameter of the solute.
4. Polarity is just one factor controlling the melting temperature. Symmetry is another; the more symmetric the molecule, the higher the melting temperature (when comparing "similar" molecules).

11

SURFACES AND INTERFACES

Up to this point in our study of thermodynamics we have dealt with bulk phases only; that is, we have ignored possible influences of the surfaces of these phases. This attitude is justified when the surface constitutes a very small fraction of the system. In some circumstances, however, the surface : volume ratio of the system becomes relatively large, and then the properties of the surface may dominate the behavior of the system. In the pharmaceutical field, the dosage forms called *emulsions*, *suspensions*, and *foams* exemplify such circumstances; collectively these are known as *disperse systems*; emulsions are dispersions of liquid droplets in an immiscible liquid, suspensions are dispersions of solid particles in a liquid, and foams are dispersions of gases in liquids.

Let us begin with a clarification of terminology. Strictly speaking, the boundary between any two phases constitutes an interface, but it is conventional to call this interface a "surface" when one of the phases is a vapor or gas (especially, and usually, when it is air). We therefore have these identifications:

Surfaces	Interfaces
Solid–gas	Solid–solid
Liquid–gas	Solid–liquid
	Liquid–liquid

Despite these definitions, it is common to use the word "surface" in a generic sense to embrace all such phase boundaries.

11.1. THERMODYNAMIC PROPERTIES

Surface Tension and Interfacial Tension. Let us carry out this thought-experiment. Figure 11.1a illustrates a column of a liquid, constituting a single phase, and having a cross-sectional area of 1 cm^2. Now imagine this column to be pulled apart cleanly into two parts, as shown in Fig. 11.1b. The result of this imagined experiment has been to create two surfaces of the liquid, each of area 1 cm^2.

Energy was required to create these surfaces, because molecules had to be pulled apart, and the forces of intermolecular interaction had to be overcome. The work of carrying out this process is called the *work of cohesion*, w_c, and it is set equal to the energy of the surfaces that were created. (Because we can neither create nor destroy energy, the work w_c done on the system is now possessed by the system in the form of surface energy.) We write

$$w_c = 2\gamma \tag{11.1}$$

where γ is the surface energy per square centimeter, and is called the *surface tension*. (The factor 2 appears because 2 cm^2 of surface were created in Fig. 11.1.)

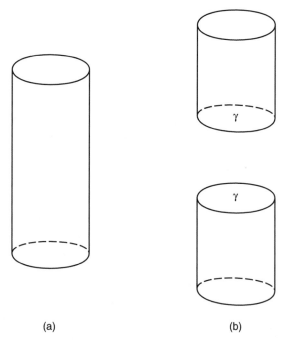

(a)   (b)

Figure 11.1. (a) A column of liquid 1 cm^2 in cross section; (b) the column separated to create two surfaces, each with area 1 cm^2 and surface tension γ.

We can now connect this concept of surface energy to other kinds of energy by recalling (Chapter 1) that work (or energy) can be expressed as the product of an intensity factor and a capacity factor. For surface work or energy we have

$$\text{Surface energy} = \text{surface tension} \times \text{change in surface area}$$
$$\Delta G = \gamma \, \Delta A \tag{11.2}$$

If ΔA is positive (surface area is created), ΔG is positive and the process is non-spontaneous; work must be done to create new surface area. If ΔA is negative, ΔG is negative and the process is spontaneous. The surface energy is identified with the change in Gibbs free energy if the temperature and pressure are constant.

Table 11.1 lists the surface tensions of some liquids. First consider the units of γ, which is an energy per unit area. Thus in SI units, $J\,m^{-2}$ is a correct designation for the units of γ. Moreover, since work (energy) is the product of force and length, and $1\,J = 1\,N\,m$, the units $N\,m^{-1}$ are also acceptable. In the older cgs system, in which most of the literature values of γ are recorded, the corresponding units are $erg\,cm^{-2}$ and $dyn\,cm^{-1}$. However, in order that the numerical values of γ be identical in the cgs and SI systems, the SI units are multiplied by 10^3. Thus we can state the surface tension of water in these equivalent units:

$$\gamma = 71.8\,\frac{erg}{cm^2} = 71.8\,\frac{dyn}{cm} = 71.8\,\frac{mJ}{m^2} = 71.8\,\frac{mN}{m}$$

Inasmuch as the surface tension is a measure of the energy required to create unit area of surface, we might expect γ to be larger for solvents having stronger inter-molecular forces of interaction, and generally we see that this expectation is borne out. Very polar molecules and those capable of hydrogen bonding tend to have higher values of γ than do nonpolar substances.

As the temperature of a liquid is increased, the liquid acquires more thermal energy, and so less additional energy needs to be supplied to create new surface. As a consequence, the surface tension is smaller at higher temperatures.

Table 11.1. Surface tensions at 25°C

Solvent	γ (dyn cm^{-1})	Solvent	γ (dyn cm^{-1})
n-Hexane	17.9	Acetone	22.9
Cyclohexane	19.8	Ethanol	21.8
Benzene	28.2	Methanol	22.4
Diethyl ether	16.5	Acetonitrile	28.5
Chloroform	26.5	Glycerol	62.5
Ethyl acetate	23.2	Dimethylsulfoxide	42.8
n-Butyl alcohol	24.2	Water	71.8
n-Propyl alcohol	23.4	Mercury	485.5

Another point of view may be helpful in visualizing the physical nature of the surface tension. The properties of a system consisting of a liquid in contact with its vapor do not change discontinuously at the surface, but rather change in a smooth continuous fashion. Another way to say this is to point out that the surface is not a mathematical boundary, but is a region having a thickness of several molecular diameters. Consider the density as a property that varies from a relatively high value in the bulk liquid (expressed as g mL^{-1} or as number of molecules per unit volume) to a very low value in the vapor. Evidently the density will have an intermediate value in the surface region. Taking a slice coplanar with the surface, then, the number of molecules per unit area in the surface is smaller than in the bulk. In other words, the surface is analogous to an extended spring; energy is required to create the surface (or to stretch the spring), and this energy is manifested as a tension in the plane of the surface; this is the surface tension (Fowkes 1964).

Now we will carry out another thought experiment in the style of Fig. 11.1, this one as shown in Fig. 11.2. Here we have a column of 1 cm^2 cross-sectional area, but consisting of two immiscible liquid phases, 1 and 2, in contact. We now imagine the phases separated at their boundary. According to our earlier analysis, we can expect an amount of work to be required equal to the sum $\gamma_1 + \gamma_2$, for 1 cm^2 of surface of each 1 and 2 is created in this process. But there is a further factor to consider, for in the initial state of the system there existed an interface between 1 and 2, and this

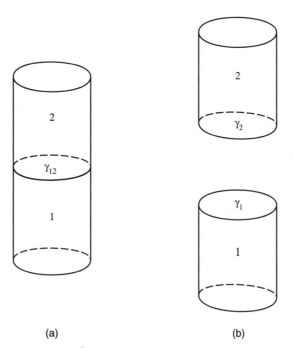

(a)   (b)

Figure 11.2. (a) A column of 1 cm^2 cross-sectional area of phases 1 and 2 in contact; (b) the phases are separated to create two surfaces, one of liquid 1, the other of liquid 2.

Table 11.2. Interfacial tensions at 20°C

Liquids	γ (dyn cm^{-1})	Liquids	γ (dyn cm^{-1})
Water/mercury	375	Water/n-hexane	51.1
Water/n-octane	50.8	Water/CCl$_4$	45
Water/benzene	35.0	Water/ether	10.7
Mercury/benzene	375		

interface itself possesses surface (or interface) energy, labeled γ_{12}. In the final state of the system this interface no longer exists, so neither does its energy, which has, in effect, been applied to defray the energetic cost of creating the two new surfaces. The work involved in passing from the initial state in Fig. 11.2a to the final state in Fig. 11.2b is called the *work of adhesion*, w_a, and is given by

$$w_a = \gamma_1 + \gamma_2 - \gamma_{12} \tag{11.3}$$

The quantity γ_{12} is the *interfacial tension*. It has the same units and the same physical significance as the surface tension. Table 11.2 gives some interfacial tensions. It must be realized that in such systems the two liquids are mutually saturated.

The interfacial tension can be measured, or it can be calculated with reasonable accuracy by means of

$$\gamma_{12} = \gamma_1 + \gamma_2 - 2(\gamma_1^d \gamma_2^d)^{1/2} \tag{11.4}$$

where γ_1^d and γ_2^d are the London dispersion force contributions to γ_1 and γ_2 (Fowkes 1964). The dispersion force is an attractive force (sometimes called the van der Waals force) between all molecules. For nonpolar molecules such as saturated hydrocarbons it is the only attractive force, so $\gamma^d = \gamma$ for such liquids. For mercury γ^d is 200 dyn cm^{-1} and for water $\gamma^d = 21.8$ dyn cm^{-1}. Equation (11.4) incorporates the geometric mean approximation of regular solution theory (Section 10.5); see Eq. (10.23) in particular.

Example 11.1. Estimate the interfacial tension at the water/n-hexane interface. We use Eq. (11.4):

$$\gamma_{12} = 71.8 + 17.9 - 2(21.8 \times 17.9)^{1/2}$$
$$= 50.2 \text{ dyn cm}^{-1}$$

The experimental value (Table 11.2) is 51.1 dyn cm^{-1}.

Because a surface is of relatively high energy compared to the bulk, there is a thermodynamic driving force for minimization of surface area. A sphere is the geometric form having the minimum surface : volume ratio, so that under the influence of surface tension alone units of matter will tend to assume a spherical shape, as with droplets of liquids. This tendency may be opposed by other forces, such as the gravitational force. The trend to surface minimization also accounts for the tendency of a dispersion of liquid drops in a liquid (an emulsion) to coalesce into two bulk phases.

Spreading of Liquids on Liquids.   Picture a small volume of liquid 2 placed on the planar surface of liquid 1. What will happen? Will it just sit there as a globule (flattened by gravity into a "lens" shape), or will it spread out into a very thin film? This question can be answered by considering the work of adhesion (which measures the attraction between 1 and 2) and the work of cohesion (which measures the attraction within 2) (Adamson 1960, p. 107; Bummer 2000). The *spreading coefficient* $S_{2/1}$ for the spreading of 2 on 1 is defined as

$$S_{2/1} = w_a - w_{c(2)} \tag{11.5}$$

where $w_{c(2)}$ is the work of cohesion of liquid 2. Similarly, the spreading coefficient $S_{1/2}$ for the spreading of 1 on 2 is

$$S_{1/2} = w_a - w_{c(1)} \tag{11.6}$$

Incorporating Eqs. (11.1) and (11.3) into these definitions gives

$$S_{2/1} = \gamma_1 - (\gamma_2 + \gamma_{12}) \tag{11.7}$$
$$S_{1/2} = \gamma_2 - (\gamma_1 + \gamma_{12}) \tag{11.8}$$

Let us try to anticipate the possible outcomes of numerical calculations of spreading coefficients. If $w_a \gg w_{c(2)}$, evidently the attraction between 1 and 2 is greater than the self-attraction of liquid 2, so the spreading coefficient will be positive and we may expect 2 to spread on 1. Compare the rather extreme cases in Example 11.2.

Example 11.2. Calculate the spreading coefficients of water on mercury and of mercury on water and interpret the results. (Ignore the density difference!)
    Let mercury be liquid 1 and water liquid 2. From Eqs. (11.7) and (11.8) and data in Tables 11.1 and 11.2, we have

$$S_{2/1} = 485.5 - (71.8 + 375) = +38.7$$
$$S_{1/2} = 71.8 - (485.5 + 375) = -788.7$$

Thus water will spread on mercury but mercury will not spread on water.

In general a liquid of lower surface tension will spread on a liquid of higher surface tension. However, spreading does not continue indefinitely, because the phenomenon in which liquid 2 spreads on liquid 1 creates a new surface tension, leading to a situation in which the spreading coefficient is negative and addition of further 2 leads to formation of a lens rather than continued spreading.

Wetting of Solids by Liquids. Consider the system of a drop of liquid L on a planar surface of a solid S, where the system is at equilibrium with the vapor V of the liquid. The shape of the drop can be specified in terms of the angle θ that a tangent makes to the surface of the liquid at its point of contact with the solid. This angle is called the *contact angle*. It can be measured experimentally.

A simple relationship can be obtained connecting θ with the system surface and interfacial tensions. Figure 11.3 shows the construction, the lengths of the arrows (vectors) being proportional to the indicated tensions. At equilibrium, the force associated with tension γ_{SV} is exactly balanced by the sum of the forces due to γ_{SL} and the component of γ_{LV} lying in the same plane and direction as γ_{SL}. This component has the magnitude ab in the figure, and is seen to be equal to $\gamma_{LV} \cos\theta$. Thus Eq. (11.9) can be written.

$$\gamma_{SV} = \gamma_{SL} + \gamma_{LV} \cos\theta \tag{11.9}$$

The tension γ_{LV} is, of course, simply the surface tension of the liquid. γ_{SL} is the liquid/solid interfacial tension, and γ_{SV} is the surface tension of the solid.

If the liquid wets the solid, the liquid spreads out on the surface, reducing the angle θ; commonly a liquid that wets a solid is considered to have a contact angle of $0°$. If $\theta > 90°$, the liquid does not wet the solid. Examination of Fig. 11.3 shows that θ will be reduced under the influence of these factors: a larger value of γ_{SV}, or smaller values of γ_{LV} and of γ_{SL}. For a given solid, wetting will be favored by liquids with lower surface tensions. For a given liquid, wetting will be favored by solids with higher surface tensions.[1]

Pressure Difference across Spherical Surfaces. A *bubble* is a region of vapor (often including air) surrounded by a thin film of liquid. A *cavity* is a hole (containing vapor) in a liquid. A *droplet* is a small volume of liquid. Bubbles,

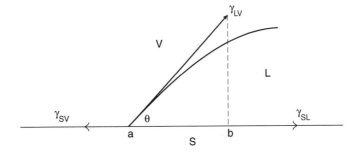

Figure 11.3. Contact angle θ of a solid on a solid.

cavities, and droplets are approximately spherical; they would be spheres if surface forces only were active, but other forces distort their shape. We will assume that they are spheres. Bubbles actually have double walls, an inner film and an outer film, so they have twice the surface area of a sphere their size. Cavities and droplets have single surfaces.

An interesting property of these systems has been known for a long time. Consider a spherical system (we may think of a bubble, while neglecting the double wall), of radius r. There is a driving force for reducing r as a consequence of two factors. One of these is the external pressure on the bubble, and the other is the surface energy. At equilibrium this combined force is just balanced by that due to the internal pressure. We seek the condition of equilibrium balance. First we write the external and internal work terms, then differentiate these with respect to r (giving forces), and then equate the forces.

The external work is a sum of a work of expansion contribution and a surface work term:

$$dw_{ext} = P_{ext}\,dV + \gamma\,dA$$

The force is dw_{ext}/dr, or

$$\frac{dw_{ext}}{dr} = P_{ext}\frac{dV}{dr} + \gamma\frac{dA}{dr}$$

For a sphere $V = (4/3)\pi r^3$ and $A = 4\pi r^2$, so we get

$$\frac{dw_{ext}}{dr} = 4\pi r^2 P_{ext} + 8\pi r\gamma \tag{11.10}$$

The internal work is $dw_{int} = P_{int}dV$, giving in the same way

$$\frac{dw_{int}}{dr} = 4\pi r^2 P_{int} \tag{11.11}$$

Equating Eqs. (11.10) and (11.11) yields

$$P_{int} = P_{ext} + \frac{2\gamma}{r} \tag{11.12}$$

According to this surprising result, the pressure inside the bubble or cavity is greater than that outside by the amount $2\gamma/r$.

Example 11.3. Calculate the pressure difference inside and outside a cavity in water whose radius is 0.01 mm.

We use eq. (11.12) with $r = 10^{-5}$ m and $\gamma = 71.8\,\text{mN m}^{-1}$, finding

$$P_{int} - P_{ext} = 1.436 \times 10^7\,\text{mN m}^{-2}$$

This quantity can be converted to more familiar units by using the identities

$$1\,Pa = 1\,N\,m^{-2}$$
$$1\,atm = 101325\,Pa$$

The result is 0.142 atm.

For a planar surface, r is infinite, so the pressure difference vanishes.

Two practical consequences of eq. (11.12), which we will not develop here, are (1) the vapor pressure of very small droplets is greater than that of large droplets, so the small droplets evaporate; (2) the solubility of very small particles is greater than that of larger particles (Glasstone 1947, p. 247).

11.2. ADSORPTION

The Surface Phase. To the eye a surface or interface at equilibrium appears to be a quiescent, two-dimensional element, but since matter is atomic or molecular in structure we have to consider the nature of the surface in molecular terms. We know that molecules possess thermal energy; in particular, they possess translational energy and are incessantly in motion. Thus at the boundary between a liquid and its vapor, molecules are passing from the liquid state to the vapor state, and vice versa. If the system is at thermodynamic equilibrium, these two rates are equal, so the net transport between the phases is zero, but the extent of molecular traffic is prodigious. The molecules within the liquid phase are also in thermal motion. We noted earlier that the surface region extends several molecular diameters in thickness into the liquid phase. This surface region or phase cannot be sharply demarcated at either of its boundaries (with the bulk liquid or with the vapor) because of the molecular motion. Far from being a quiescent two-dimensional construction, the surface region is a turbulent three-dimensional "interphase."

Molecules in the surface region experience a force field different from that experienced by those in the bulk. A molecule within a bulk liquid is enveloped in a homogeneous force field (on average), because its molecular environment is the same in every direction. Consequently the forces on the molecule are everywhere balanced out, so it experiences no net force. At the surface, on the other hand, the molecule's environment is disymmetric; it experiences more intermolecular forces from the bulk liquid side than from the vapor side. (This disymmetric nature of the forces is treated by some authors as the source of the surface tension.)

Notwithstanding our recognition that the surface region is ill-defined geometrically on the molecular scale, we find it convenient, and also justifiable, as we will see, to treat the surface as a two-dimensional mathematical abstraction. First, treating the surface region realistically as a phase, we may conclude from standard thermodynamics that the chemical potentials of all constituents in a system at equilibrium are identical in all phases, including the surface phase. Next, turning to the surface region treated abstractly as a mathematical surface dividing two phases,

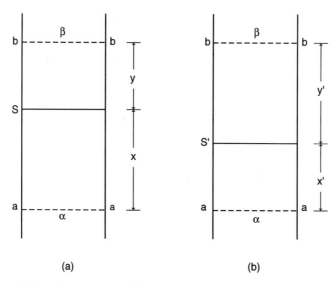

Figure 11.4. (a) Two-phase system, with aa and bb located within bulk phases α and β, and s the dividing boundary within the surface phase; (b) same as (a) but with the dividing boundary moved to s'.

refer to Fig. 11.4a, which depicts two phases, α and β, divided by surface s, whose location is arbitrarily chosen to separate chemically bulk α from chemically bulk β; that is, s is located *somewhere* within the surface region. Suppose the system consists of two components, 1 and 2. The element shown in the figure has cross-sectional area A. If n_1 and n_2 are the total numbers of moles of 1 and 2 contained between the limits aa and bb, respectively, we can write these mass balances:

$$n_1^\alpha + n_1^\beta + n_1^s = n_1 \qquad (11.13a)$$

$$n_2^\alpha + n_2^\beta + n_2^s = n_2 \qquad (11.13b)$$

Now since the molar concentration of 1 in phase α is $c_1^\alpha = n_1^\alpha/V^\alpha$, where $V^\alpha = xA$, and so on, we expand Eq. (11.13) to

$$xAc_1^\alpha + yAc_1^\beta + n_1^s = n_1 \qquad (11.14a)$$

$$xAc_2^\alpha + yAc_2^\beta + n_2^s = n_2 \qquad (11.14b)$$

We divide by A and define $\Gamma = n^s/A$, obtaining

$$xc_1^\alpha + yc_2^\beta + \Gamma_1 = \frac{n_1}{A} \qquad (11.15a)$$

$$xc_2^\alpha + yc_2^\beta + \Gamma_2 = \frac{n_2}{A} \qquad (11.15b)$$

This quantity Γ is called the *surface excess* of the specified constituent. Referring to Eq. (11.13a), we can write

$$\Gamma_1 = \frac{n_1}{A} - \frac{n_1^\alpha + n_1^\beta}{A}$$

which shows that Γ_1 can be zero, positive, or negative. If Γ_1 is positive, an excess of constituent 1 (relative to the bulk) is located at the surface, whereas a negative value of Γ_1 indicates a deficiency at the surface (although it is still called the surface excess).

Returning to our mathematical treatment, let us suppose that phase β is a vapor phase, and that c_2^β is negligible. We then have

$$xc_1^\alpha + \Gamma_1 = \frac{n_1}{A} \tag{11.16a}$$

$$xc_2^\alpha + \Gamma_2 = \frac{n_2}{A} \tag{11.16b}$$

Next we construct Fig. 11.4b for the same system, altering the construction only by displacing boundary s to position s' (but still within the surface region). Repeating the treatment gives the following, by analogy with Eq. (11.16):

$$x'c_1^\alpha + \Gamma_1' = \frac{n_1}{A} \tag{11.17a}$$

$$x'c_2^\alpha + \Gamma_2' = \frac{n_2}{A} \tag{11.17b}$$

Since n_1 and n_2 are fixed and independent of the choice of s or s', we write from (11.16) and (11.17)

$$xc_1^\alpha + \Gamma_1 = x'c_1^\alpha + \Gamma_1' \tag{11.18a}$$
$$xc_2^\alpha + \Gamma_2 = x'c_2^\alpha + \Gamma_2' \tag{11.18b}$$

These two equations combine to give

$$\frac{\Gamma_1' - \Gamma_1}{c_1^\alpha} = \frac{\Gamma_2' - \Gamma_2}{c_2^\alpha}$$

which further rearranges to

$$\Gamma_1' c_2^\alpha - \Gamma_2' c_1^\alpha = \Gamma_1 c_2^\alpha - \Gamma_2 c_1^\alpha = \text{constant} \tag{11.19}$$

That is, the left-hand portion of Eq. (11.19) refers solely to dividing line s', whereas the right-hand portion refers solely to dividing line s, and these are equal. If we created yet more dividing surfaces (within the surface region), say, s'', s''', and so on, the corresponding terms would all be the same. The conclusion is that the choice of dividing surface is arbitrary and irrelevant, provided it lies within the surface region. Of course, the numerical values of the surface excesses depend on the location of the dividing line, so practical issues may lead to a preferred location, but there is no fundamental issue involved (Adamson 1960, pp. 73–79).

This consideration leads to a very convenient simplification in our next development, for, if we can place the dividing surface as we wish, why not place it so that one of the surface excesses is equal to zero?

The Gibbs Adsorption Equation. We are going to develop a famous equation of Gibbs by following a path used earlier in analyzing an open system without consideration of a surface phase. Where we earlier wrote the free energy as the general function [Eq. (3.19)]

$$G = f(T, P, n_1, n_2, \ldots)$$

we now expand the description, writing

$$G = f(T, P, \gamma, n_1, n_2, \ldots) \tag{11.20}$$

In order to simplify the treatment, we will consider that the temperature and pressure are constant, and that only two components are present. Carrying through the earlier development gives the surface phase analog to the Gibbs–Duhem equation [Eq. (3.28)]

$$A \, d\gamma + n_1^s \, d\mu_1 + n_2^s \, d\mu_2 = 0 \tag{11.21}$$

where μ_1 and μ_2 are the chemical potentials of the two components in the surface phase (but we do not need to distinguish them as surface potentials because at equilibrium the potential is the same everywhere).

Now dividing through by A and recalling the definition of surface excess gives

$$d\gamma + \Gamma_1 \, d\mu_1 + \Gamma_2 \, d\mu_2 = 0 \tag{11.22}$$

Next we make use of the demonstration of the preceding analysis, where we saw that the dividing surface can be arbitrarily placed, and we choose to place it such that Γ_1, the surface excess of component 1 (which we can take as the solvent) is zero. Thus

$$d\gamma = -\Gamma_2 \, d\mu_2 \tag{11.23}$$

At low solute concentrations, where the solute activity coefficient may be taken as essentially unity, we have

$$\mu_2 = \mu_0 + RT \ln c_2 \tag{11.24}$$

Combining Eqs. (11.23) and (11.24) gives the *Gibbs adsorption equation:*[2]

$$\Gamma_2 = -\frac{c_2}{RT}\left(\frac{d\gamma}{dc_2}\right) \tag{11.25}$$

The great value of the adsorption equation is that it connects the readily measurable quantities on the right-hand side with the somewhat abstract concept of the surface excess. Qualitatively we can see that if the surface tension of a solution of solute 2 in solvent 1 decreases as the concentration of 2 increases, then Γ_2 is positive, meaning that solute 2 is more concentrated at the surface than in the bulk of the solution. Substances that exhibit positive surface excesses, and therefore produce surface tension decreases, are called *surface active agents,* or *surfactants.* Soaps and detergents are surfactants. Such agents tend to be fairly large molecules, having one end of the molecule polar (and therefore attracted to a polar solvent like water) and the other end nonpolar (and therefore preferring to reside in a nonpolar phase). Even quite small molecules with these molecular attributes exhibit positive surface excesses. Organic solvents such as alcohols, acetone, acetonitrile, and dimethylsulfoxide decrease the surface tension of water.[3] Inorganic salts, on the other hand, increase the surface tension of water.

Equation (11.25) can be written in the equivalent form

$$\Gamma_2 = -\frac{1}{RT}\left(\frac{d\gamma}{d\ln c_2}\right) \tag{11.26}$$

or

$$d\gamma = -RT\,\Gamma_2\,d\ln c_2 \tag{11.27}$$

Of course Γ_2 is a function of concentration, so simple integration is unwarranted, but Eqs. (11.26) and (11.27) suggest that plots of γ against $\ln c_2$ may be fruitful forms of data analysis. Such plots are curved, but their slopes (tangents to the curve) yield estimates of Γ_2 as a function of concentration (Bummer 2000).

Adsorption Isotherms. Adsorption is that process in which a substance develops a positive surface excess at a surface or interface. In our present discussion we will restrict attention to those systems in which a component of a gas or vapor phase is adsorbed to a solid surface, or in which a component of a liquid solution is adsorbed to a solid surface. The substance that is adsorbed is called the *adsorbate,*[4] and the solid is called the *adsorbent.* It might seem that the Gibbs surface excess Γ is the quantity that should be sought experimentally in a study of adsorption, but usually some more accessible measure of the extent of adsorption is determined. A graph of this measure of extent of adsorption against the partial pressure of the adsorbate in the vapor (for vapor–solid systems) or against its solution concentration (for liquid–solid systems) is called an *adsorption isotherm.* (The term *isotherm* simply means that the temperature is held constant.)

Many shapes of adsorption isotherms have been found experimentally, but we will consider only one of these in detail. This function, called the *Langmuir adsorption isotherm*, is widely observed, its physical basis is simple, and its mathematics turn out also to be applicable to other types of systems involving noncovalent interactions, such as enzyme–substrate complexing and molecular complex formation. To focus attention, suppose that we have a two-component solution of solvent 1 and solute (adsorbate) 2 in contact, and at equilibrium, with solid. The process can be portrayed as

$$\text{Adsorbate in solution} \underset{\text{desorption}}{\overset{\text{adsorption}}{\rightleftharpoons}} \text{adsorbate on surface}$$

Our approach, oddly, is a kinetic one. At equilibrium the rate at which molecules of adsorbate adsorb to the surface is just equal to the rate at which they desorb from the surface. We write these expressions for these rates:

$$\text{Rate of adsorption} = k_a c_2 A_f \tag{11.28}$$

$$\text{Rate of desorption} = k_d A_b \tag{11.29}$$

In these equations c_2 is the solution concentration of adsorbate; k_a and k_d are rate constants for adsorption and desorption, respectively; A_f is the solid surface area per unit mass (usually per gram) that is "free," namely, unoccupied by adsorbate molecules; and A_b is the solid surface area per unit mass that is "bound," or occupied by adsorbate molecules. Equation (11.28) postulates that the rate of adsorption is directly proportional to the concentration (actually activity) of adsorbate and to the amount of space available for adsorption on the surface. Equation (11.29) says that the rate of desorption is directly proportional to the extent of surface already covered by adsorbate molecules. It is important to recognize that, for any given system, Eqs. (11.28) and (11.29) a priori may or may not be valid; they constitute hypotheses, to be justified by subsequent testing against experimental data.

At equilibrium these two rates are equal. Let us work out the ramifications of this equality:

$$k_a c_2 A_f = k_d A_b \tag{11.30}$$

Define the total surface area per unit mass as A_t, so

$$A_t = A_f + A_b \tag{11.31}$$

Eliminating A_f, defining $K = k_a/k_d$ (K is an equilibrium constant), and rearranging gives

$$K c_2 = \frac{A_b}{A_t - A_b} \tag{11.32}$$

We now define θ, the *degree of saturation*, by

$$\theta = \frac{A_b}{A_t} \tag{11.33}$$

Combining Eqs. (11.32) and (11.33) gives

$$Kc_2 = \frac{\theta}{1 - \theta} \tag{11.34}$$

which is one form of the Langmuir adsorption isotherm. More commonly it is encountered in this rearranged form:

$$\theta = \frac{Kc_2}{1 + Kc_2} \tag{11.35}$$

Equation (11.35) is equivalent to

$$A_b = \frac{KA_tc_2}{1 + Kc_2} \tag{11.36}$$

Now let σ be the area occupied per molecule on the surface, so A_b/σ is the number of molecules adsorbed per gram of solid, and $n_b = A_b/\sigma N_A$ (where N_A is Avogadro's number) is the number of moles of adsorbate bound per gram of solid. Similarly, $A_t/\sigma N_A = n_{max}$ is the maximum number of moles that can be bound per gram of solid. Making substitutions in Eq. (11.36) gives finally

$$n_b = \frac{Kn_{max}c_2}{1 + Kc_2} \tag{11.37}$$

This is a very practical form of the Langmuir adsorption isotherm. Experimentally we know c_2, the solution concentration of adsorbate, and we measure n_b, the number of moles of adsorbate per gram of solid.

Two practical problems remain. We wish to test the hypothesis against the data (i.e., we wish to establish whether the system is described by the Langmuir isotherm), and, if Eq. (11.37) is in fact descriptive of the system, we wish to evaluate the model parameters K and n_{max}. Both problems have traditionally been solved by rearranging Eq. (11.37) to this form:

$$\frac{c_2}{n_b} = \frac{c_2}{n_{max}} + \frac{1}{Kn_{max}} \tag{11.38}$$

This is the equation of a straight line. If the Langmuir isotherm is obeyed, a plot of c_2/n_b against c_2 should be linear, with slope $= 1/n_{max}$ and intercept $= 1/Kn_{max}$. Thus $n_{max} = 1/\text{slope}$, and $K = \text{slope/intercept}$.

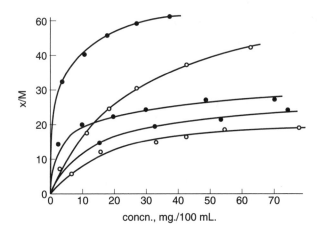

Figure 11.5. Plots of milligrams of dye absorbed per gram of cornstarch $[x(\mathrm{M})]$, versus milligrams of dye per 100 ML of solution at equilibrium for FD&C Red No. 3 (◓), FD&C Blue No. 2 (⊖), Ext. D&C Red No. 15 (⊙), FD&C Yellow No. 5 (⊕), and FD&C Green No. 1 (○). [Reproduced with permission from Zografi and Mattocks (1963).]

From Eq. (11.37) we can analyze Langmuirian behavior. If c_2 is very low, so that $Kc_2 \ll 1$, then $n_b \approx Kn_{max}c_2$; the isotherm is nearly linear at very low adsorbate concentrations. At relatively high c_2 values, where $Kc_2 \gg 1$, then $n_b \approx n_{max}$; the extent of adsorption reaches a maximum value and becomes independent of the solution concentration. The physical interpretation of this result is that the surface is completely covered with adsorbate molecules, and that no further adsorption can occur because no more solid surface is accessible. This is interpreted to mean that the surface is covered with a layer of adsorbate one molecule thick (a monomolecular layer). This is one of the physical implications of the Langmuir isotherm. Another implication is that adsorption "sites" on the solid surface are independent in the sense that the energy of adsorption of an adsorbate molecule to a surface site is independent of whether an adjacent site is already occupied.

These physical restrictions are rather severe, so it may seem unlikely that the Langmuir isotherm will be followed by real systems, yet many adsorption systems fit the equation well or at least reasonably so as a good approximation. Figure 11.5 shows some isotherms for the adsorption of dyes on cornstarch (Zografi and Mattocks 1963). The shapes of these curves are typical of Langmuirian adsorption, and the plots according to Eq. (11.38), in Fig. 11.6, confirm the validity of Eq. (11.37) as a description of the phenomenon.

Example 11.4. Figure 11.7 is the isotherm for the adsorption of indolinospiropyran from cyclohexane solution onto alumina of specific area $155\,\mathrm{m^2\,g^{-1}}$ (Connors and Jozwiakowski 1987; Jozwiakowski 1987). The quantity y is the amount adsorbed in $\mathrm{mg\,g^{-1}}$. From the plot according to Eq. (11.38) these parameters were found: $K = 810\,\mathrm{M^{-1}}$ and $y_{max} = 53.9\,\mathrm{mg\,g^{-1}}$. The molecular weight of the adsorbate is

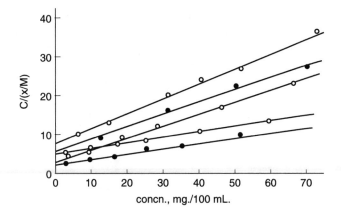

Figure 11.6. Plots according to Eq. (11.38) for the isotherms shown in Fig. 11.5. [Reproduced with permission from Zografi and Mattocks (1963).]

327. Calculate the area occupied per molecule of adsorbate on the surface of the solid.

The area we want is σ, which appears in the relationship $A_t/\sigma N_A = n_{max}$. We therefore first convert y_{max} to n_{max}; $y_{max} = 53.9 \, \mathrm{mg \, g^{-1}} = 0.0539 \, \mathrm{g \, g^{-1}}$; dividing by the molecular weight gives us $n_{max} = 1.65 \times 10^{-4} \, \mathrm{mol \, g^{-1}}$.

We solve for σ in $\sigma = A_t/N_A n_{max}$, where $A_t = 155 \, \mathrm{m^2 g^{-1}}$, finding $\sigma = 1.56 \times 10^{-18} \, \mathrm{m^2 molecule^{-1}}$, which is equivalent to $156 \, \mathrm{\mathring{A}^2 \, molecule^{-1}}$. Incidentally, the specific area A_t is itself determined by a gas adsorption method.

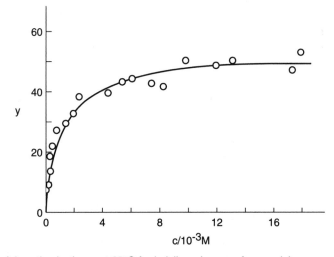

Figure 11.7. Adsorption isotherm at 25°C for indolinospiropyran from cyclohexane onto alumina. The smooth line was drawn with Eq. (11.37) and the parameters given in Example 11.4. [Reproduced by permission from Connors and Jozwiakowski (1987).]

Solids as adsorbents have limited but important application as pharmaceutical agents; they serve mainly to adsorb toxic agents in the gastrointestinal tract. Activated charcoal is used for this purpose, being administered as soon as possible after ingestion of a toxic dose of a drug or poison, which on adsorption to the solid is effectively inactivated and is excreted. Besides this emergency application, adsorbents are widely used in the purification of chemicals, because they are effective in adsorbing colored impurities (colored molecules tend to have large surface areas and numerous polar groups) and in separation processes such as chromatography.

PROBLEMS

11.1. Calculate the work of adhesion at the water-diethyl ether interface.

11.2. Calculate the spreading coefficients of water on ether and of ether on water, and interpret the results.

11.3. Calculate the surface work required to enlarge a cavity in water from a diameter of 0.1 mm to a diameter of 1 mm.

11.4. Equation (11.38) is a linearized version of Eq. (11.37). There exist two additional linearized forms of Eq. (11.37). Find these linear equations, and show how the model parameters can be obtained from the slope and intercept of the plots.

11.5. These are data for the adsorption of 6-methoxybenzoindolinopyran from cyclohexane solution onto silica gel of specific area $300 \, m^2 \, g^{-1}$. The quantity y is the amount of adsorbate adsorbed in $mg \, g^{-1}$. The molecular weight of the adsorbate is 307. Analyze the data; that is, determine if the data fit the Langmuir isotherm and, if so, evaluate the model parameters (Connors and Jozwiakowski 1987; Jozwiakowski 1987).

$10^3 \, c_2 \, (M)$	$y \, (mg \, g^{-1})$
1.18	58.2
2.08	60.6
4.26	94.7
5.75	103.5
8.65	105.8
10.62	107.4
12.27	119.7
14.13	123.8
16.06	124.8
16.98	127.6
19.81	134.3

NOTES

1. Solids with higher surface tensions are said to be higher energy solids. Such solids tend to possess polar functional groups. A solid such as paraffin, which is a saturated hydrocarbon, is a low-energy solid. Silica (glass) is of higher energy.

2. See Gibbs (1876, 1878). Equations (11.23) and (11.25) are obtained on pp. 232 and 235, respectively, of the Dover (1961) edition. Much of Gibbs' massive work on thermodynamics is difficult for the modern reader to follow, in part because his symbolism differs from our usage, but two of the symbols Gibbs introduced, μ for chemical potential and Γ for surface excess, are still used, so his surface equations are more accessible. Incidentally, Gibbs would write Eqs. (11.23) and (11.25) with the symbol $\Gamma_{2(1)}$, thus explicitly noting that this is the value of Γ_2 given that Γ_1 is set to zero.

3. Equations have been described with which the surface tensions of binary aqueous–organic solvent mixtures can be modeled over the entire composition range; see Connors and Wright (1989) and Khossravi and Connors (1993).

4. In *adsorption* the adsorbate adheres to the surface of the solid. In *absorption* the solute is taken up throughout the volume of the solid. When the nature of the process is unknown, the generic term *sorption* may be used.

THERMODYNAMICS OF CHEMICAL PROCESSES

Parts I and II of this book provide most of the concepts and quantitative relationships that we will need in our treatment of chemical processes. Occasional reference will be made to passages or equations in earlier chapters so as to minimize repetition of material. For brevity we state here that, except when indicated otherwise, constant temperature and pressure may be assumed; thus minimization of the Gibbs free energy is the criterion for equilibrium. Commonly the fixed pressure is the ambient (atmospheric) pressure and the fixed temperature is 25°C or "room temperature." Usually solute concentrations are given in moles per liter (molarity), symbolized either c_A *or* [A]; these represent concentrations at equilibrium unless noted otherwise. The solute reference state is the infinitely dilute solution, and very often we will suppose that the solute is in its reference state so that its activity coefficient is unity and its activity is equal to its concentration; this condition will allow us to focus on the essential chemistry of the process without being needlessly distracted by considering corrections for nonideal behavior. Such corrections can always be brought into the description as they are found to be required.

12

ACID–BASE EQUILIBRIA

Most drug molecules and biomolecules include one or more acidic or basic functional groups, so acid–base chemistry is pervasive in pharmaceutical systems. Acid–base equilibria therefore deserve detailed attention.

12.1. ACID–BASE THEORY

Definitions. Acid–base phenomena were observed very early in the development of chemical science, but their systematic understanding is a twentieth-century accomplishment. The Arrhenius theory of acids and bases, dating from the close of the 19th century, postulated that an acid is a substance that in water gives rise to hydronium ions, and that a base is a substance that in water gives rise to hydroxide ions. Thus HCl is an acid and NaOH is a base. The admittedly basic properties of compounds like amines, which do not contain the elements of the hydroxide ion, were proposed to result from reaction with water (hydrolysis) to generate hydroxide ions, as in

$$RNH_2 + H_2O \rightleftharpoons RNH_3^+ + OH^-$$

The Arrhenius theory provided a satisfactory conceptual basis for understanding acid–base behavior in aqueous solution, but it was limited by its dependence on water as a solvent.

Acid–base behavior is observable in many solvents other than water, and such systems became comprehensible with the introduction, in 1923, of an acid–base theory by Bronsted (and independently by Lowry) based on these definitions; an

157

acid is a species that can donate a proton, and a *base* is a species that can accept a proton. In reaction form this is

$$HA \rightleftharpoons H^+ + A^- \tag{12.1}$$
$$\text{acid}$$

$$H^+ + B \rightleftharpoons BH^+ \tag{12.2}$$
$$\text{base}$$

Observe that the Bronsted definitions are built on the proton, and not the hydronium ion, so the new definition is independent of the solvent. We now proceed to explore the ramifications of this powerful definition.[1]

The Conjugate Pair Concept. Observe in Eq. (12.1), on reading it from right to left, that the species A^- is accepting a proton, and so it must, by definition, be a base. Similarly, in Eq. (12.2) read from right to left, BH^+ is donating a proton, so it must be an acid. The Bronsted acid–base definitions can be generally represented by

$$\text{Acid} \rightleftharpoons H^+ + \text{base} \tag{12.3}$$

An acid–base pair related by Eq. (12.3) is called a *conjugate acid–base pair*. Thus, referring to Eq. (12.1), we speak of A^- as the conjugate base of acid HA; from Eq. (12.2), BH^+ is the conjugate acid of base B.

Equation (12.3) and the associated definitions make no mention of the charge types of the acid or base; the only requirement is that an acid be one positive charge greater than its conjugate base. Here are examples of equilibria that fit Eq. (12.3), showing acids and bases of various charge types:

Acid	Base
$CH_3CH_2COOH \rightleftharpoons$	$H^+ + CH_3CH_2COO^-$
$HCO_3^- \rightleftharpoons$	$H^+ + CO_3^{2-}$
$CH_3CH_2NH_3^+ \rightleftharpoons$	$H^+ + CH_3CH_2NH_2$
$H_3^+N{-}C_6H_4{-}NH_3^+ \rightleftharpoons$	$H^+ + H_2N{-}C_6H_4{-}NH_3^+$

The proton of Eq. (12.3), which is a naked nucleus, is a species of extremely high reactivity, a reactivity so high that in ordinary chemical systems the proton will not be detectable (because it will certainly combine with some other species in its vicinity). Consequently we never actually observe Eq. (12.3) by itself. But if we combine two conjugate pairs, the proton donated by the acid of one pair can be accepted by the base of the other pair, and we observe an overall *proton transfer reaction*. Writing the conjugate pair reactions separately and adding them to give the net reaction:

Pair 1: $\underset{\text{acid 1}}{\text{HA}} \rightleftharpoons H^+ + \underset{\text{base 1}}{A^-}$

Pair 2: $\underset{\text{base 2}}{B} + H^+ \rightleftharpoons \underset{\text{acid 2}}{BH^+}$

Overall: $HA + B \rightleftharpoons A^- + BH^+$

The net result is that a proton has been transferred from the first pair to the second pair (reading from left to right), or vice versa when reading from right to left.

Next suppose that one of the pairs is the solvent. In particular, let it be water, our most important solvent. Water reacts in the pattern of Eq. (12.3):

$$\underset{\text{acid}}{H_2O} \rightleftharpoons H^+ + \underset{\text{base}}{OH^-} \tag{12.4}$$

Thus H_2O is an acid, and OH^- is its conjugate base. But water is also capable of functioning in this version of Eq. (12.3):

$$\underset{\text{acid}}{H_3O^+} \rightleftharpoons H^+ + \underset{\text{base}}{H_2O} \tag{12.5}$$

Thus H_2O is the conjugate base of H_3O^+. A substance that (like water) can be either an acid or a base is said to be *amphoteric*. The amphoteric nature of water allows it to play the role of the second conjugate pair for either acids or bases. If the solute is an acid (say, HA), then H_2O functions as a base:

$$HA + H_2O \rightleftharpoons A^- + H_3O^+ \tag{12.6}$$

whereas if the solute is a base (say, B), then H_2O functions as an acid:

$$B + H_2O \rightleftharpoons BH^+ + OH^- \tag{12.7}$$

Throughout most of Chapter 12 we will be concerned with reactions like those in Eqs. (12.6) and (12.7).

Dissociation Constants. Consider the system described by Eq. (12.6) at equilibrium.[2] We can apply the thermodynamic concept of the equilibrium constant (Section 4.3) to define the quantity K_a:

$$K_a = \frac{[H_3O^+][A^-]}{[HA]} \tag{12.8}$$

where we assume that activity coefficients are unity. (The activity of water is equal to its mole fraction, essentially unity in dilute solution.) Very commonly, when water is understood to be the solvent, Eq. (12.6) is abbreviated to

$$HA \rightleftharpoons H^+ + A^-$$

and Eq. (12.8) becomes

$$K_a = \frac{[H^+][A^-]}{[HA]} \qquad (12.9)$$

The equilibrium constant K_a is known as the *acid dissociation constant* (also called the *acid ionization constant* or the *acidity constant*). In like manner, from Eq. (12.7) we define the *base dissociation constant* K_b:

$$K_b = \frac{[BH^+][OH^-]}{[B]} \qquad (12.10)$$

We can apply the same formalism to water. From Eq. (12.4), we have

$$K_w = [H^+][OH^-] \qquad (12.11)$$

where again the activity of water in the denominator is unity. K_w is called the *ion product* or *autoprotolysis constant* of water.

We are now prepared to develop the most powerful quantitative result of the Bronsted acid–base theory. Consider the equilibria of HA as an acid and of A^- as its conjugate base:

$$HA \rightleftharpoons H^+ + A^-; \qquad K_a = \frac{[H^+][A^-]}{[HA]} \qquad (12.12)$$

$$A^- + H_2O \rightleftharpoons HA + OH^-; \qquad K_b = \frac{[HA][OH^-]}{[A^-]} \qquad (12.13)$$

Now multiply together the K_a of eq. (12.12) and the K_b of Eq. (12.13). The result is $[H^+]$ $[OH^-]$, or

$$K_w = K_a K_b \qquad (12.14)$$

where the K_a and K_b of Eq. (12.14) refer to a conjugate acid–base pair. Since K_w is a constant (at a given temperature), Eq. (12.14) says that K_a and K_b are reciprocally related; that is, $K_b = K_w/K_a$. Values of K_w are known over the entire practical temperature range, so a result of Eq. (12.14) is that if we know either K_a or K_b, we can calculate the other. It is not necessary to measure both quantities.

We will subsequently see that K_a is a measure of acid strength and that K_b is a measure of base strength. Thus Eq. (12.14) shows that the strengths of an acid and its conjugate base are not independent; on the contrary, the stronger the acid, the weaker the base, and vice versa. Because of this relationship, we commonly specify acid strength in terms of K_a, but we do not use K_b to describe the strength of a base. Instead we use the K_a of the conjugate acid of the base. This may seem illogical, but it is traditional, and we will return to the issue in Section 12.7.

As it happens, K_a and K_b values are usually very small numbers, so for convenience (as one motive) we define

$$pK = -\log K \tag{12.15}$$

where K may be K_a, K_b, or K_w. The symbol p is a mathematical operator that turns a quantity into its negative logarithm. Applying Eq. (12.15) to Eq. (12.14) gives

$$pK_w = pK_a + pK_b \tag{12.16}$$

which is a very convenient form.

Conventionally we divide acids and bases into the classes of strong acids and bases and of weak acids and bases. Strong acids and bases are strong electrolytes, essentially completely dissociated in water; HCl, H_2SO_4, HNO_3, $NaOH$, and KOH are examples. Weak acids and bases are incompletely dissociated in water; carboxylic acids, phenols, and amines are examples. The concept of the equilibrium constant is usefully applied only to the weak acids and bases.

pH. Let us apply the p operator to the hydrogen ion concentration. We write

$$pH = -\log [H^+] \tag{12.17}$$

Extending this formalism to Eq. (12.11) gives

$$pK_w = pH + pOH \tag{12.18}$$

from which we see that the acidity of a solution (measured by pH) and its alkalinity (measured by pOH) are coupled, so we do not need to measure both quantities. In the laboratory it is much easier to measure pH, so this is the quantity that we use to describe solution acidity or alkalinity. Table 12.1 lists pK_w values at several temperatures (Harned and Owen 1958, p. 638). Note that $pK_w = 14.00$ at 25°C.

Table 12.1. Ion product of water as a function of temperature

$t\,(^\circ C)$	pK_w
0	14.94
10	14.54
20	14.17
25	14.00
30	13.83
40	13.54
50	13.26
60	13.02

A solution in which $pH = pOH$ is said to be *neutral*; hence a neutral solution has $pH = 7.00$ (but only at $25°C$). The practical pH range in water is essentially defined by the value of pK_w, or 14 pH units. The lower the pH the more acidic the solution; the higher the pH, the more alkaline the solution.[3]

Example 12.1

(a) Convert $K_a = 2 \times 10^{-4}$ to pK_a.

$$pK_a = -\log K_a$$
$$= -(\log 2 + \log 10^{-4})$$
$$= -(0.30 - 4)$$
$$= -(-3.70)$$
$$= 3.70$$

(b) If $pK_a = 5.30$, what is K_a?

$$-\log K_a = 5.30$$
$$\log K_a = -5.30$$
$$= -6.00 + 0.70$$
$$K_a = 5.0 \times 10^{-6}$$

Example 12.2. $pK_a = 4.75$ for acetic acid at $25°C$. What is K_b of acetate ion?
From $pK_a = 4.75$ we find $K_a = 1.78 \times 10^{-5}$. Using either Eq. (12.14) or Eq. (12.16), we find $pK_b = 9.25$ or $K_b = 5.62 \times 10^{-10}$.

Example 12.3. What is the hydroxide ion concentration of a solution having $pH = 6.50$ at $25°C$?
From Eq. (12.18), $pOH = 14.00 - 6.50 = 7.50$, so $[OH^-] = 3.16 \times 10^{-8}$ M.

Example 12.4. The pK_a of the conjugate acid of methylamine is 10.64 at $25°C$. Calculate the standard free energy change for the acid dissociation process.
From the basic thermodynamic result

$$\Delta G° = -RT \ln K$$

and the definition $pK_a = -\log K_a$ we derive

$$\Delta G° = 2.303 \, RT \, pK_a$$
$$= (2.303)(1.987 \, \text{cal mol}^{-1} \, \text{K}^{-1})(298.15 \, \text{K})(10.64)$$
$$= 14517 \, \text{cal mol}^{-1}$$
$$= 14.5 \, \text{kcal mol}^{-1}$$
$$= 60.7 \, \text{kJ mol}^{-1}$$

$\Delta G°$ is positive because K_a is smaller (much smaller) than one. pK_a is seen to be directly proportional to $\Delta G°$.

12.2. pH DEPENDENCE OF ACID–BASE EQUILIBRIA

Fractional Distribution of Acid–Base Species. Some of the treatment described here follows Connors (1982). Picture a very dilute solution of a given weak acid or base in an aqueous medium whose pH can be controlled, independently of the solute of interest, by the experimenter. Such pH control is easy to accomplish. We now assert, and will shortly demonstrate, that the fractions of solute present in the conjugate acid and base forms depend only on the pH of the solution and the pK_a of the acid. Thus the pH is a "master variable" that controls all acid-base equilibria in the solution.

Consider acid HA (whose charge type is irrelevant in what follows), having acid dissociation constant K_a. Let c be its total molar concentration, so that the mass balance expression Eq. (12.19) can be written.

$$c = [HA] + [A^-] \tag{12.19}$$

We introduce the fractions of solute in the conjugate acid and base forms with these definitions:

$$F_{HA} = \frac{[HA]}{c} \tag{12.20}$$

$$F_A = \frac{[A^-]}{c} \tag{12.21}$$

Algebraic combination of Eqs. (12.9) and (12.19)–(12.21) gives

$$F_{HA} = \frac{[H^+]}{[H^+] + K_a} \tag{12.22}$$

$$F_A = \frac{K_a}{[H^+] + K_a} \tag{12.23}$$

which relate the fractions of solute in the conjugate acid and base forms to the acid dissociation constant and the hydrogen ion concentration of the medium. Equations (12.22) and (12.23) confirm the earlier assertion that the solution pH (which we recall can be established independently of the solute acid) is the only variable controlling the position of the acid–base equilibrium. Figure 12.1 is a plot of F_{HA} and F_A against pH, calculated with Eqs. (12.22) and (12.23) for a hypothetical acid having $pK_a = 4.0$. This curve is called a *sigmoid curve* because of its shape.

From Eqs. (12.22) and (12.23) we can deduce these general properties of such distribution curves. At any given pH, $F_{HA} + F_A = 1$ [a conclusion implicit

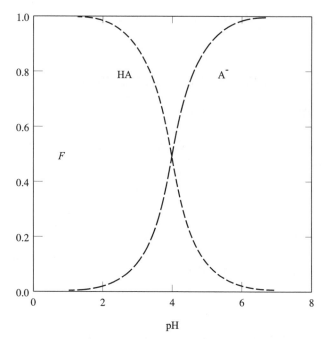

Figure 12.1. Variation with pH of the fraction F_{HA} (conjugate acid) and F_A (conjugate base) for an acid with $pK_a = 4.0$. [Reproduced by permission from Connors (1982).]

in Eq. (12.19)]. At the point where the two curves cross, $F_{HA} = F_A = 0.5$, and at this point $[H^+] = K_a$, or $pH = pK_a$. At pH values much less than pK_a, F_{HA} approaches unity and F_A approaches zero; at pH values much greater than pK_a, F_A approaches unity and F_{HA} approaches zero. The curves in Fig. 12.1 apply to any monoprotic acid–base pair (i.e., one having only a single acid–base group and therefore only a single pK_a value) merely by sliding the curves along the pH axis until their pH of intersection matches the solute pK_a. From Fig. 12.1 we also can see that most of the interesting acid–base chemistry of this system takes place in the approximate pH range of $pK_a \pm 2$ units; outside this range the solute exists largely either as HA (at low pH) or as A^- (at high pH).

Rearrangement of Eqs. (12.20) and (12.21) gives $[HA] = cF_{HA}$ and $[A^-] = cF_A$; if, therefore, the total concentration c is known (c is sometimes called the *analytical concentration*), and if the pH and pK_a are known, the individual conjugate acid and base species concentrations are easily calculated.

Example 12.5. The pK_a of benzoic acid is 4.20. Calculate the concentrations of benzoic acid and benzoate ion in a solution whose $pH = 5.20$ and which was prepared to contain 0.005 M benzoic acid.

The preceding wording may seem confusing, but it is a fair example of the terminology that might be used in a laboratory. Its meaning is that $c = 0.005$ M.

From the pK_a we find $K_a = 6.31 \times 10^{-5}$ and from the pH we find $[H^+] = 6.31 \times 10^{-6}$. Equations (12.22) and (12.23) then give $F_{HA} = 0.0909$ and $F_A = 0.909$. Thus $[HA] = 0.005 \times 0.0909 = 4.55 \times 10^{-4}$ M and $[A^-] = 0.005 \times 0.909 = 4.55 \times 10^{-3}$ M. The slight discrepancy between the given value of c and the value obtained by summing $[HA]$ and $[A^-]$ results from rounding errors (and is probably experimentally negligible). Notice that $pH = pK_a + 1$ and that at this condition $[A^-] = 10[HA]$.

A diprotic acid (sometimes called a dibasic acid) possesses two acidic groups and two pK_a values. We can symbolize such an acid as H_2A and write the acid–base equilibria as follows:

$$H_2A \overset{K_1}{\rightleftharpoons} H^+ + HA^-$$

$$HA^- \overset{K_2}{\rightleftharpoons} H^+ + A^{2-}$$

The placement of K_1 and K_2 over the arrows effectively defines these constants. We proceed to define fractions as before, except that now we have three solute species

$$F_{H_2A} = \frac{[H_2A]}{c}$$

$$F_{HA} = \frac{[HA^-]}{c}$$

$$F_A = \frac{[A^{2-}]}{c}$$

where $c = [H_2A] + [HA^-] + [A^{2-}]$. Combining these relations with the two dissociation constants gives

$$F_{H_2A} = \frac{[H^+]^2}{[H^+]^2 + K_1[H^+] + K_1K_2} \qquad (12.24)$$

$$F_{HA} = \frac{K_1[H^+]}{[H^+]^2 + K_1[H^+] + K_1K_2} \qquad (12.25)$$

$$F_A = \frac{K_1K_2}{[H^+]^2 + K_1[H^+] + K_1K_2} \qquad (12.26)$$

Obviously $F_{H_2A} + F_{HA} + F_A = 1$. Observe how the three terms that make up the denominator constitute in turn the numerators of Eqs. (12.24)–(12.26). At high values of the hydrogen ion concentration the term $[H^+]^2$ dominates; as $[H^+]$ decreases the middle term, $K_1[H^+]$, takes over as the largest contributor, and finally at small values of $[H^+]$ the last term, K_1K_2, becomes the largest. Again some general relationships can be derived from Eqs. (12.24)–(12.26). Where the curves for F_{H_2A} and F_{HA} cross, equating Eqs. (12.24) and (12.25) gives $pH = pK_1$.

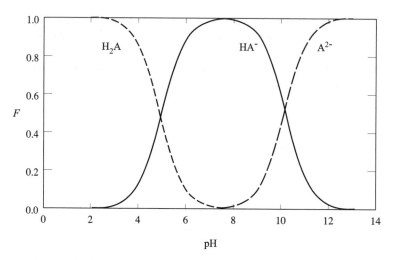

Figure 12.2. Species distribution diagram for a dibasic acid H_2A with $pK_1 = 5.0$ and $pK_2 = 10.0$. [Reproduced by permission from Connors (1982).]

Similarly, where F_{HA} and F_A are equal, $pH = pK_2$. The pH at which the maximum in F_{HA} appears is found by differentiating Eq. (12.25) with respect to $[H^+]$ and setting the derivative equal to zero; the result is

$$pH_{max} = \frac{pK_1 + pK_2}{2} \tag{12.27}$$

Figure 12.2 is a plot of Eqs. (12.24)–(12.26) for a hypothetical diprotic acid having $pK_1 = 5.0$ and $pK_2 = 10.0$. Note that the fraction F_{HA} rises essentially to unity at a pH given by Eq. (12.27).

Now compare Fig. 12.3 with Fig. 12.2. Again the curves are calculated with Eqs. (12.24)–(12.26), but now $pK_1 = 7.0$ and $pK_2 = 8.0$. Equation (12.27) is still obeyed, but now the fraction F_{HA} fails to rise to anywhere near unity. The behavior seen here is closely connected with the observation, in Fig. 12.1, that the essential acid–base chemistry occurs largely in the pH region $pK_a \pm 2$ units. In Fig. 12.2 the pK_1 and pK_2 values differ by 5 units, so the two acid–base equilibria described by K_1 and K_2 act essentially independently. In Fig. 12.3, however, $\Delta pK_a = pK_2 - pK_1$ is only 1 unit. As, in imagination, the pH is raised, swept from left to right across Fig. 12.3, H_2A is converted to HA^-; this transformation commences at about $pK_1 - 2$ units, or pH 5. But before it can be carried to completion (which would not occur until $pK_1 + 2$, or pH 9), the system has been brought to within the range $pK_2 - 2$, or pH 6, so the second transformation, of HA^- to A^{2-}, must take place. The consequence is that F_{HA} cannot rise as high as it did in Fig. 12.2, where ΔpK_a was 5 units. Generally one may expect successive pK_a values to control essentially independent equilibria if $\Delta pK_a \geq 4$. The consequence in Fig. 12.2 is that the system contains essentially only two acid–base species $(H_2A + HA^-$ *or*

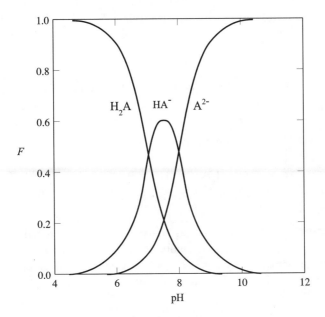

Figure 12.3. Species distribution diagram for a dibasic acid H_2A with $pK_1 = 7.0$ and $pK_2 = 8.0$. [Reproduced by permission from Connors (1982).]

$HA^- + A^{2-}$) at any given pH. In Fig. 12.3, however, the three species coexist in a wide pH range.[4]

These principles can be extended to acids and bases with any number of acid–base groups. The form of the expressions for the fractions is seen to take on a predictable pattern, and it is possible to write these expressions down without derivation. For the tribasic acid H_3A these expressions become

$$F_{H_3A} = \frac{[H^+]^3}{[H^+]^3 + K_1[H^+]^2 + K_1K_2[H^+] + K_1K_2K_3}$$

$$F_{H_2A} = \frac{K_1[H^+]^2}{[H^+]^3 + K_1[H^+]^2 + K_1K_2[H^+] + K_1K_2K_3}$$

and so on.

Example 12.6. Calculate the concentration of monoanion in an aqueous solution 0.01 M in phthalic acid at pH 5.00. $pK_1 = 2.95$; $pK_2 = 5.41$.

Phthalic acid is

1

The two ionizable groups are obviously equivalent. We calculate $K_1 = 1.12 \times 10^{-3}$ and $K_2 = 3.89 \times 10^{-6}$. From Eq. (12.25), we obtain

$$F_{HA} = \frac{(1.12 \times 10^{-3})(1 \times 10^{-5})}{(1 \times 10^{-5})^2 + (1.12 \times 10^{-3})(1 \times 10^{-5}) + (1.12 \times 10^{-3})(3.89 \times 10^{-6})}$$
$$= 0.713$$

Then from $[HA^-] = cF_{HA}$, we have

$$[HA^-] = 0.01 \times 0.713$$
$$= 7.13 \times 10^{-3} \, M$$

Buffer Solutions. Suppose that an aqueous solution is prepared to contain a mol L^{-1} of a weak acid HA and b mol L^{-1} of its conjugate base A^-. (Of course A^- will be accompanied by b mol L^{-1} of its counterion, a cation.) As we have done earlier, the K_a for this system is defined

$$K_a = \frac{[H^+][A^-]}{[HA]} \tag{12.28}$$

and we now apply the p operator to Eq. (12.28) to obtain the convenient form

$$pK_a = pH - \log \frac{[A^-]}{[HA]} \tag{12.29}$$

The quantities a and b are the *formal* concentrations of HA and A^-; the actual equilibrium concentrations are somewhat different from these values because *both* of these equilibria must be mutually satisfied:

$$HA \rightleftharpoons H^+ + A^-$$
$$H_2O \rightleftharpoons H^+ + OH^-$$

We can find exact expressions for these concentrations by making use of mass balance and electroneutrality relationships. To be specific, suppose that the cationic counterion is labeled M^+. Then these two mass balance expressions can be written as follows:

$$b = [M^+] \tag{12.30}$$
$$a + b = [HA] + [A^-] \tag{12.31}$$

The electroneutrality principle asserts that any macroscopic volume of solution is electrically neutral. This means that the sum of positive charges equals the sum of negative charges. For the aqueous solution under discussion

$$[H^+] + [M^+] = [OH^-] + [A^-] \tag{12.32}$$

Algebraic combination of Eqs. (12.30)–(12.32) gives the desired relationships:

$$[HA] = a - [H^+] + [OH^-] \tag{12.33}$$

$$[A^-] = b + [H^+] - [OH^-] \tag{12.34}$$

Combining Eqs. (12.29), (12.33), and (12.34), we obtain

$$pK_a = pH - \log \frac{b + [H^+] - [OH^-]}{a - [H^+] + [OH^-]} \tag{12.35}$$

If the solution pH is in the approximate range 4–10, the contributions of $[H^+]$ and $[OH^-]$ in Eq. (12.35) are usually negligible, and Eq. (12.35) becomes

$$pK_a = pH - \log \frac{b}{a} \tag{12.36}$$

In this form Eq. (12.36) is known as the *Henderson–Hasselbalch equation*. This is a very convenient form for carrying out calculations.

A solution that contains comparable and appreciable concentrations of a conjugate weak acid–base pair is called a *buffer solution* because it resists a change in pH on the addition of a small amount of acid or base. This phenomenon can be demonstrated with an example. Suppose a solution is prepared to be 0.1 M in acetic acid $(pK_a 4.76)$ and 0.1 M in sodium acetate. Then $b/a = 1.00$ and, according to Eq. (12.36), $pH = pK_a$, or $pH = 4.76$. Now let 1.0 mL of 0.1 M NaOH be added to 100 mL of this solution; what will be the new value of pH? It may be assumed that the sodium hydroxide converts an equivalent amount of acetic acid to sodium acetate. The solution therefore contains, after addition of the sodium hydroxide, $(100)(0.1) - (1)(0.1) = 9.9$ mmol of acetic acid, and $(100)(0.1) + (1)(0.1) = 10.1$ mmol of acetate, all in 101 mL of solution. The ratio b/a is now 1.02, its logarithm is 0.01, and Eq. (12.36) shows that the new pH is 4.77. Addition of the alkali has resulted in a pH change of only 0.01 unit. If the same volume of the sodium hydroxide solution had been added to 100 mL of pH 4.76 strong acid, the pH would have changed to about 11.

Equation (12.36) will sometimes be encountered in different guises, because some authors consider that a weak acid, on treatment with a strong base, is converted to its salt; thus the equation could be written $pH = pK_a + \log$ (salt/acid); when a weak base is treated with a strong acid to form its salt, the equivalent form is $pH = pK_a + \log$ (base/salt). Because of the possible confusion resulting from this terminology, we will use the Bronsted terminology by speaking of conjugate acid and base species. Thus Eq. (12.36) and equivalent versions always can be written in the form

$$pH = pK_a + \log \frac{[\text{conjugate base}]}{[\text{conjugate acid}]} \qquad (12.37)$$

This equation relates the three quantities pH, pK_a, and the ratio b/a. Often two of these are known and the third may then be calculated.

Example 12.7. Calculate the pH of a buffer solution prepared by dissolving 242.2 mg of tris(hydroxymethyl)aminomethane in 10.0 mL of 0.170 M HCl and diluting to 100 mL with water. The molecular weight of the solute is 121.1. It is a primary amine of structure $(HOCH_2)_3CNH_2$, with $pK_a = 8.08$ for the conjugate acid.

A total of 2.00 mmol of solute was weighed out, and 1.70 mmol of HCl was added. Since the HCl reacts with the amine to convert an equivalent amount to its conjugate acid (protonated) form, this means that $a = 1.7/100$ M and $b = (2.0 - 1.7)/100$ M. Using these figures in the Henderson–Hasselbalch equation, we obtain

$$pH = pK_a + \log \frac{0.003}{0.017} = 8.08 - \log \frac{0.017}{0.003}$$

$$= 8.08 - \log 5.67 = 7.25$$

In this calculation the ratio was inverted merely to give a value greater than unity, for ease in taking the logarithm.

Example 12.8. Calculate the pH of a buffer prepared to contain 0.09 M NaH_2PO_4 and 0.01 M K_2HPO_4. $pK_1 = 2.23$, $pK_2 = 7.21$, $pK_3 = 12.32$ for phosphoric acid.

In general a buffer of a polyprotic acid may be a very complex mixture, and a species distribution diagram is helpful in clarifying the problem. Figure 12.4 shows this diagram for phosphoric acid. The pK values of this acid are widely spaced, and phosphoric acid behaves essentially as if it were an equimolar mixture of three monobasic acids of the given pK values. From the experimental values $a = 0.09$ M and $b = 0.01$ M, Fig. 12.4 clearly shows that the pH will be approximately 6.3 and that the solution contains practically no H_3PO_4 or PO_4^{3-} at this pH. We have now simplified the problem to that of a monobasic acid $(H_2PO_4^-)$ and its conjugate base (HPO_4^{2-}), with the dissociation constant $pK_2 = 7.21$. Applying the Henderson–Hasselbalch equation gives pH $= 7.21 - \log 9 = 6.26$.

Table 12.2 was constructed by means of Eq. (12.36). Table 12.2 illustrates the symmetry and simplicity provided by the logarithmic form of the dissociation constant expression. The table also confirms the suggestion derived from Fig. 12.1 that most of the acid–base "action" takes place in the approximate pH range $pK_a \pm 2$.

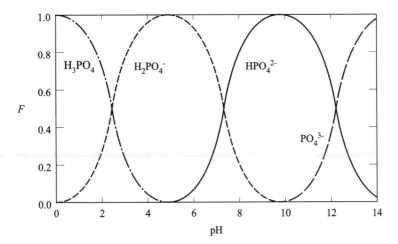

Figure 12.4. Species distribution diagram for phosphoric acid: $pK_1 = 2.23$, $pK_2 = 7.21$, $pK_3 = 12.32$. [Reproduced by permission from Connors (1982).]

Inasmuch as the function of a buffer is to minimize changes in pH, it is useful to have a measure of the "buffering capacity" of a buffer solution. This is provided by the *buffer index* β. Let b be the concentration of strong base added to a solution containing total concentration c of a weak acid. Then β is defined by

$$\beta = \frac{db}{d\text{pH}} \tag{12.38}$$

Thus β is the concentration of strong base required to change the pH by a given amount; the larger the value of β, the greater is the buffer capacity of the solution. Since the strong base converts the weak acid to its conjugate base, b has the meaning given to it earlier, and we write from Eqs. (12.21) and (12.23), $F_A = b/c = K_a/[H^+] + K_a)$, or

Table 12.2. Relationship of pH, pK_a, and the conjugate base/acid ratio

b/a	pH
$0.001(10^{-3})$	$pK_a - 3$
$0.01(10^{-2})$	$pK_a - 2$
$0.1(10^{-1})$	$pK_a - 1$
$1(10^0)$	pK_a
$10(10^1)$	$pK_a + 1$
$100(10^2)$	$pK_a + 2$
$1000(10^3)$	$pK_a + 3$

$$b = \frac{cK_a}{[H^+] + K_a}$$

Therefore

$$\frac{db}{d[H^+]} = \frac{-cK_a}{([H^+] + K_a)^2}$$

and

$$\frac{db}{d\,pH} = -2.3[H^+]\frac{db}{d[H^+]}$$

$$\beta = 2.3\,cF_{HA}\,F_A$$

Equation (12.39) shows that β is directly proportional to total buffer concentration c, as well as to the product $F_{HA}F_A$. It is easy to show (e.g., by inserting numbers for the fractions) that this product is maximal when $F_{HA} = F_A = 0.5$, which, we have seen, occurs when $pH = pK_a$. This result, together with extensive laboratory experience, leads to the guideline that buffer capacity is maximal when $pH = pK_a$ and is acceptable in the approximate range of $pH = pK_a \pm 1$. This is the information needed to design effective buffer solutions.[5]

12.3. CALCULATION OF SOLUTION pH

We have already seen some calculations of solution pH, but here the treatment will be more systematic. There are two kinds of aqueous solutions to consider: (1) a solution prepared with a single solute, whether a strong acid, strong base, weak acid, or weak base; and (2) a solution prepared to contain two conjugate species, namely a weak acid and its conjugate base. Obviously all acid–base systems contain both species; the distinction being made is that in (1) one of these arises solely from the operation of the solution equilibria, whereas in (2) the experimenter ensures by manipulation that appreciable concentrations of both are present.

Any aqueous acid–base system can be completely described by carrying through the following procedure:

1. Write the electroneutrality equation for the solution.
2. Write the mass balance expressions for each solute.
3. Define all pertinent K_a values.
4. Define K_w.
5. Algebraically combine the preceding expressions.

Seldom is it necessary to carry through the system in its full generality, and we will see that shortened versions, often employing chemically reasonable approximations, will usually suffice. The level of accuracy sought is determined by the typical accuracy in an experimental measurement, which is, at best, about 0.01 pH unit.

Strong Acid or Base. A strong acid or base is essentially completely dissociated in dilute aqueous solution. The common strong acids are hydrochloric (HCl), sulfuric (H_2SO_4), nitric (HNO_3), and perchloric ($HClO_4$); the common strong bases are sodium and potassium hydroxides (NaOH, KOH).

Let c be the total (analytical) molar concentration of strong acid HX. According to the electroneutrality principle applied to this solution

$$[H^+] = [OH^-] + [X^-] \qquad (12.40)$$

The source of the hydroxide ion is the dissociation of water. The mass balance expression for this solution is

$$c = [X^-] \qquad (12.41)$$

Equations (12.40) and (12.41) can be combined with the definition of K_w to give a quadratic equation, which can be solved for $[H^+]$. However, if the concentration c is greater than $\sim 10^{-6}$ M, then $[X^-]$ will be much greater than $[OH^-]$, and we can write the acceptable approximation $[H^+] = [X^-]$, or

$$[H^+] = c \qquad (12.42)$$

which states that the hydrogen ion concentration is numerically equal to the total concentration of strong acid. Similarly for a strong base MOH the electroneutrality equation is

$$[H^+] + [M^+] = [OH^-] \qquad (12.43)$$

which simplifies to $c = [OH^-]$, where c is the analytical concentration of the strong base.

These calculations have ignored nonideality effects, which, we have seen, set in at fairly low ionic strengths for ionic species (Chapter 8). For example, the calculated pH of 0.10 M HCl is 1.00, whereas the measured pH is 1.10.

Example 12.9

(a) What is the pH of 0.005 M H_2SO_4? Sulfuric acid dissociates according to $H_2SO_4 \rightarrow 2H^+ + SO_4{}^{2-}$. Thus in this solution $[H^+] = 2c = 0.010$ M, and pH = 2.00.

(b) What is the pH of 0.025 M NaOH? We have $[OH^-] = 0.025$ M, so pOH = 1.60 and pH = $14.00 - 1.60 = 12.40$.

Weak Acid. Let HA be a monoprotic weak acid at total concentration c. The dissociation reaction is

$$HA \overset{K_a}{\rightleftharpoons} H^+ + A^-$$

From the electroneutrality principle we write

$$[H^+] = [OH^-] + [A^-] \tag{12.44}$$

and the mass balance expression is

$$c = [HA] + [A^-] \tag{12.45}$$

An exact solution combines Eqs. (12.44) and (12.45) with the definitions of K_a and K_w. Usually, however, it is reasonable to approximate Eq. (12.44) by $[H^+] = [A^-]$. Using this equality in the definition of K_a yields

$$K_a = \frac{[H^+]^2}{c - [H^+]} \tag{12.46}$$

which can be rearranged to the quadratic form

$$[H^+]^2 + K_a[H^+] - K_a c = 0 \tag{12.47}$$

Application of the quadratic formula gives

$$[H^+] = \frac{-K_a \pm \sqrt{K_a^2 + 4K_a c}}{2} \tag{12.48}$$

One uses the physically meaningful solution.

Suppose that $[H^+] \ll c$; then the denominator in Eq. (12.46) can be approximated by $c - [H^+] \approx c$. If this is acceptable, we obtain $K_a = [H^+]^2/c$, or

$$[H^+] = \sqrt{K_a c} \tag{12.49}$$

This equation offers an extremely simple solution to the problem. Whether this approximation is reasonable can be assessed by comparing the results calculated by Eqs. (12.48) and (12.49).

The preceding derivations are applicable to aqueous solutions of monoprotic acids regardless of charge type, so Eqs. (12.48) and (12.49) apply to neutral acids (such as RCOOH), to positively charged acids (like RNH_3^+), and to negatively charged acids (like HPO_4^{2-}).

Example 12.10

(a) Calculate the pH of 0.02 M *trans*-cinnamic acid ($pK_a = 4.30$). We can use Eq. (12.49) with $c = 0.02$ and $K_a = 5.0 \times 10^{-5}$; the result is $[H^+] = 1.0 \times 10^{-3}$ M, or pH = 3.00. Assessing the validity of the approximation leading to Eq. (12.49), we see that $c = 0.020$ M and $[H^+] = 0.001$ M (as calculated), so $[H^+]$ is about 5% of c. Let us repeat the calculation with Eq. (12.48):

$$[H^+] = \frac{-5 \times 10^{-5} \pm \sqrt{(5 \times 10^{-5})^2 + (4)(0.02)(5 \times 10^{-5})}}{2}$$

$$= \frac{-5 \times 10^{-5} \pm \sqrt{25 \times 10^{-10} + 0.4 \times 10^{-5}}}{2}$$

$$= \frac{-5 \times 10^{-5} \pm \sqrt{4 \times 10^{-6}}}{2}$$

$$= \frac{0.002 - 0.00005}{2}$$

$$= 0.975 \times 10^{-3}$$

so pH = 2.99. The approximate solution, Eq. (12.49), gave pH = 3.00, which usually would be considered acceptable, because pH seldom can be measured to better than 0.01 unit.

(b) Calculate the pH of 0.05 M ammonium chloride ($pK_a = 9.25$). Ammonium chloride is a salt. It dissociates completely according to

$$NH_4Cl \rightarrow NH_4^+ + Cl^-$$

The ammonium ion NH_4^+ is a weak acid:

$$NH_4^+ \overset{K_a}{\rightleftharpoons} H^+ + NH_3$$

Therefore we anticipate that the solution will be acidic.[6] The given pK_a is for the acid NH_4^+. Using Eq. (12.49) with $c = 0.05$ and $K_a = 5.62 \times 10^{-10}$ gives $[H^+] = 5.30 \times 10^{-6}$ M, or pH = 5.28. Our experience with Example 12.10(a) convinces us that this is an acceptably accurate solution.

Weak Base. The base dissociation reaction is

$$B + H_2O \overset{K_b}{\rightleftharpoons} BH^+ + OH^-$$

and by reasoning identical with that applied to the weak acid case, we derive

$$K_b = \frac{[OH^-]^2}{c - [OH^-]} \tag{12.50}$$

When $[OH^-] \ll c$, Eq. (12.50) becomes

$$[OH^-] = \sqrt{K_b c} \qquad (12.51)$$

where c is the total base concentration. Equations. (12.50) and (12.51) apply to neutral bases (like RNH_2), to positively charged bases (like $H_2NCH_2CH_2NH_2^+$), and to negatively charged bases (like $RCOO^-$).

Example 12.11. What is the pH of 0.10 M potassium acetate? ($pK_a = 4.76$).

We will use Eq. (12.51) with $c = 0.10$. The pK_a that is given is for the conjugate acid, namely, acetic acid. The chemistry of this system mimics what we saw in Example 12.10(b). First the salt potassium acetate (symbolized KOAc) completely dissociates:

$$KOAc \rightarrow K^+ + OAc^-$$

The potassium ion is neutral, but OAc^- is a weak base; it is the conjugate base of acetic acid, and it makes the solution basic because of the equilibrium

$$OAc^- + H_2O \rightleftharpoons HOAc + OH^-$$

From pK_a 4.76 we find $pK_b = 14.00 - 4.76 = 9.24$, or $K_b = 5.75 \times 10^{-10}$. Applying Eq. (12.51), we obtain

$$[OH^-] = \sqrt{(5.75 \times 10^{-10})(0.1)}$$
$$= \sqrt{5.75 \times 10^{-11}}$$
$$= \sqrt{57.5 \times 10^{-12}}$$
$$= 7.6 \times 10^{-6}$$

so pOH = 5.12 and pH = 8.88. It is helpful to check that the calculated pH is on the correct side of neutrality.

Mixture of Weak Acid and Its Conjugate Base. We have already treated this case under *Buffer solutions*. The appropriate relationship is

$$pK_a = pH - \log \frac{[A^-]}{[HA]} \qquad (12.52)$$

and we have seen how this equation can be applied to calculate the pH of buffers. Of course, if we wish to prepare a buffer of given pH, we use the equation in an alternative manner. First a buffer substance is selected according to the criterion that the desired pH be in the range $pK_a \pm 1$. Then we use Eq. (12.52) to find the ratio $[A^-]/[HA]$ that is needed to deliver this pH. Finally we decide on a total buffer concentration c. Then, since we have the sum $c = [HA] + [A^-]$ and the ratio $[A^-]/[HA]$, we solve for the individual concentrations $[HA]$ and $[A^-]$, and prepare the solution to contain these concentrations.

Some mixtures of acids and bases can be quite complex, consisting of polyprotic acids or bases, or of a weak acid and a weak base (not its conjugate). A complete analytic description can always be obtained by means of the general scheme outlined at the beginning of this section, but the solution of the final equation will usually require approximations of the type we have made use of above.[7]

12.4. ACID–BASE TITRATIONS

A titration is an experimental operation in which a solution of one reactant (the *titrant*), this solution having an accurately known concentration, is added to a solution of a substance (the sample or *analyte*) with which it will stoichiometrically and quantitatively react, until chemically equivalent amounts of titrant and sample have been mixed. From the stoichiometry of the known reaction between the titrant and sample substances, and the known concentration of titrant, the amount or concentration of the sample substance can be calculated. The theoretical point at which the amounts of titrant and sample are equivalent is called the *equivalence point*, and its experimental estimate is the *endpoint* of the titration. If the titrant is an acid and the sample a base, or the reverse, the operation is called *acid–base titration*. The analytic calculations, which are simple, lie outside our present concern. Here we are interested in how the pH of the sample solution varies, throughout the course of the titration, as increasing volumes of titrant solution are added to it. A plot of this pH [on the vertical axis (ordinate; y axis)] against the volume of titrant added [on the horizontal axis (abscissa; x axis)] is called an *acid–base titration curve*. We will see how it is possible to calculate such a titration curve, and the information to be derived from it.

Strong Acid–Strong Base Titration. A strong acid is completely dissociated into H^+ and its anion, which is neutral; a strong base is completely dissociated into OH^- and its cation, which is neutral. Consequently the reaction that occurs in the sample solution is

$$H^+ + OH^- \rightleftharpoons H_2O$$

This is the reverse of the autoprotolysis of water, so its equilibrium constant is $1/K_w$, or 1×10^{14}. The reaction is obviously quantitative; in casual terms, "it goes completely to the right." At each stage in the titration the sample solution consists of a solution of a strong acid or a strong base, so the calculation of the titration curve involves no new concepts.

Example 12.12. Calculate the titration curve for the titration of 25.0 mL of 0.05 M HCl with 0.10 M NaOH.

In this titration HCl is the sample and NaOH is the titrant. Before any titrant has been added, the solution consists of 0.05 M HCl, so $[H^+] = 0.05$ M and pH $= 1.30$. Now suppose we add 1.0 mL of titrant. We can arrange the work in tabular form:

Initially the sample had $(25)(0.05) = 1.25$ mmol H^+
We have added $(1)(0.10) = 0.10$ mmol OH^-
_____

Remaining in the solution are 1.15 mmol H^+

This 1.15 mmol of H^+ is contained in 26 mL of solution, so the new concentration is $[H^+] = 1.15$ mmol$/26$ mL $= 0.04423$ M, and the new pH is 1.35. Obviously the pH has risen because we have added a strong base to the solution.

This calculation is repeated with increasing volumes of titrant. Here are some results: at 5 mL of titrant, pH $= 1.60$; at 8 mL, pH $= 1.87$; at 10 mL, pH $= 2.15$; at 12 mL, pH $= 2.87$; at 12.2 mL, pH $= 3.09$; at 12.4 mL, pH $= 3.57$.

The equivalence point occurs at 12.5 mL of titrant, because at this volume the number of millimoles (mmol) of NaOH added exactly matches the number of mmol of HCl initially present; and at this point the foregoing method of calculation gives an embarrassing result, for it leads to the conclusion that the number of mmol of H^+ remaining is zero. But of course there always will be hydrogen ions in water. At the equivalence point we simply have a solution of sodium and chloride ions, and (neglecting impurities from the atmosphere) the solution is neutral, so pH $= 7.00$.

Let us continue to add titrant; suppose that 13 mL has been added. All that is happening is that the titrant is being diluted. Since the first 12.5 mL of titrant was consumed in the titration reaction, we have added 0.5 mL in excess, or $(0.5)(0.1) = 0.05$ mmol of OH^-. This is contained in 38 mL of solution, so $[OH^-] = 0.05/38 = 0.001316$ M, pOH $= 2.88$, and pH $= 11.12$.

It is left as an exercise to plot the titration curve and to locate the equivalence point. The calculation of a few more points in the titration, especially after the equivalence point, may be helpful in defining the shape of the curve.

Weak Acid–Strong Base Titration. We could apply the systematic treatment outlined at the beginning of Section 12.3 to obtain a general equation applicable throughout the course of the titration, but it is simpler to recognize that at any stage in the titration the solution consists of an example of a type that we have already considered. For the titration of a weak acid HA with a strong base MOH, here are the four such stages into which we divide the titration:

Stage 1: Before the Titration Begins. The sample solution is simply a solution of a weak acid, and Eq. (12.48) or (12.49) is applicable.

Stage 2: During Titration. Since some strong base has been added and has converted an equivalent amount of weak acid to its conjugate base according to

$$HA + OH^- \rightleftharpoons A^- + H_2O$$

the solution contains appreciable quantities of both HA and A$^-$. It is a buffer solution throughout much of this stage, and Eq. (12.36) applies.

Stage 3: At the Equivalence Point. Now the weak acid HA has been quantitatively converted to A$^-$. The sample solution consists of this weak base in water, and Eq. (12.50) or Eq. (12.51) may be used.

Stage 4: After the Equivalence Point. The solution contains excess strong base and the weak base A$^-$, whose dissociation is repressed by the common ion effect of the hydroxide from the strong base. We therefore ignore the contribution of A$^-$, and calculate the concentration of hydroxide exactly as in Example 12.12.

Example 12.13. Calculate the titration curve for the titration of 10.0 mL of 0.2 M weak acid (pK_a = 5.0) with 0.2 M sodium hydroxide.

Stage 1. We have $K_a = 1 \times 10^{-5}$ and $c = 0.02$, so, from Eq. (12.49),

$$[H^+] = \sqrt{(1 \times 10^{-5})(0.2)}$$
$$= 1.41 \times 10^{-3}$$

or pH = 2.85.

Stage 2. Let 2.0 ml of titrant be added. This is the situation:

Initially in the sample:	$(10.0)(0.2) = 2.00$ mmol HA
Strong base added:	$(2.0)(0.2) = 0.40$ mmol OH$^-$
Weak acid remaining	1.60 mmol HA

Using Eq. (12.36), we have

$$pH = 5.00 + \log\frac{0.40}{1.60}$$
$$= 4.40$$

Of course, the logarithmic term is strictly a ratio of *concentrations*, so we should have written

$$pH = 5.00 + \log\frac{0.40/12}{1.60/12}$$

where 12 mL is the total volume, but these volumes cancel, so we effectively calculate a ratio of *amounts*. Using the same calculational method, we obtain these further results: at 5.0 mL, pH = 5.00; at 7.0 mL, pH = 5.37.

Stage 3. The equivalence point obviously corresponds to 10.0 mL of titrant added. Initially we had $(10.0)(0.2) = 2.00$ mL of HA, and this has now been converted to 2.00 mL of A^-, which is contained in 20.0 mL of solution. Using Eq. (12.51), with $K_b = 1 \times 10^{-9}$ and $c = 0.10$ M, we obtain

$$[OH^-] = \sqrt{(1 \times 10^{-9})(0.1)}$$
$$= 1 \times 10^{-5} \text{ M}$$

so pOH = 5.00, and pH = 9.00. Obviously the solution is basic at the equivalence point, since it contains only a weak base.

Stage 4. Let 12.0 mL of titrant be added. This constitutes an excess of 2.0 mL of 0.2 M strong base in a total volume of 22.0 mL, so $[OH^-] = (2.0)(0.2)/22 = 0.0182$ M, giving pOH = 1.74 and pH = 12.26.

Figure 12.5 is a plot of the full titration curve. Three important lessons are to be learned from this graphical display:

Detection of the Endpoint. Observe the relatively sharp "break" in the curve corresponding to the equivalence point at 10.0 mL of titrant. The point at which the slope has its maximum value gives us our experimental estimate of the endpoint. In the laboratory we make use of this information in either of two ways: (1) if we know the pH at the endpoint by either calculation or experience, we can titrate to that pH (usually as detected with a visual indicator); or (2) we can experimentally measure the pH, plot the curve, and establish the endpoint graphically.

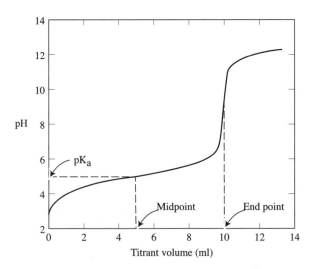

Figure 12.5. Calculated curve for the titration of 10.0 mL of 0.2 N weak acid ($pK_a = 5.00$) with 0.2 N strong base. [Reproduced by permission from Connors (1982).]

Buffer Properties. We have seen that the sample solution throughout much of the titration is a buffer, and this property is manifested in the slope of the titration curve, which is seen to be the reciprocal of β, the buffer index [Eq. (12.38)]. Thus the shallower the slope, the greater the buffer capacity. Recall our earlier claim that buffer capacity is acceptable in the range pH $= pK_a \pm 1$, and observe how this range is reflected on the titration curve.[8]

Determination of pK_a. We will subsequently learn how to measure the pH experimentally, so the titration curve can be determined. Writing Eq. (12.37) again

$$pH = pK_a + \log \frac{[\text{conjugate base}]}{[\text{conjugate acid}]}$$

we see that if we know the ratio appearing in the logarithmic term and can measure the pH of the solution, we can calculate pK_a. In particular, consider the point in the titration corresponding to one-half way to the endpoint, as measured in titrant volume. At this point (call it the midpoint), one-half of the weak acid has been converted to its conjugate base, so the ratio [conjugate base]/[conjugate acid] $=$ 1.00, and pH $= pK_a$. This relationship is shown on Fig. 12.5. (Of course, the pK_a thus determined is not a "thermodynamic pK_a" because we have not yet applied activity coefficient corrections; these are discussed in Chapter 13.) An interesting capability of this technique is that it allows us to determine the pK_a of an acid whose identity is unknown; we merely need to determine the titration curve, read off the endpoint volume, and then by interpolation to establish the pH corresponding to one-half the endpoint volume.

This equality pH $= pK_a$ at the titration midpoint is yet another manifestation of a condition we have encountered before, notably in discussing Eqs. (12.22) and (12.23), Eqs. (12.24)–(12.26), Table 12.2, and Eq. (12.39).

Calculation of the titration curve for the titration of a weak base with a strong acid is analogous to the preceding treatment. For such a titration the pH will initially be on the alkaline side of neutrality and will decrease throughout the titration. At the endpoint the solution contains the conjugate acid of the sample base, so the solution is acidic.

The titration curves of polyfunctional acids and bases, if their successive pK_a values differ by about 4 or more units, show a "break" at each endpoint for the successive titration of the groups (in the order strongest to weakest). If, however, the successive pK_a values are not widely spaced, the successive breaks are less distinct because the phenomenon seen in Fig. 12.3, in which more than two solute species coexist at some pH values, intrudes. Such systems can be algebraically described, and in this manner the experimental data can be fitted to the equation to extract the pK_a values. We will not pursue this analysis.

Acid–Base Indicators. An acid–base indicator is a compound whose conjugate acid and base forms exhibit different colors. There is no limitation on the charge type of the indicator. Indicators are used to detect the endpoint in a titration; the selection of an indicator is based on the simple principles to be discussed here.

Consider the indicator acid HI. This acid will undergo dissociation in aqueous solution:

$$HI \rightleftharpoons H^+ + I^-$$

The acid dissociation constant has the form of K_a, but it is often symbolized K_I:

$$K_I = \frac{[H^+][I^-]}{[HI]} \tag{12.53}$$

The acid form HI is responsible for the acid color of the indicator solution, and I^- shows the base color. The color that our eyes see is related to the relative concentrations of these two forms of the indicator. Rearranging Eq. (12.53) gives

$$\frac{[I^-]}{[HI]} = \frac{K_I}{[H^+]} \tag{12.54}$$

Two important conclusions follow from Eq. (12.54). The color is controlled by the pH of the solution; and the color change during a titration is not abrupt but occurs in a continuous manner, since the pH changes continuously, as we saw earlier.

It is characteristic of the typical human eye that in order to detect the first deviation from the pure acid color in a solution of the indicator, the ratio $[I^-]/[HI]$ must be at least $\frac{1}{10}$; that is, about 10% of the indicator must be in the base form. Similarly, about 10% of the indicator must be in the acid form to detect any acid color. (These statements apply to two-color indicators.) In between these limits the eye recognizes that a mixture of colors is present, and that the indicator color change is taking place if a titration is being carried out. These limits for $[I^-]/[HI]$ of 0.1 to 10 have no theoretical chemical significance but are related to the sensitivity of the observer's eyes and to the particular indicator used; some colors are more readily detected than others.

The pH values at which these limits of observable color change occur are easily calculated. From Eq. (12.54):

$$pH = pK_I + \log \frac{[I^-]}{[HI]} \tag{12.55}$$

For the limit on the acid side, $[I^-]/[HI] = 0.1$, or $pH = pK_I - 1$. For the limit on the base side, $[I^-]/[HI] = 10$, or $pH = pK_I + 1$. The pH range within which the indicator can be observed to be changing color is thus given approximately by $pH = pK_I \pm 1$. This is called the *transition interval* of the indicator, and it clearly

Table 12.3. Acid–base indicators

Indicator	Transition Interval	Acid Color	Base Color
Methyl violet	0.15–3.2	Yellow	Violet
Thymol blue	1.2–2.8	Red	Yellow
Quinaldine red	1.4–3.2	Colorless	Red
2,4-Dinitrophenol	2.4–4.0	Colorless	Yellow
Methyl yellow	2.9–4.0	Red	Yellow
Bromphenol blue	3.0–4.6	Yellow	Blue
Methyl orange	3.1–4.4	Red	Yellow
Bromcresol green	3.8–5.4	Yellow	Blue
Methyl red	4.4–6.2	Red	Yellow
Bromcresol purple	5.2–6.8	Yellow	Purple
4-Nitrophenol	5.6–7.6	Colorless	Yellow
Bromothymol blue	6.0–7.6	Yellow	Blue
Phenol red	6.4–8.2	Yellow	Red
Cresol red	7.2–8.8	Yellow	Red
Thymol blue	8.0–9.6	Yellow	Blue
Phenolphthalein	8.2–10	Colorless	Red
Thymolpthalein	9.3–10.5	Colorless	Blue
α-Naphtholbenzein	9.8–11.0	Yellow	Blue

depends on the pK_I of the indicator. This is why indicators of different structure change color at different pH values.

Table 12.3 gives the colors and transition intervals of some useful acid–base indicators. Many of the intervals are less than 2 pH units, suggesting that the limits $pK_I \pm 1$ are rather conservative. One-color indicators, in which only one of the conjugate forms possesses a visible color, will not behave visually in accordance with the above mentioned treatment, although of course their equilibria will be described by the same equations. The pK_I of an indicator, and therefore its transition interval, can be affected by the salt concentration of the solution and by organic solvents incorporated into the aqueous medium.

In order to achieve an accurate visual detection of the endpoint in an acid–base titration, evidently the pH of the solution must change by about 2 units in the immediate vicinity (say, ±0.2%) of the endpoint. Whether this condition is satisfied in any given circumstance can be determined by calculating the titration curve. Figure 12.5 shows the results of such a calculation, indicating that this would be a feasible titration with visual endpoint detection because of the sharp break in the region of the theoretical equivalence point. Calculations show that this break is greater, the more concentrated the solution and the stronger the acid (for titrations with base).

An indicator should now be chosen such that the pH at the titration equivalence point falls within the transition interval of the indicator. In the titration of a weak acid with a strong base, at the endpoint the solution contains the conjugate base of the acid, so its pH is in the alkaline range, as shown in Fig. 12.5. Weak acids therefore are usually titrated using thymol blue, phenolphthalein, or thymolphthalein as indicators. In titrations of weak bases with strong acids the endpoint pH will be in the acidic range, and methyl red, methyl orange, and bromcresol green are commonly used indicators.

Without some understanding of the relationship of molecular structure to optical absorption spectra a full accounting for the color changes of indicators is not possible, but an approximate treatment is feasible. The essential fact about acid–base indicators is that the acid and base forms have different colors. All acid–base indicators in common use are organic compounds. Apparently the reason for the different colors must be sought in the different structures of the acid and base forms of the indicator. It is possible to account for the fact of color differences on this basis; if two forms of the indicator differ markedly in their electronic distribution, and particularly in their extents of resonance delocalization, two colors will be observed. Color is associated with the capability of the compound to absorb visible light, and this capability can be related to the electronic structure. In the resonance hybrid several factors may contribute, but we can simplify and say that a change in the length of conjugation path or in extent of electronic delocalization will result in absorption of a different color component of white light, with a resultant color change. For a simple example we take 4-nitrophenol, one of the indicators in Table 12.3. The acid–base dissociation is

2   3

The acid form is colorless, but the base form is yellow. This yellow color can be correlated with electron delocalization in the base form as indicated in this conventional depiction of a resonance hybrid:

4   5

Possibilities for such electron delocalization increase with the size of the molecule, and most indicators are quite large molecules. Here is the kind of electron distribution responsible for the color change in methyl orange:

Base (yellow)

6

$$(CH_3)_2N-\!\!\!\bigcirc\!\!\!-N=\overset{H}{\underset{+}{N}}-\!\!\!\bigcirc\!\!\!-SO_3^-$$

7

$$(CH_3)_2\overset{+}{N}=\!\!\!\bigcirc\!\!\!=N-\overset{H}{N}-\!\!\!\bigcirc\!\!\!-SO_3^-$$

Acid (red)

8

12.5. AQUEOUS SOLUBILITY OF WEAK ACIDS AND BASES

Many acidic and basic drugs possess a limited solubility in water, and we have a practical interest in being able to increase their solubility. We can often accomplish this by means of pH control. The pH of an aqueous solution can usually be adjusted independently of the acid–base equilibrium of the solute drug by means of a buffer solution.

This is the general principle that we apply—the total solubility is limited by the intrinsic solubility of the uncharged (nonionic) form of the drug. We can assume that the ionic form has unlimited solubility; this is not strictly true, but the assumption carries no practical drawbacks. Notice that for the first time in our consideration of acid–base chemistry we are directing our attention to the charge types of the species.

The experimental approach is to place enough of the solute in its ionic (charged) form to achieve the desired total concentration. This is accomplished either by raising the pH if the drug is an acid (thus deprotonating it) or lowering the pH if the drug is a base (thus protonating it). We therefore must recognize whether the drug is an acid or a base, and we require the pK_a in order to calculate the needed pH of the solution.

As noted in the preceding paragraph, we have two cases to consider: (1) a neutral weak acid, such as a carboxylic acid, to be symbolized HA; and (2) a neutral weak base, such as an amine, symbolized B. For the present, concentrations will be in molar units. We make these definitions:

Let s_0 be the equilibrium solubility of the neutral (uncharged) form of the drug.
Let S_t be the total (apparent) solubility of the drug at any given pH of the solution.

We take it that the pH of the solution is under our control, for example by adding a buffer. Also note that we are restricting attention to compounds having a single ionizable group. Then we can write in general

Total concentration = solubility of uncharged form + concentration of charged form

We will develop the two cases in parallel:

Neutral Acid, HA	Neutral Base, B

$$S_t = [HA] + [A^-] = s_0 + [A^-] \qquad\qquad S_t = [B] + [BH^+] = s_0 + [BH^+]$$

$$K_a = \frac{[H^+][A^-]}{[HA]} = \frac{[H^+](S_t - s_0)}{s_0} \qquad\qquad K_a = \frac{[H^+][B]}{[BH^+]} = \frac{[H^+]s_0}{S_t - s_0}$$

$$pK_a = pH - \log\frac{S_t - s_0}{s_0} \quad (12.56a) \qquad pK_a = pH - \log\frac{s_0}{S_t - s_0} \quad (12.56b)$$

Observe that Eqs. (12.56a) and (12.56b) are simply forms of the familiar Henderson–Hasselbalch equation. The physical interpretation of these equations is that S_t is the maximum concentration of drug that can be achieved *at the given pH*. An alternative view is that the pH given by the equation is the limit beyond which precipitation of the uncharged drug will occur *at the given* S_t; the pH directional change that will produce such precipitation depends on the solute; acids will precipitate as the pH is lowered, bases will precipitate as the pH is raised.

Equations (12.56) contain two parameters (pK_a and s_0) and two variables (pH and S_t). In the most desirable situation pK_a and s_0 will be available as experimentally measured quantities; otherwise they must be estimated. Methods for estimating the solubilities of nonelectrolytes are available (Chapter 10).

Let us examine Eqs. (12.56) more closely. As noted above, these equations contain the four quantities pK_a, pH, S_t, s_0. In most applications we will know pK_a and s_0, and will either set a "target" S_t value and calculate pH, or set a target pH and calculate S_t. The concentrations appear as the ratio $(S_t - s_0)/s_0$ or its reciprocal, so it makes no difference whether molar units or physical units (such as $mg\,mL^{-1}$) are used, so long as S_t and s_0 are expressed in the same units.

The nonlogarithmic form of Eq. (12.56a) can be arranged to Eq. (12.57):

$$S_t = s_0 + \frac{K_a}{[H^+]} s_0 \qquad\qquad (12.57)$$

When $[H^+] \gg K_a$ (i.e., when $pH \ll pK_a$), for this neutral acid, Eq. (12.57) becomes $S_t = s_0$. Essentially all of the solute is in the conjugate acid form. When $[H^+] \ll K_a (pH \gg pK_a)$, Eq. (12.57) approaches

$$S_t = \frac{K_a}{[H^+]} s_0$$

which can be written

$$\log S_t = \log s_0 + pH - pK_a \qquad\qquad (12.58)$$

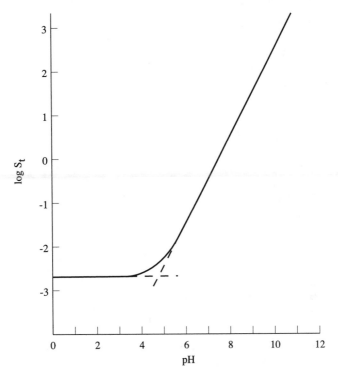

Figure 12.6. Plot of Eq. (12.56a); $pK_a = 5.0$, $s_0 = 2 \times 10^{-3}$ M.

Under these conditions the slope of a plot of $\log S_t$ versus pH is unity; that is, for each unit increase in pH the concentration increases tenfold. At the point where $pH = pK_a$, $\log S_t = \log s_0$ [but this is an extrapolated condition, because Eq. (12.58) does not hold when $pH = pK_a$]. The reverse pH dependence (slope of the plot of $\log S_t$ vs. pH is -1.00) will be seen for a neutral base. Figure 12.6 shows this behavior for a hypothetical weak acid having $pK_a = 5.00$ and $s_0 = 2.10^{-3}$ M.

In applying either Eq. (12.56a) or (12.56b) we must first establish whether the drug is a neutral acid or a neutral base. Consider sodium benzoate, useful as a preservative. We recognize this as the sodium salt of benzoic acid, prepared by reacting benzoic acid with sodium hydroxide. The solute in this case is a neutral weak acid, even though we weigh it out and dissolve it as the salt (the charged conjugate base). Benzoic acid has a limited water solubility whereas sodium benzoate is quite soluble. But we realize that sodium benzoate, in solution, is in equilibrium with benzoic acid, as the position of equilibrium is determined solely by the pK_a of benzoic acid and the pH of the solution. Despite the high solubility of sodium benzoate, if at the experimental pH the concentration placed in solution exceeds the S_t value given by Eq. (12.56a), free benzoic acid will precipitate until the equation is satisfied. We reiterate: the original form of the solute is irrelevant; this is an equilibrium situation entirely controlled by pK_a, pH, and s_0.

We mentioned earlier that the pH is under our control, but this may not always be so, and in some cases the pH may be established by a complex mixture of buffers or other formulation components. Calculation of the pH may not be feasible in such circumstances; instead the pH should be measured. Even pH indicator paper may be adequate to this purpose.

Example 12.14

(a) Suppose a drug is available as the sodium salt of a carboxylic acid whose molecular weight is 150, $pK_a = 5.00$, and solubility of the unionized acid form is 2×10^{-3} M. What is the maximum concentration of drug that can be dissolved at pH 5.00? Applying Eq. (12.56a) with $s_0 = 2 \times 10^{-3}$ M gives $S_t = 4 \times 10^{-3}$ M. Compare this with Fig. 12.6, which was calculated with these same parameters. Note that in this problem $pH = pK_a$, so equal concentrations of the ionized and unionized forms are present.

(b) Can 0.5% of the sodium salt described in Example 12.14(a) be dissolved at pH 4.00? Using Eq. (12.56a) gives $S_t = 2.2 \times 10^{-3}$ M. The desired concentration is $0.5 \, \text{g}/100 \, \text{mL} = 5 \, \text{g/L} = 3.3 \times 10^{-2}$ M, which far exceeds the calculated S_t. All drug exceeding 2.2×10^{-3} M will precipitate as the free acid, at pH 4.00.

(c) For the drug of Examples 12.14(a) and 12.14(b), what pH range will permit 0.5% to be dissolved? Now we let $S_t = 3.3 \times 10^{-2}$ M, $s_0 = 2 \times 10^{-3}$ M, and $pK_a = 5.00$, applying Eq. (12.56a) to get $pH = 6.19$. Thus any pH equal to 6.19 *or higher* will allow 0.5% to be dissolved. (See Fig. 12.6; $\log 0.033 = -1.48$.)

Example 12.15. In what pH range is it possible to prepare an aqueous solution of chlordiazepoxide (**9**) at a concentration of 10 mg/5 mL?

Chlordiazepoxide, pK_a 4.6, MW 299.8, solubility 1 g/10,000 mL H_2O

9

Chlordiazepoxide is obviously a neutral weak base. It is not obvious to which nitrogen atom the pK_a should be assigned, but its value is reasonable for an aromatic amine. The reported aqueous solubility corresponds to 0.01%. (The drug is also available as the hydrochloride salt, which is quite soluble, but as noted in the earlier discussion, this is entirely irrelevant to the problem.)

The desired concentration of 10 mg/5 mL is equivalent to 200 mg/100 mL or 0.2%. We can use Eq. (12.56b) with $s_0 = 0.01$ and $S_t = 0.2$. The result is $pH = 3.3$; that is, at any pH of 3.3 or below (more acidic), this concentration of drug can be dissolved.

We have emphasized that the form (neutral molecule or its salt) used experimentally is irrelevant, the total achievable concentration depending solely on the parameters pK_a and s_0 and on the assigned pH. This is true when the pH is fixed by the experimentalist, by means of a buffer. But if control of pH is not important, then the simplest procedure is merely to dissolve the salt form, which is usually very soluble, to the desired concentration. The pH will shift to a value determined by pK_a and concentration. [And we know how to calculate this pH by using either Eq. (12.49) or Eq. (12.51).] But this procedure may be unacceptable if the resulting pH is outside the desired range. Such a solution, moreover, is unbuffered and is susceptible to perturbation of its pH by other ingredients.

12.6. NONAQUEOUS ACID–BASE BEHAVIOR

Although water is our most important solvent, in some applications we often make use of nonaqueous solvents. Acid–base behavior (reaction of acids with bases, attainment of acid–base equilibrium, acid–base indicator color changes) is widely observable in nonaqueous media, and here we survey this very large class of substances. It would be possible to develop quantitative acid–base theories for these solvents, but the results would be much more complicated than the acid–base theory of aqueous solutions owing to the lower dielectric constants of organic solvents. This circumstance leads to the formation of ion pairs (and even of ion triplets and higher aggregates), whose existence complicates the description, so we will be satisfied with a qualitative treatment.

Dissociating Solvents. Let us take water as our model of a dissociating solvent. Omitting the molecule of water that hydrates the hydrogen ion:

$$H_2O \rightleftharpoons H^+ + OH^-$$

A large number of *dissociating solvents* fit this pattern. Methanol and other alcohols give alkoxide ions, analogous to hydroxide in water:

$$MeOH \rightleftharpoons H^+ + OMe^-$$

It is important to realize that the symbol H^+ represents a different species in these two equations; in water it means H_3O^+ and in methanol it means $MeOH_2^+$.

Liquid carboxylic acids, of which glacial acetic acid is the most important, also are dissociating solvents. Letting Ac represent CH_3CO, the acetyl group, we obtain

$$HOAc \rightleftharpoons H^+ + OAc^-$$

(glacial acetic acid simply denotes pure acetic acid). In this equation H^+ represents H_2OAc^+. The proton is not a necessary product of solvent dissociation. Here is how acetic anhydride dissociates:

$$Ac_2O \rightleftharpoons Ac^+ + OAc^-$$

The symbol Ac^+ represents the acetylium ion, CH_3CO^+.

There are also many nondissociating solvents, such as hydrocarbons, ethers, and carbon tetrachloride. Actually the distinction between dissociating and nondissociating solvents is a matter of degree, for with sufficiently sensitive techniques we might detect some level of dissociation by nearly any solvent. We adopt a practical viewpoint based on ordinary laboratory experience.

Let us generally represent a dissociating solvent by the symbol CA, where C is the cationic component and A is the anionic component. Then the solvent dissociation is

$$CA \rightleftharpoons C^+ + A^-$$

and, just as we did for water, we define an ion product, K_s:

$$K_s = [C^+][A^-] \tag{12.59}$$

Table 12.4 lists some ion products as $pK_s = -\log K_s$.

Here is an interesting consequence of the pK_s value. We will compare water and ethanol. In water, in order to pass from an acidic solution in which pC (i.e., pH) = 1 to an alkaline solution in which pA (i.e., pOH) = 1, a range of acidity corresponding to 12 pH units must be traversed, since pC + pA = 14 for water. For ethanol, however, pC + pA = 19.1, so to go from pC = 1 to pA = 1 requires that 17.1 orders of magnitude be covered. Very roughly we may expect that the smaller is K_s for a solvent, the greater the range of the acidity scale available for studying or titrating sample solutes.

Acid–Base Properties. Solvents may be discussed as acids or bases just as are any other substances. The Bronsted theory forms the basis of the discussion, and the terms used are given in Table 12.5. Very generally we recognize that protogenic and amphiprotic solvents are dissociating solvents, whereas protophilic and aprotic solvents are nondissociating solvents.

A useful analogy may now be made between water, whose acid–base properties we understand, and several nonaqueous solvents. The dissociating solvent CA

Table 12.4. Properties of some solvents

Solvent	pK_s	Dielectric Constant
Water	14.00	78.5
Methanol	16.70	32.6
Ethanol	19.10	24.3
Acetic acid	14.45	6.19
Formic acid	6.20	58
Acetic anhydride	14.5	21
Acetonitrile	26.5	36.2

Table 12.5. Solvent classifications

Class	Characteristics	Examples
Protogenic	Acidic; donate a proton	Glacial HOAc; H_2SO_4
Protophilic	Basic; accept a proton	Amines; ethers; esters
Amphiprotic	Both acidic and basic; can donate or accept a proton	Water; alcohols
Aprotic	Neither acidic nor basic.	Hydrocarbons, CCl_4, CH_3CN, dioxane

yields the cation C^+, which is called the *lyonium ion*, and the anion A^-, called the *lyate ion*:

Solvent	$\rightleftharpoons$	Lyonium ion	+ Lyate ion
$2\,H_2O$	$\rightleftharpoons$	H_3O^+	$+ OH^-$
$2\,MeOH$	$\rightleftharpoons$	$MeOH_2^+$	$+ OMe^-$
$2\,HOAc$	$\rightleftharpoons$	H_2OAc^+	$+ OAc^-$
Ac_2O	$\rightleftharpoons$	Ac^+	$+ OAc^-$
$2\,NH_3$ (liq)	$\rightleftharpoons$	NH_4^+	$+ NH_2^-$

With water as the solvent we are accustomed to regarding its lyonium ion, H_3O^+, as the strongest possible acid, and OH^-, the lyate ion, as the strongest possible base. Let us extend this concept to the other solvents. In glacial acetic acid as a solvent, we would conclude that the acetate ion OAc^- is the strongest possible base. In other words, sodium acetate (which we recall is a weak base in water) should be a strong base in glacial acetic acid, just as sodium hydroxide is a strong base in water. This expectation is borne out by experiment. Similarly we predict that ammonium chloride should be a strong acid in liquid ammonia. This analogy is a powerful concept for the design of experiments.

The Leveling and Differentiating Effects. Since solvents can be acids or bases, an acidic or basic solute reacts with such a solvent to a degree determined by their relative strengths. We can distinguish two possibilities. Let S represent a basic solvent and HX a strongly acidic solute. Then one possibility is that the reaction

$$HX + S \rightarrow SH^+ + X^-$$

goes essentially completely to the right. Thus, the solute is quantitatively transformed into the lyonium ion of the solvent, which is the strongest acid that can exist in this solvent. (Any acid stronger than SH^+, such as HX, will be transformed to SH^+; this lowers the free energy of the system.) We say that the solvent S is a *leveling solvent* for HX, or that HX is leveled by S. If we also had a second very strong acid HY that was leveled by S, the acids HX and HY would appear to be of the same strength, because they both have been converted to SH^+. This is what happens when the familiar strong acids (HCl, HNO_3, H_2SO_4, $HClO_4$) are dissolved in water; they are levelled to H_3O^+ and all appear to be of the same acid strength. Glacial acetic acid as a solvent, which is fairly acidic, levels many bases, such as amines, by quantitatively transforming them to its lyate ion:

$$RNH_2 + HOAc \rightarrow RNH_3^+ + OAc^-$$

The other possibility, of course, is that the reaction between solvent and solute does not go to completion. Imagine the acid HA reacting with solvent S:

$$HA + S \rightleftharpoons SH^+ + A^-$$

If the reaction does not go completely to the right, we can measure an equilibrium constant for it, and this constant is a quantitative measure of the extent of reaction. Now if we take a second comparable acid HB and measure its equilibrium constant, we can compare the acid strengths of HA and HB with respect to the reference base S. We call S a *differentiating solvent* for HA and HB. This is just what we do in water when we measure K_a values for weak acids and bases.

Figure 12.7 is a schematic representation of these ideas. Here we have supposed that there exists for every solute an innate absolute acidity or basicity (which is not true, but is a reasonable practical approximation), and as solutes we have taken, in order of decreasing acidity and increasing basicity, $HClO_4$, HOAc, ArOH (a phenol), H_2O, $ArNH_2$ (an aromatic amine), RNH_2 (an aliphatic amine), NaOH. These are spread out on scales, which may be taken as proportional to pH or pK_a.

The key idea is that the pure solvent is taken as the neutral point of the scale. Thus in the upper scale, showing H_2O as the solvent, H_2O is the neutral point. Any

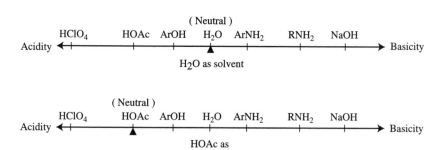

Figure 12.7. Illustrating acidity/basicity relative to the solvent, and the leveling and differentiating effects.

solute, acid or base, lying very far from this point, will be leveled by water, because the difference in their acid-base properties is great. Those solutes not falling very distant from the neutral point are differentiated by water, as we know that HOAc, ArOH, ArNH$_2$, and RNH$_2$ are differentiated, because we can measure their K_a values.

Now turn to the scale for glacial acetic acid as solvent. Acetic acid now becomes our neutral point, and we may question whether even such a strong acid as perchloric acid (HClO$_4$) is leveled by acetic acid. On the other hand, we readily accept that aliphatic amines are leveled, because they lie distant from the neutral point.

These considerations of acid–base strength are somewhat complicated by the concomitant phenomenon of limited dissociation as a result of the low dielectric constant of some nonaqueous solvents, but as a qualitative guide they are useful. The role of dielectric constant and the distinction between ionization and dissociation was treated earlier, in Chapter 8.

12.7. ACID–BASE STRUCTURE AND STRENGTH

Principles. We should be able to look at a molecular structure and to make reasonable, even though approximate, estimates of the acid or base strengths of functional groups. The ability to do this from fundamental theoretical principles is almost nonexistent at present, and need not be considered. Quite sophisticated yet practical empirical techniques are available, but they are beyond our present requirements (Perrin et al. 1981). Our treatment will be very brief.

We begin with Eq. (12.16), repeated here

$$pK_w = pK_a + pK_b$$

and the insight provided by the Bronsted theory that acid and base strength, *for a conjugate pair*, are reciprocally related, that is, $K_a = K_w/K_b$ or $K_b = K_w/K_a$. Now, it is the essence of the acid–base definitions that we can make these statements:

1. As K_a increases, pK_a decreases, and acid strength increases.
2. As K_b increases, pK_b decreases, and base strength increases.

For a conjugate pair, a smaller pK_a (stronger acid) must be accompanied by a larger pK_b (weaker base); this is the reciprocal effect. Observe in Table 12.6, these pairs of pK_a and pK_b values for (hypothetical) conjugate acid-base pairs.

It is obvious that pK_a is a reasonable quantitative measure of acid strength. What is not so obvious is that it has become conventional to use the pK_a of the conjugate acid to specify base strength! And Table 12.6 shows that a stronger base is associated with a larger pK_a (of its conjugate acid—but this parenthetical addition is seldom stated). So our chemical problem is twofold: (1) we must be able to recognize, by examination of the molecular structure, whether a functional group is acidic or basic and (2) we must estimate its pK_a value. Alternatively, if the pK_a is

Table 12.6. Measures of acid and base strength for hypothetical conjugate pairs

	Conjugate Acid, pK_a	Conjugate Base, pK_b	
	3	11	
↑	4	10	
	5	9	Stronger base
Stronger acid	6	8	
	7	7	
	8	6	
	9	5	
	10	4	↓
	11	3	

known, we must examine the structure to determine whether the pK_a describes an acid or a base.

Table 12.7 gives data for some important acid–base pairs. Thus we see that acetic acid is a stronger acid than is dihydrogen phosphate, which is stronger than ammonium ion. It follows inevitably that ammonia is a stronger base than monohydrogen phosphate, which is stronger than acetate ion. To find this set of data in the literature, one looks for the pK_a of acetic acid; the *second* pK_a (pK_2) of phosphoric acid, H_3PO_4; and the pK_a of *ammonia*.

A very simplified view of pK_a prediction is often adequate. First we note that these commonly seen functional groups can be considered to have essentially no acidic or basic character in aqueous solution:

Alcohols and sugars, ROH
Amides, $RCONH_2$
Ethers, ROR′
Esters, RCOOR′
Carbonyls, RCOR′; RCHO

Table 12.8 gives pK_a ranges that will include many of the commonly encountered acidic and basic functional groups. Recall that an aromatic amine has the nitrogen

Table 12.7. pK_a and pK_b of some acids and bases

Conjugate Acid	pK_a	Conjugate Base	pK_b
CH_3COOH	4.76	CH_3COO^-	9.24
$H_2PO_4^-$	7.21	HPO_4^{2-}	6.79
NH_4^+	9.25	NH_3	4.75

Table 12.8. pK_a Ranges of Acids and Bases

Type	pK_a
Acids	
Carboxylic acids, RCOOH	2–6 (3–5 typical)
Sulfonic acids, RSO$_3$H	−1 to 1
Phenols, ArOH	7–11
Thiols, RSH	7–10
Imides—CONHCO—	8–11
Bases	
Aliphatic amines	8–11
Aromatic amines	4–7
Guanidines, (RNH)$_2$C=NH	11–14

either as part of the ring system (as in pyridine) or directly attached to an aromatic ring (aniline).

It is valuable to memorize, (or otherwise keep readily available) a few typical pK_a values to serve as reference points. Here are some examples:

Acetic acid, CH$_3$COOH	pK_a 4.76
Benzoic acid, C$_6$H$_5$COOH	pK_a 4.20
Phenol, C$_6$H$_5$OH	pK_a 10.00
4-Nitrophenol, O$_2$N-C$_6$H$_4$OH	pK_a 7.14
Triethylamine, Et$_3$N	pK_a 10.78
Aniline, C$_6$H$_5$NH$_2$	pK_a 4.69

Bearing in mind the definitions of acid (proton donor) and base (proton acceptor), it is clear that a structural change that increases the electron density at a functional group will weaken an acid (raise its pK_a) by making it more difficult for the proton to leave; and will strengthen a base (raise its pK_a) by more avidly attracting the proton, and vice versa for electron withdrawal from the functional group. This is why 4-nitrophenol is a much stronger acid than is phenol. With the few pK_a values given here and the ranges of Table 12.8, quite useful estimates can be made by analogy.

Structural Effects. We have seen that electron-withdrawing structural features are acid-strengthening and base-weakening, whereas electron-donating structural features are acid-weakening and base strengthening. Discrete charges display these effects very clearly. Compare these data:

$$H_3^+N-CH_2COOH \rightleftharpoons H_3^+N-CH_2COO^- + H^+ \qquad pK_a = 2.31$$
$$H_3C-CH_2COOH \rightleftharpoons H_3C-CH_2COO^- + H^+ \qquad pK_a = 4.88$$
$$^-O_2C-CH_2COOH \rightleftharpoons {}^-O_2C-CH_2COO^- + H^+ \qquad pK_a = 5.69$$

Table 12.9. pK_a values of benzoic acids at 25°C

	Position		
Substituent	Ortho	Meta	Para
—H	4.20	4.20	4.20
—NO_2	2.17	3.45	3.44
—Cl	2.94	3.83	3.99
—OCH_3	4.09	4.09	4.47
—CH_3	3.91	4.24	4.34
—$C(CH_3)_3$	3.46	4.28	4.40
—COOH	2.95	3.54	3.51
—COO^-	5.41	4.60	4.82
—OH	2.98	4.08	4.58
—NH_2	4.98	4.79	4.92

Taking propionic acid as our reference, the pK_a of the positively substituted acid lies as expected, because a simple electrostatic argument states that like charge repulsion will facilitate the departure of the proton, thus enhancing acid strength. Just the opposite effect is seen with the negative substituent, which through unlike charge attraction inhibits the dissociation of the proton, weakening the acid. This is why pK_2 of a diprotic acid is always larger than pK_1.

More subtle effects are seen with substituents capable of exerting electron release or electron withdrawal by inductive or resonance mechanisms. The aromatic ring provides good examples of such effects, and in fact much of our information on the electronic effects of substituents has come from pK_a measurements. Table 12.9 lists pK_a values for monosubstituted benzoic acids.

Some of the effects are easy to rationalize. For example, the nitro group is electron-withdrawing from any position. (The ortho substituent often is atypical because steric as well as electronic effects operate.) Similarly the amino group is electron-releasing from every position. But some of the results may seem anomalous. Thus methoxy is acid-weakening in the para position but acid-strengthening in the meta position. How can this be explained?

Recall that both the inductive and resonance effects are present. The inductive effect (a through-bond displacement of electron density) is governed mainly by the electronegativity difference of the bonded atoms. The resonance effect is an electron delocalization resulting from molecular orbital overlap. These two effects may operate in the same directions, thus largely adding their effects; or they may oppose each other. In the methoxy case such opposition occurs; the methoxy group is electron-releasing by the resonance effect but electron-withdrawing by the inductive effect. In the para position the resonance effect dominates, but in the meta position resonance is largely ineffective, and the inductive effect dominates.

Table 12.10 gives pK_a values for phenols. The substituent effects on phenolic pK_a values are more marked than those on the benzoic acid series because the

Table 12.10. pK_a values for monosubstituted phenols in water

Substituent	Ortho	Meta	Para
		Position	
$-H$	10.00	10.00	10.00
$-NO_2$	7.23	8.35	7.14
$-Cl$	8.48	9.02	9.35
$-OCH_3$	9.93	9.65	10.20
$-CH_3$	10.28	10.08	10.19
$-NH_2$	9.71	9.87	10.30

phenolic group can enter into direct conjugation with the substituent (as we saw in describing 4-nitrophenol as an acid-base indicator).

Table 12.11 lists a few pK_a values of amines. These display the range of pK_a values typically seen with this class of compound, although even more dramatic substituent effects may be encountered; for example, p$K_a = 1.11$ for 4-nitroaniline. Comparison of the aromatic amine aniline **10** with its saturated analog cyclohexylamine **11** shows that the aromatic ring decreases base strength by a millionfold ($\Delta pK_a = 6.06$):

10   **11**

Table 12.11. Amine pK_a values

Amine	pK_a	
Ammonia, NH_3	9.25	
Methylamine	10.64	
Ethylamine	10.67	
Dimethylamine	10.73	
Ethanolamine, $HOCH_2CH_2NH_2$	9.50	
Hydroxylamine, $HONH_2$	5.96	
Hydrazine, H_2NNH_2	8.12	
Aniline	4.58	$\Delta pK_a = 6.06$
Cyclohexylamine	10.64	
Pyridine	5.17	$\Delta pK_a = 5.96$
Piperidine	11.13	

The same effect is seen with the pair pyridine and piperidine:

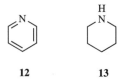

| 12 | 13 |

Although it may seem counterintuitive, the only conclusion that can be drawn is that the aromatic ring is responsible for reducing the electron density on the nitrogen, and therefore must be functioning as an electron-withdrawing substituent (Brown et al. 1955). This is a resonance delocalization effect.

The appearance of the imide structure as an acid in Table 12.8 may be surprising, so let us view an imide as a product of successive acylations of ammonia:

$$
\begin{array}{ccc}
& \overset{\displaystyle O}{\underset{\displaystyle \|}{}} & \overset{\displaystyle O}{\underset{\displaystyle \|}{}}\ \ \overset{\displaystyle }{}\ \ \overset{\displaystyle O}{\underset{\displaystyle \|}{}} \\
NH_3 & CH_3C-NH_2 & CH_3C-N-CCH_3 \\
Basic & Neutral & Acidic \\
\mathbf{14} & \mathbf{15} & \mathbf{16}
\end{array}
$$

It follows that the acyl group is electron-withdrawing, reducing the electron density on nitrogen to such an extent that the basic ammonia molecule is converted to the neutral acetamide, with a second acetyl group producing an imide, which has an ionizable hydrogen. Many drug molecules, including the barbituric acid derivatives and the hydantoins, include the imide group. The sulfonamide drugs contain the functional group

$$
Ar\ \overset{\displaystyle O}{\underset{\displaystyle O}{S}}\ NHR
$$

17

which bears some relationship to the imide group, and is likewise acidic.

Assignment of pK_a Values. To this point we have been considering the problem of predicting, to a semiquantitative level, the pK_a of a molecule from knowledge of its molecular structure, the method being based on analogy with pK_a values of model compounds. Now we face a related but distinctly different problem. Suppose a compound of known structure is studied experimentally and its pK_a value or values are measured. The problem is to associate these pK_a values with the functional groups responsible for them. This is called assigning the pK_a values.

If only a single pK_a is measurable, the problem is usually trivial, because there will be only a single reasonable choice of functional group to associate with the experimental value.[9] We therefore turn to the more interesting case of a diprotic acid, which we symbolize HABH. In general the two ionizable hydrogens are associated with chemically different functional groups, so we must expand our description of the acid-base equilibria to accommodate two possible pathways:

$$
\begin{array}{ccc}
& \text{HAB}^- & \\
{\scriptstyle k_1}\nearrow & & \searrow{\scriptstyle k_3} \\
\text{HABH} & & \text{AB}^{2-} \\
{\scriptstyle k_2}\searrow & & \nearrow{\scriptstyle k_4} \\
& {}^-\text{ABH} &
\end{array}
\qquad (12.60)
$$

Here HAB^- and ^-ABH represent the two possible monoprotic species. The constants are called *microscopic dissociation constants* and are obviously defined as follows:

$$
k_1 = \frac{[\text{HAB}^-]}{[\text{HABH}]}
$$

$$
k_2 = \frac{[^-\text{ABH}]}{[\text{HABH}]}
$$

$$
(12.61)
$$

$$
k_3 = \frac{[\text{AB}^{2-}]}{[\text{HAB}^-]}
$$

$$
k_4 = \frac{[\text{AB}^{2-}]}{[^-\text{ABH}]}
$$

The observed stepwise acid dissociation constants are given by

$$
K_1 = \frac{[\text{H}^+]([\text{HAB}^-] + [^-\text{ABH}])}{[\text{HABH}]} \qquad (12.62)
$$

$$
K_2 = \frac{[\text{H}^+][\text{AB}^{2-}]}{[\text{HAB}^-] + [^-\text{ABH}]} \qquad (12.63)
$$

Algebraic combination of Eqs. (12.61)–(12.63) gives

$$
K_1 = k_1 + k_2 \qquad (12.64)
$$

$$
\frac{1}{K_2} = \frac{1}{k_3} + \frac{1}{k_4} \qquad (12.65)
$$

From Eqs. (12.61) we find

$$
k_1 k_3 = k_2 k_4 \qquad (12.66)
$$

showing that only three of the four microscopic constants are independent. We might even define a fifth microscopic constant according to

$$HAB^- \overset{k_{iso}}{\rightleftharpoons} {}^-ABH$$

and further manipulation results in

$$k_{iso} = \frac{k_2}{k_1} = \frac{k_3}{k_4} \tag{12.67}$$

Before continuing with this general case, let us pause to analyze the special case in which the two ionizable groups are chemically identical and are independent of each other. The fact that they are identical means that $k_1 = k_2$ and that $k_3 = k_4$. The fact that they are independent means that $k_1 = k_3$ and $k_2 = k_4$. Inserting these special conditions into Eqs. (12.64) and (12.65) gives $K_1 = 2k$ and $1/K_2 = 2/k$, or, combining these

$$\frac{K_1}{K_2} = 4 \tag{12.68}$$

This result is usually described as a statistical effect. Equation (12.68) is not closely obeyed by long-chain dicarboxylic acids because of the superimposed electrostatic effects of the anionic charges (Brown et al. 1955); in other words, the two groups, although identical, are not independent.

We now return to the general case in which the two functional groups are different. From Eqs. (12.64), (12.65), and (12.67) we get

$$K_1 = k_1(1 + k_{iso}) \tag{12.69}$$

$$K_2 = \frac{k_3}{1 + k_{iso}} \tag{12.70}$$

Now suppose that k_{iso} is very much smaller than one. From Eq. (12.67), this means that $k_2 \lll k_1$ and $k_3 \lll k_4$, or from Eqs. (12.69)–(12.70)

$$K_1 = k_1 \tag{12.71}$$

$$K_2 = k_3 \tag{12.72}$$

In this case the observed K_a values can be equated to microscopic constants. Chemically this means that essentially only the uppermost pathway in Eq. (12.60) is followed, and the only monoprotic species is HAB^-. The condition $k_{iso} \lll 1$ (or the reverse, $k_{iso} \ggg 1$), which leads to a single ionization pathway, is satisfied if the observed pK_a values are widely spaced.

We now turn to specific chemical compounds. In making pK_a assignments, begin by writing the compound in its fully protonated form, whether this is uncharged or cationic. First consider 4-hydroxybenzoic acid. We place this in the center, with its measured pK_1 and pK_2 values, and flank it with very obvious model compounds and their pK_a values:

4.2	4.6; 9.3	10.0
18	**19**	**20**

It is reasonable and even obvious to assign pK_1 to the carboxylic acid and pK_2 to the phenolic group. Moreover, since $K_1 \ggg K_2$, we can expect that only a single pathway is followed, and that the only monoprotic species present in significant concentration is the carboxylate. Thus for this compound the ionization pathway is

$$(12.73)$$

Incidentally, the differences between 4.6 and 4.2, and 9.3 and 10.0, are to be ascribed to electronic substituent effects.

Next consider 3-aminophenol:

4.9	4.4; 9.8	10.0
21	**22**	**23**

By analogy we assign the pK_1 to the amine and pK_2 to the phenol. Again the two dissociation constants are widely spaced, and this is the sequence:

$$(12.74)$$

Finally consider glycine, **25**:

$$CH_3NH_3^+ \qquad H_3^+NCH_2COOH \qquad CH_3COOH$$

$$10.7 \qquad\qquad 2.4; 9.8 \qquad\qquad 4.8$$

$$\textbf{24} \qquad\qquad\qquad \textbf{25} \qquad\qquad\qquad \textbf{26}$$

Once again by using model compounds as guides we make our assignment, this time of pK_1 to ionization of the carboxylic acid and pK_2 to the amine function. The ionization sequence is therefore

$$H_3^+NCH_2COOH \overset{K_1}{\rightleftharpoons} H_3^+NCH_2COO^- \overset{K_2}{\rightleftharpoons} H_2NCH_2COO^- \qquad (12.75)$$

The intermediate species, carrying both a positive charge and a negative charge, is called a *zwitterion*.

What is the difference between 3-aminophenol (which does not yield a zwitterion) and glycine? Representing both molecules in this scheme

we see that 3-aminophenol follows the $k_1 \rightarrow k_3$ pathway, because the protonated amine, which is the conjugate acid of an aromatic amine, is a stronger acid than is the phenol. For glycine, on the other hand, the carboxylic acid is stronger than is the protonated amine (which in this compound is the conjugate acid of an aliphatic amine), so the $k_2 \rightarrow k_4$ route predominates.

If K_1 and K_2 are not widely separated, then both ionization routes are followed, and both monoprotic species may be present in the solution in significant concentration. Unique assignment of the pK_1 and pK_2 values then is not possible, and the interesting problem, which we will not pursue here, is to determine the values of the microscopic constants.

PROBLEMS

12.1. Calculate the pH of each of these aqueous solutions at 25°C.
   (a) 2.50×10^{-4} M HCl
   (b) 2.50×10^{-4} M H_2SO_4
   (c) 0.04 M ammonia
   (d) 0.04 M ammonium chloride
   (e) 3.0×10^{-3} M KOH

12.2. A buffer was prepared by mixing 25.0 mL of 0.10 M acetic acid and 15.0 mL of 0.075 M KOH, and diluting to 50.0 mL with water. Calculate its pH ($pK_a = 4.76$).

12.3. Give directions for the preparation of 500 mL of 0.10 M pH 8.35 tris buffer, starting with pure tris and 0.10 M HCl. (See Example 12.7 for needed information.)

12.4. Sorensen buffer solutions are prepared by mixing appropriate volumes of these stock solutions:

Stock solution A. 9.91 g of $NaH_2PO_4 \cdot H_2O$ (MW 138.0) is dissolved in water to make 1 L.
Stock solution B. 9.47 g of Na_2HPO_4 (MW 142.0) is dissolved in water to make 1 L.

(a) Calculate the molar concentrations of stock solutions A and B.
(b) Calculate the pH of a Sorensen's buffer prepared by mixing 40 mL of A and 60 mL of B. Use $pK_2 = 6.80$ as the effective pK_2 of phosphoric acid.

12.5. Calculate the titration curve for the titration of 24.0 mL of 0.20 M n-butylamine ($pK_a = 10.60$) with 0.30 M HCl when the following volumes of titrant have been added: 0 mL, 2 mL, 5 mL, 8 mL, 12 mL, 16 mL, 18 mL. Suggest a suitable indicator for the titration.

12.6. Calculate and plot the species distribution curves for these solutes.
(a) Phenol, $pK_a = 10.00$.
(b) Hydroxylamine, $pK_a = 5.96$.
(c) Phthalic acid, $pK_1 = 2.95$, $pK_2 = 5.41$.
(d) Citric acid, $pK_1 = 3.06$, $pK_2 = 4.74$, $pK_3 = 5.40$.
(e) Is there any pH range within which significant concentrations of the uncharged forms of phenol and hydroxylamine can coexist in solution?

12.7. Give numerical values for the equilibrium constants of these reactions.
(a) $C_6H_5COOH + CH_3NH_2 \rightleftharpoons C_6H_5COO^- + CH_3NH_3^+$
(b) $C_6H_5OH + OH^- \rightleftharpoons C_6H_5O^- + H_2O$

12.8. Assign the pK_a values of these compounds. (Look up the structures as necessary.)
(a) Salicylic acid; $pK_1 = 2.98$, $pK_2 = 13.00$.
(b) Arginine; $pK_1 = 2.17$, $pK_2 = 9.04$, $pK_3 = 12.48$.
(c) Quinine; $pK_1 = 6.66$, $pK_2 = 9.48$.
(d) Theophylline; $pK_a = 8.77$.

12.9. For the titration of weak acid HA with strong base MOH, let $b = [M^+]$ and $c = [HA] + [A^-]$. Derive an *exact* equation relating $[H^+]$, K_a, K_w, b, and c throughout the entire titration. (*Hint*: Apply the systematic procedure outlined at the beginning of Section 12.3.)

12.10. Write the electroneutrality equation for aqueous solutions of each of these solutes.

(a) Ammonium chloride.

(b) The triprotic neutral acid H_3A.

(c) A pH 7 phosphate buffer (assume sodium ion is the counterion).

12.11. What is the pH of a 2.00% solution of ephedrine hydrochloride (MW 211.7, pK_a 9.60)?

12.12. Given: 5.444 g of KH_2PO_4 (MW 136.1) was dissolved in 100.0 mL of 0.300 M KOH and the solution was diluted to 1000 mL. Calculate the pH ($pK_1 = 2.23$, $pK_2 = 7.21$, $pK_3 = 12.32$).

12.13. Given: 50.0 mL of an aqueous solution of ammonia (pK_a 9.25) titrated with 0.100 M HCl, 9.50 mL of titrant being required.

(a) What was the pH of the solution when 4.75 mL of titrant had been added?

(b) What was the pH of the solution at the endpoint?

12.14. Calculate the standard free-energy change at 25°C for the dissociation of phenol in water ($pK_a = 10.00$).

12.15. What weight of anhydrous sodium acetate (MW 82.0) must be added to 1.00 L of pH 3.75 acetate buffer containing a total buffer concentration of 0.055 M in order to change the pH to 3.90 ($pK_a = 4.75$)?

12.16. Show how a fraction and a ratio are related; in particular, how are the fraction $F = [HA]/c$ and the ratio $R = [HA]/[A^-]$ related (c is the total concentration)?

12.17. What is the concentration of benzoate ion in a solution prepared to be 0.10 M in acetic acid, 0.10 M in potassium acetate, and 5×10^{-4} M in (total) benzoic acid ($pK_a = 4.75$ for acetic acid; $pK_a = 4.20$ for benzoic acid)?

12.18. Suppose that the pH of a solution of a diprotic weak acid H_2A is adjusted to be equal to $(pK_1 + pK_2)/2$.

(a) Will the concentration of the monoanion HA^- increase or decrease when some HCl is added?

(b) Will the concentration of the monoanion HA^- increase or decrease when some KOH is added?

12.19. What is the pH at the midpoint of the titration of 15.0 mL of 0.050 M HCl with 0.10 M NaOH?

12.20. You wish to prepare 1.00 L of pH 7.00 phosphate buffer containing a total phosphate concentration of 0.100 M. You have available crystalline $NaH_2PO_4 \cdot H_2O$ (MW 138.0) and Na_2HPO_4 (MW 142.0). For phosphoric acid, $pK_1 = 2.23$, $pK_2 = 7.21$, $pK_3 = 12.32$. Neglecting activity coefficient effects, what weights of the two solutes must be taken?

12.21. What is the standard free energy change of this reaction at 25°C?

$$H^+ + OH^- \rightleftharpoons H_2O$$

NOTES

1. G. N. Lewis, also in 1923, proposed an even more general acid–based theory. Just as Bronsted improved on the Arrhenius theory by eliminating the hydroxide ion as a defining feature, so Lewis generalized the Bronsted theory by eliminating the proton. Lewis defined an *acid as an electron pair acceptor*, and a *base as an electron pair donor*. Thus every Bronsted base is also a Lewis base, but the Lewis acid concept greatly expands our ideas of acid character. In the reaction

$$BF_3 + NH_3 \rightleftharpoons F_3B : NH_3$$

   boron trifluoride is a Lewis acid.

2. Proton transfer reactions are extremely fast, so as soon as the solution has been made macroscopically homogeneous by mixing, the system is at equilibrium.

3. It is important to appreciate a critical difference in the meanings of Eq. (12.16), $pK_w = pK_a + pK_b$; and of Eq. (12.18), $pK_w = pH + pOH$. Equation (12.16) refers to a *conjugate acid–base pair*; pK_a and pK_b are *constants*, although mutually dependent. Equation (12.18) refers to a *solution*; pH and pOH are *variables*, although mutually dependent.

4. Of course, these are equilibria, and all species are, strictly speaking, present in all solutions. From the practical point of view, however, we are often justified in neglecting the presence of a species if it is experimentally undetectable or exhibits no detectable influence.

5. Buffers are commonly described in an abbreviated terminology that must be understood. For example, a 0.10 M pH 5.00 acetate buffers means that the total buffer concentration c is 0.10 M and the pH is 5.00; obviously the solution contains both acetate and acetic acid, in concentrations that can be worked out from the Henderson–Hasselbalch equation. Similarly, a 0.05 M pH 7.0 phosphate buffer contains both dihydrogen phosphate ($H_2PO_4^-$) and monohydrogen phosphate (HPO_4^{2-}), usually taken as their salts.

6. The chloride ion is neutral, as may be deduced by noting that HCl is a strong acid; that is, its "conjugate base" Cl^- is so weak that it is completely ineffectual at capturing the proton.

7. The exact equation obtained by applying this general scheme will be a polynomial in $[H^+]$, whose highest power will be equal to the number of dissociation constants (including K_w) plus one.

8. Figure 12.5 also shows that fairly high concentrations of a strong base (seen well beyond the endpoint in Fig. 12.5) constitute good buffers. The same is true of strong acids.

9. The choice is not always obvious, however, as is illustrated by the data in Example 12.15 for chlordiazepoxide.

13

ELECTRICAL WORK

13.1. INTRODUCTION

In Chapter 1 we saw that work can be expressed as the product of an intensive property and an extensive property

$$\text{Work (energy)} = \text{intensity factor} \times \text{capacity factor}$$

and these four examples were given:

$$\text{Mechanical work} = \text{mechanical force} \times \text{distance}$$
$$\text{Work of expansion} = \text{pressure} \times \text{volume change}$$
$$\text{Surface work} = \text{surface tension} \times \text{area change}$$
$$\text{Electrical work} = \text{electric potential} \times \text{charge}$$

Mechanical work is dealt with in classical mechanics. In earlier chapters we treated expansion work and surface work. The present section develops the idea of electrical work. Recall from Chapter 3 that the Gibbs free-energy change in a reversible process when carried out reversibly is equal to the maximum work obtainable from the system (exclusive of work of expansion). One kind of useful work measured by the free-energy change is electrical work. We routinely exploit this application of thermodynamics when we use batteries.

The essential phenomenon that we will study consists of a transfer of charge between an electrolyte solution and another phase (usually a solid). There are two ways in which this charge can be transferred: by electron-transfer (the subject of Sections 13.2–13.4) and by ion transfer (Section 13.5), commonly called *ion exchange*.

13.2. OXIDATION–REDUCTION REACTIONS

Inorganic Redox Reactions. We saw in Chapter 12 that acid–base reactions are manifested as proton transfers from one conjugate acid–base pair to another. Now we encounter a formal analogy in the phenomenon of electron transfer. First we define an oxidation–reduction (*redox*) half-reaction:

$$\text{Red} \underset{\text{reduction}}{\overset{\text{oxidation}}{\rightleftharpoons}} \text{Ox} + n(\text{e}) \tag{13.1}$$

where "Red" is the reduced form of the reacting species (also known as the *reductant* or *reducing agent*), "Ox" is the oxidized form (the *oxidant* or *oxidizing agent*), "e" is the electron, and n is the number of electrons in the balanced half-reaction. Of course, in ordinary chemical systems we do not observe the half-reaction; instead two half-reactions are coupled, and the net process consists of one or more electrons being transferred from one redox pair to another:

$$\text{Red}(1) \rightleftharpoons \text{Ox}(1) + n(\text{e})$$

$$n(\text{e}) + \text{Ox}(2) \rightleftharpoons \text{Red}(2)$$

$$\text{Net: } \text{Red}(1) + \text{Ox}(2) \rightleftharpoons \text{Ox}(1) + \text{Red}(2)$$

Equation (13.1) shows that oxidation is the process in which a substance loses electrons and reduction is the process in which a substance gains electrons. Here are some simple examples of redox half-reactions.

$$H_2 \rightleftharpoons 2H^+ + 2e$$
$$Na \rightleftharpoons Na^+ + e$$
$$Fe^{2+} \rightleftharpoons Fe^{3+} + e$$
$$2Cl^- \rightleftharpoons Cl_2 + 2e$$

As in other types of chemical processes, redox reactions must be written in balanced form in order to express the experimental stoichiometry and to define equilibrium constants. For the simple examples shown above, it is easy to combine half-reactions into balanced net reactions, such as

$$H_2 + 2Na^+ \rightleftharpoons 2H^+ + 2Na$$
$$2Fe^{2+} + Cl_2 \rightleftharpoons 2Fe^{3+} + 2Cl^-$$

Observe that a balanced redox reaction (whether a half-reaction or a net reaction) is balanced both chemically and electrically.

Some inorganic redox species take part in more complicated processes, and the balancing of their reactions is not intuitively obvious. For example, $Cr_2O_7^{2-}$ is reduced to Cr^{3+}. There is a systematic balancing procedure that serves to generate balanced redox reactions in all instances.

Step 1. Balance each half-reaction both chemically and electrically, using water and hydrogen ions where necessary. (We assume that the solvent is water.)

Step 2. Equate the electron yield in the oxidation to the electron consumption in the reduction.

Step 3. Add the balanced half-reactions, thus canceling electrons.

Step 4. If necessary, reduce stoichiometric coefficients to whole numbers, and, if desired, express the balanced equation in molecular rather than ionic form.

Example 13.1. Balance the reaction in which potassium dichromate oxidizes ferrous ion. The unbalanced dichromate half-reaction is $Cr_2O_7^{2-} \rightleftharpoons Cr^{3+}$.

$$6e + Cr_2O_7^{2-} + 14H^+ \rightleftharpoons 2Cr^{3+} + 7H_2O$$
$$Fe^{2+} \rightleftharpoons Fe^{3+} + e$$

(Step 1)

In balancing the dichromate half-reaction, two Cr^{3+} are placed on the right side. Then $7H_2O$ are added to make up the oxygens in dichromate, and $14H^+$ are added to the left side to balance the water. Finally the 6 electrons balance the half-reaction electronically.

$$6e + Cr_2O_7^{2-} + 14H^+ \rightleftharpoons 2Cr^{3+} + 7H_2O$$
$$6Fe^{2+} \rightleftharpoons 6Fe^{3+} + 6e$$

(Step 2)

$$Cr_2O_7^{2-} + 6Fe^{2+} + 14H^+ \rightleftharpoons 2Cr^{3+} + 6Fe^{3+} + 7H_2O \qquad \text{(Step 3)}$$
$$K_2Cr_2O_7 + 6FeCl_2 + 14HCl \rightleftharpoons 2CrCl_3 + 6FeCl_3 + 7H_2O + 2KCl \qquad \text{(Step 4)}$$

Very effective analytic methods have been based on redox reactions. In redox titrations a reductant is titrated with an oxidant (or vice versa). The endpoint can be detected with a redox indicator, which is a substance whose oxidized and reduced forms exhibit different colors. Alternatively an instrumental method of detection, to be described in Section 13.3, may be applied.

Organic Redox Reactions. The oxidation of organic compounds can be extremely complicated, and many of these reactions are not effectively reversible. Nevertheless, this kind of reaction is important pharmaceutically because many drug molecules undergo degradative oxidation (Connors et al. 1986), and a brief discussion is appropriate. The essential concept is that the oxidation state of a carbon atom is a result of the number of bonds from carbon to oxygen; the more carbon–oxygen bonds, the more highly oxidized the carbon atom is.[1] The simplest example of this concept is provided by these one-carbon compounds:

oxidation
$\longrightarrow$

$$
\underset{\overset{|}{H}}{\overset{\overset{H}{|}}{H-C-H}}
\qquad
\underset{\overset{|}{H}}{\overset{\overset{H}{|}}{H-C-OH}}
\qquad
\underset{H}{\overset{H}{\diagdown}}C{=}O
\qquad
H-C{\overset{\diagup O}{\diagdown OH}}
\qquad
O{=}C{=}O
$$

$\longleftarrow$
reduction

Now, if oxidation is the addition of oxygen, then the reverse reaction must be reduction. This leads to the identification of reduction with the addition of hydrogen. Let us broaden this idea to consider the addition of hydrogen to an olefin:

$$
H_2 + RCH{=}CHR \underset{\text{oxidation}}{\overset{\text{reduction}}{\rightleftarrows}} RCH_2CH_2R
$$

Since the hydrogenation reaction is a reduction, the reverse of this, a dehydrogenation, must be an oxidation. And now we see that we have an organic oxidation process that does not involve oxygen. We can apply the same idea to other reactions, as in the formal conversion of a sulfhydryl (mercaptan) group to a disulfide:

$$
2RSH \underset{\text{reduction}}{\overset{\text{oxidation}}{\rightleftarrows}} RSSR + H_2
$$

In the presence of oxygen (as the oxidizing agent) this reaction proceeds according to

$$
2RSH + \tfrac{1}{2}O_2 \rightleftharpoons RSSR + H_2O
$$

The mechanisms of organic redox reactions are seldom simple. Mechanisms (the detailed pathways from the initial to the final states) are investigated by the methods of kinetics, and do not form part of the field of classical thermodynamics.

We have now seen oxidation described as an electron loss, as an addition of oxygen, or as a loss of hydrogen, with reduction as the reverse process. Here is a yet broader context. We noted that a reducing agent is a substance that yields electrons, and, from Chapter 12, that a base is a substance that donates an electron pair. More generally we label as a *nucleophile* ("nucleus lover") a substance that furnishes electrons; thus reducing agents and bases are special cases of nucleophiles. Similarly, the class of *electrophiles* ("electron lovers") includes oxidizing agents and Lewis acids.

13.3. ELECTROCHEMICAL CELLS

Electrodes. In the present context, an electrode is a conductor of electricity immersed in an electrolyte solution. A transfer of charge may take place at the interface between the electrode surface and the solution. This charge transfer may result from the transfer either of electrons or of ions across the interface. Our present concern is with electron transfer, which arises from the occurrence of oxidation–reduction reactions.

Suppose that we assemble a system consisting of two electrodes, one each of two different redox half-reactions. One of these might be a piece of zinc metal partly immersed in a solution of zinc sulfate, with the other a piece of copper metal partly immersed in a solution of cupric sulfate. Assume that the solutions are in electrical contact but prevented from mixing and the metal electrodes are connected externally by a conductor, such as a length of copper wire. This assembly is an example of an *electrochemical cell*, this particular example being known as the *Daniell cell*. Figure 13.1 shows the Daniell cell.

If we prepare the solutions each to be about 1 M, the redox half-reactions that take place in this cell will be

$$Zn \rightleftharpoons Zn^{2+} + 2e$$
$$2e + Cu^{2+} \rightleftharpoons Cu$$

Thus, oxidation occurs at the zinc electrode (removing metal from the solid zinc) and reduction occurs at the copper electrode (plating copper metal onto the solid copper). We will shortly learn how the direction of reaction can be predicted. On atomic and subatomic scales, electrons are being released at the zinc electrode, they flow through the external conductor, constituting an electric current, and are

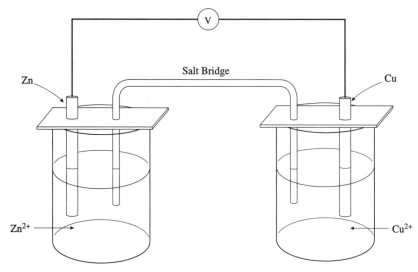

Figure 13.1. The Daniell cell. The salt bridge is a gel containing an electrolyte; it permits the passage of current, but prevents mixing of the solutions. [Reproduced by permission from Connors (1982).]

consumed at the copper electrode by reduction of cupric ions. If a voltmeter is introduced to the external circuit, it will indicate a voltage difference between the electrodes. The *electric potential* between the electrodes is the source of this measured voltage. [Electric potential is also called *electromotive force* (emf).] Electric potential is a consequence of a difference in charge between two points; it is the electrical analog of the chemical potential.

There are two ways to operate an electrochemical cell:

1. If we simply connect the external leads, thus creating a closed circuit, the redox reactions at the electrodes occur as we have described, and the cell generates an emf, which we can use to do work. In fact, the cell is a battery. In this mode of operation the cell half-reactions are occurring spontaneously. The cell is called a *galvanic* or *voltaic cell* when it is operating spontaneously. The essential thermodynamic phenomenon taking place is that chemical energy is being transformed to electrical energy.
2. The second mode of operation of a cell opposes the cell potential with a greater external potential, thus reversing the cell reactions. Now we are converting electrical energy to chemical energy. This is how we recharge a battery. In this type of operation the cell is called an *electrolytic cell*. The cell reactions are occurring nonspontaneously, provided with energy from an external source to drive them in reverse.

Whether an electrochemical cell is operating as a galvanic cell (spontaneously) or as an electrolytic cell (nonspontaneously), the electrode at which oxidation occurs is called the *anode* and the electrode at which reduction occurs is called the *cathode*. In the Daniell cell of Fig. 13.1, for example, when operating spontaneously the zinc electrode is the anode and the copper electrode is the cathode, whereas in the nonspontaneous mode the copper electrode is the anode and the zinc electrode is the cathode.

All electrochemistry takes place at interfaces between phases. This is explicitly indicated in a shorthand notation for describing electrochemical cells. The physical state (gas, liquid, solid) may be shown if not obvious, and solution activities or concentrations or gas pressure may be indicated. Here is the designation of the cell in Fig. 13.1:

$$Zn \mid ZnSO_4(1\,M) \parallel CuSO_4(1\,M) \mid Cu$$

A single vertical line represents an interface across which a potential difference exists. This potential difference is called an *electrode potential*. The potential of the cell as a whole, which is what we measure, is the sum of the two electrode potentials (we cannot measure a single electrode potential because a single electrode does not constitute a closed electric circuit). The double vertical line signifies a *salt bridge*, which is an electrolyte solution (usually in a viscous medium like agar or gelatin) that establishes electrical contact between the electrode solutions while keeping them physically separated. The existence of the salt bridge introduces a complication, for at each end of the salt bridge there is another interface, and across these interfaces there are compositional differences. This means that charge differences must exist across each solution/salt bridge interface, and therefore electric potentials must exist. This *liquid junction potential* is small but is measurable, and it is difficult to account for theoretically in a rigorous and accurate way, so an experimental approach is taken to render it negligible. Since the source of the liquid junction potential is known to be the different mobilities of cations and anions, salt bridges are constructed with high concentrations of KCl as the electrolyte, because K^+ and Cl^- have nearly the same mobility; thus the bulk of the current is carried by these ions, and the liquid junction potential is minimized. In extremely accurate work cells without liquid junctions may be used, but in usual laboratory situations our cells possess liquid junctions. We will not need to take the liquid junction potential into account.

The Nernst Equation.   Consider the generalized chemical reaction

$$aA + bB \rightleftharpoons mM + nN$$

In Chapter 4, Section 4.3 we derived Eq. (13.2) for this system

$$\Delta G = \Delta G^\circ + RT \ln \frac{a_M^m a_N^n}{a_A^a a_B^b} \tag{13.2}$$

where a_i represents the activity of substance i, ΔG is the free-energy change (per mole), and ΔG° is the standard free-energy change. It is important to realize that the activities in Eq. (13.2) do not necessarily represent the values at equilibrium. If, however, we now impose the equilibrium condition, meaning that $\Delta G = 0$, we obtain the important relationship (which we have used frequently in earlier developments)

$$\Delta G^\circ = -RT \ln K \tag{13.3}$$

where K is the equilibrium constant:

$$K = \frac{(a_M^n)_{eq}(a_N^n)_{eq}}{(a_A^a)_{eq}(a_B^b)_{eq}} \tag{13.4}$$

All the foregoing is familiar. We now make a connection to the electrochemical cell, in which the reaction is an oxidation–reduction reaction, and the chemical process results in electron transfer across the electrode–solution interfaces. The key idea is that if the cell operates reversibly (in the thermodynamic meaning of this term), the electrical work produced will be the free energy change for the process, which is the maximum work (not counting work of expansion) that the system can perform. The cell will operate reversibly if an infinitesimal amount of reaction occurs, and this condition requires that zero or an infinitesimal amount of current flow through the external circuit. This is accomplished by opposing the cell potential with an external potential such that zero current flows. The measured potential is then the cell potential at zero current.

From Section 13.1, electrical work is the product of potential and charge. Let E represent the cell potential [measured in volts (V)] and F the charge of one mole of electrons [measured in coulombs (C)], so that $F = eN_A = 96,485\,C\,mol^{-1}$. The quantity F is called the *Faraday*. Then for a redox reaction in which n electrons per molecule are transferred,

$$\Delta G = -nFE \tag{13.5}$$

where the negative sign is inserted so as to achieve agreement between the sign conventions applying to free-energy changes and cell potentials, as we will later see. By analogy with Eq. (13.5) we also write

$$\Delta G° = -nFE° \tag{13.6}$$

where $E°$, called the standard cell potential, is the value of the cell potential when reactants and products are in their standard states. For convenience let us define

$$L = \frac{a_M^m a_N^n}{a_A^a a_B^b} \tag{13.7}$$

where the activities need not be equilibrium activities. Now combining Eqs. (13.2), and (13.5)–(13.7) we get

$$E = E° - \frac{RT}{nF} \ln L \tag{13.8}$$

This is the *Nernst equation*, which relates the cell potential at zero current, E, to the activities (or concentrations, when activity coefficients are essentially unity) of the reactant and product species of the electrochemical cell reaction.

Equations (13.3) and (13.6) combined give

$$E° = \frac{RT}{nF} \ln K \tag{13.9}$$

where K is the equilibrium constant of the cell reaction.

At 25°C the Nernst equation takes the form

$$E = E° - \frac{0.059}{n} \log L \tag{13.10}$$

where the final term is now expressed in base 10 logarithms.[2] According to Eq. (13.10), a change in L by a factor of 10 results in a change in the cell potential of 59/n mV. This result is said to be a "Nernstian response," and is evidence that the electrochemical system is well defined and is operating reversibly.

The foregoing equations allow us to make these associations:

1. If ΔG is negative, E is positive. The cell reaction is spontaneous; that is, with the reactant and product concentrations as specified, the reaction spontaneously proceeds from left to right.
2. If ΔG is positive, E is negative, and the reaction is nonspontaneous; it proceeds from right to left.
3. If the system is at equilibrium, then $L = K$, $\Delta G = 0$, $E = 0$. The cell can do no work.
4. If $K > 1$, E° is positive; if $K < 1$, E° is negative.

It is important to keep in mind that we have the experimental ability to arrange the reactant and product concentrations at levels far from equilibrium, and to maintain them in such a state by means of the salt bridge separation shown in Fig. 13.1, or an equivalent device; moreover, by holding the system in the zero-current condition, we achieve thermodynamic reversibility. However, if we allow current to flow, the available electrical work is less than the maximum work as measured or as calculated under conditions of reversibility.

Standard Potentials and Sign Conventions. We have seen that a functioning electrochemical cell requires a complete circuit, which means that it must possess two electrodes. We measure the cell potential. Although we cannot measure individual electrode potentials (because we would then have an open circuit), the concept of an electrode potential is so attractive that we adopt the view that a cell potential can be expressed as the sum of its electrode potentials. Consider again the Daniell cell:

$$Zn \,|\, ZnSO_4 \,\|\, CuSO_4 \,|\, Cu$$

According to this concept we write

$$E_{cell} = E_{Zn,Zn^{2+}} + E_{Cu^{2+},Cu} \tag{13.11}$$

Observe how the order of the subscripts tells which half-reaction is an oxidation and which is a reduction.[3] An analogous equation relates the standard cell potential to the standard electrode potentials:

$$E^\circ_{cell} = E^\circ_{Zn,Zn^{2+}} + E^\circ_{Cu^{2+},Cu} \tag{13.12}$$

Strictly speaking, the term *standard electrode potential* should be used only for the quantity describing the half-reaction as a reduction (IUPAC 1993, p. 61), but we will relax this nomenclature, using the direction of the subscripts to make fully explicit whether the half-reaction is an oxidation or a reduction.

We must now consider the sign conventions relating to potentials. Two different concepts are involved, and some confusion is possible because historically we have used the words *positive* and *negative* to denote both a mathematical sign and a physical characteristic (Anson 1959).

Concept 1: The Potential of the Physical Electrode. We have seen that it would be convenient to have available values of individual electrode potentials, but we have also seen that we can only measure cell potentials. This difficulty is overcome by means of the universal agreement that the standard hydrogen electrode, diagrammed as

$$\text{Pt}, \text{H}_2(1\,\text{atm})\,|\,\text{H}^+(a=1)$$

is to be assigned an electrode potential of zero volts at all temperatures. The electrode reaction is

$$\text{H}_2 \rightleftharpoons 2\text{H}^+ + 2\text{e} \qquad (E^\circ_{\text{H}_2,\text{H}^+} = 0.00\,\text{V})$$

Now, if we form a cell of the standard hydrogen electrode with any other electrode, the measured cell potential is to be assigned to the second electrode. But besides its magnitude, this potential has a sign, which is determined by whether the second electrode has an excess or a deficiency of electrons relative to the hydrogen electrode. Suppose that we construct the following cell:

$$\text{Pt}, \text{H}_2(1\,\text{atm})\,|\,\text{H}^+(a=1)\,\|\,\text{Zn}^{2+}(a=1)\,|\,\text{Zn}$$

We write the cell reaction with the left-hand electrode expressed as an oxidation and the right-hand electrode as a reduction:

$$\text{H}_2 + \text{Zn}^{2+} \rightleftharpoons 2\text{H}^+ + \text{Zn}$$

Of course, it is irrelevant to the physical system how we choose to write the reaction, and in the laboratory it is observed that, in this cell, the zinc electrode is negative relative to the hydrogen electrode; that is, oxidation occurs at the zinc electrode, releasing electrons. This is the physical characteristic alluded to earlier; it is a convention that we assign a negative charge to the electron, but it is a physical fact that in this cell oxidation occurs at the zinc electrode. The measured potential (at 25°C) is $-0.76\,\text{V}$, and since we can write

$$E^\circ_{\text{cell}} = E^\circ_{\text{H}_2,\text{H}^+} + E^\circ_{\text{Zn}^{2+},\text{Zn}} = -0.76\,\text{V}$$

Table 13.1. Standard electrode potentials at 25°C

Reduction Half-reaction	$E°$/V
$Na^+ + e = Na$	-2.71
$Zn^{2+} + 2e = Zn$	-0.76
$Fe^{2+} + 2e = Fe$	-0.44
$Ni^{2+} + 2e = Ni$	-0.25
$AgI(s) + e = Ag + I^-$	-0.15
$Sn^{2+} + 2e = Sn$	-0.14
$Pb^{2+} + 2e = Pb$	-0.13
$2H^+ + 2e = H_2$	(0.00)
$AgBr(s) + e = Ag + Br^-$	0.07
$S_4O_6^{2-} + 2e = 2S_2O_3^{2-}$	0.08
$Sn^{4+} + 2e = Sn^{2+}$	0.15
$AgCl(s) + e = Ag + Cl^-$	0.22
$Hg_2Cl_2(s) + 2e = 2Hg + 2Cl^-$	0.27
$Cu^{2+} + 2e = Cu$	0.34
$Cu^+ + e = Cu$	0.52
$I_3^- + 2e = 3I^-$	0.55
$Fe^{3+} + e = Fe^{2+}$	0.77
$Ag^+ + e = Ag$	0.80
$Cu^{2+} + I^- + e = CuI$	0.86
$Cl_2 + 2e = 2Cl^-$	1.36
$MnO_4^- + 8H^+ + 5e = Mn^{2+} + 4H_2O$	1.51
$H_2O_2 + 2H^+ + 2e = 2H_2O$	1.77

we can state that $E°_{Zn^{2+},Zn} = -0.76$ V. This is how standard electrode potentials are measured. Table 13.1 lists some standard electrode potentials. From the Nernst equation, Eq. (13.10), which can be written for either an electrode or a cell, the standard potential is equal to the potential when $L = 1$, and this condition is met when all reactant and product species are in their standard states. When determining standard potentials, the hydrogen electrode is always written on the left (as an oxidation) (IUPAC 1993, p. 61).

If a cell, or indeed a reaction mixture, is constituted of any two half-reactions listed in Table 13.1, all species being in their standard states of unit activity, then the more negative $E°$ value will represent the oxidation. Another way to say this is that the more positive the electrode potential, the greater its oxidizing power. Thus we can predict that permanganate (MnO_4^-) will oxidize Fe^{2+} to Fe^{3+}, and that iodine (as the triiodide ion I_3^-) will oxidize (i.e., will be reduced by) thiosulfate, $S_2O_3^{2-}$. This argument is made more systematic in Example 13.5 to follow.

Concept 2: The Potential of a Half-Reaction. From Eq. (13.5), $\Delta G = -nFE$, and from the thermodynamic result that a spontaneous reaction has a negative free energy change, we conclude that a spontaneous reaction has a positive potential. But we know that the reverse reaction is nonspontaneous, so its free-energy change is positive; hence its potential is negative. Therefore, in complete harmony with our practice in altering the sign of a thermodynamic quantity when we reverse the direction of the reaction, we also alter the sign of a potential when we reverse the direction of the reaction. Thus since $E^\circ_{Zn^{2+},Zn} = -0.76$ V for the half-reaction $Zn^{2+} + 2e = Zn$, we can write $E^\circ_{Zn,Zn^{2+}} = +0.76$ V for the half-reaction $Zn = Zn^{2+} + 2e$.

From Eq. (13.9), this sign change convention is equivalent to converting an equilibrium constant to its reciprocal when a reaction is written in the reverse direction.

Applications of Electrode Potentials. Electrochemical calculations are not routinely necessary in the solution of pharmaceutical problems, so our treatment will be brief; but there are two reasons to include some level of discussion. The first is that these calculations offer a perfect example of the power of thermodynamics to predict the direction of chemical change. The second reason is to provide a sound basis for the discussions in Sections 13.4 and 13.5.

We begin with the Nernst equation

$$E = E^\circ - \frac{0.059}{n} \log L \tag{13.13}$$

where

$$L = \frac{\prod a_p^v}{\prod a_r^v} \tag{13.14}$$

In Equation (13.14), $\prod$ signifies "the product of," a_p represents activity of product(s), a_r is the activity of reactant(s), and v specifies the power to which each activity is raised; v is the appropriate stoichiometric coefficient in the balanced cell reaction. The Nernst equation bears a formal resemblance to the Henderson–Hasselbalch equation, Eq. (12.36), and it is used in much the same way. The equation relates the three quantities E, E°, L, and if we know two of these, we can calculate the third. The methods will be illustrated with numerical examples.

Example 13.2. Calculate the potential of this cell at 25°C and predict the direction of the reaction. That is, will ferrous ion be oxidized or will ferric ion be reduced under these conditions?

$$Pt \,|\, Fe^{2+}(1 \times 10^{-6}\,M), Fe^{3+}(0.05\,M) \,\|\, KI(0.001\,M) \,|\, AgI, Ag$$

The Pt is inert and serves only to make electrical contact between the solution and the external conductor (as in the hydrogen electrode).

Always begin by writing the balanced cell reaction, treating the left-hand electrode as the anode (where oxidation takes place). For this cell

$$AgI + Fe^{2+} \rightleftharpoons Fe^{3+} + Ag + I^-$$

We now set up the Nernst equation:

$$E_{cell} = E_{cell}^{\circ} - 0.059 \log \frac{a_{Fe^{3+}} a_{I^-} a_{Ag}}{a_{AgI} a_{Fe^{2+}}}$$

The standard electrode potentials are found in Table 13.1:

$$E_{cell}^{\circ} = E_{Fe^{2+},Fe^{3+}}^{\circ} + E_{AgI,Ag}^{\circ}$$
$$= -0.77 - 0.15 = -0.92 \text{ V}$$

Since Ag and AgI are solids, they are in their standard states of unit activity, and activities of solutes will be approximated by concentrations:

$$E_{cell} = -0.92 - 0.059 \log \frac{(0.05)(1 \times 10^{-3})}{(1 \times 10^{-6})}$$
$$= -0.92 - 0.059 \log 50$$
$$= -0.82 \text{ V}$$

Since the calculated cell potential is negative, the reaction as it has been written is nonspontaneous. Therefore, at these concentrations, ferric ion will be reduced to ferrous ion and silver will be oxidized to Ag^+ (which precipitates as AgI).

Example 13.3. What is the solubility product of silver bromide?
    This may seem a peculiar question in the present context, because the solubility product (Chapter 10) does not describe a redox reaction.

$$AgBr(s) \rightleftharpoons Ag^+ + Br^-$$
$$K_{sp} = a_{Ag^+} a_{Br^-}$$

However, we can "compose" this reaction from two redox half-reactions as follows:

$$AgBr(s) + e \rightleftharpoons Ag + Br^-$$
$$Ag \rightleftharpoons Ag^+ + e$$

$$\overline{}$$

$$AgBr(s) \rightleftharpoons Ag^+ + Br^-$$

From Table 13.1 we find

$$E_{cell}^{\circ} = E_{AgBr,Ag}^{\circ} + E_{Ag,Ag^+}^{\circ}$$
$$= 0.07 - 0.80$$
$$= -0.73 \text{ V}$$

We now apply Eq. (13.9) at 25°C, with $n = 1$, or

$$\text{Log } K_{sp} = \frac{E^\circ_{cell}}{0.059}$$
$$= -12.37$$

or $K_{sp} = 4.3 \times 10^{-12}$. It is often more accurate to determine such equilibrium constants from potential measurements than by direct chemical analysis.

Example 13.4. Calculate the potential of this Daniell cell:

$$Zn \,|\, Zn^{2+} (0.35 \text{ M}) \,\|\, Cu^{2+} (0.001 \text{ M}) \,|\, Cu$$

The cell reaction is

$$Zn + Cu^{2+} \rightleftharpoons Zn^{2+} + Cu$$

The Nernst equation for this cell is

$$E_{cell} = E^\circ_{cell-} \frac{0.59}{n} \log \frac{a_{Zn^{2+}} a_{Cu}}{a_{Cu^{2+}} a_{Zn}}$$

where $n = 2$. We find the standard electrode potentials in Table 13.1:

$$E^\circ_{cell} = E^\circ_{Zn,Zn^{2+}} + E^\circ_{Cu^{2+},Cu}$$
$$= 0.76 + 0.34$$
$$= +1.10 \text{ V}$$

Potentials are intensive quantities, so they are independent of the amount of reaction. From the equation $\Delta G = -nFE$ we see that $E = -\Delta G/nF$; a larger n value gives a correspondingly larger ΔG, but E is unaffected. This holds because the amount of oxidation is exactly balanced by the amount of reduction. Continuing with the calculation, we have

$$E_{cell} = +1.10 - \frac{0.059}{2} \log \frac{0.35}{0.001}$$
$$= +1.02 \text{ V}$$

The cell reaction is spontaneous as written.

Example 13.5. Predict what will happen in this cell:

$$Ag, AgCl \,|\, Cl^- (1 \text{ M}), Cl_2 (p = 1 \text{ atm}) \,|\, Pt$$

The cell reaction is balanced as follows:

$$2Ag + 2Cl^- \rightleftharpoons 2AgCl + 2e$$
$$Cl_2 + 2e \rightleftharpoons 2Cl^-$$

$$\overline{}$$

$$2Ag + Cl_2 \rightleftharpoons 2AgCl$$

We recognize that all species are in their standard states, so $L = 1$ and $E_{cell} = E^\circ_{cell}$. From Table 13.1

$$E^\circ_{cell} = E^\circ_{Ag,AgCl} + E^\circ_{Cl_2,Cl^-}$$
$$= -0.22 + 1.36$$
$$= +1.14\,V$$

The reaction is spontaneous as written; that is, Cl_2 oxidizes Ag. Note that in the silver–silver chloride electrode the chloride ion does not undergo a redox process, whereas in the chlorine electrode Cl^- is a product of a reduction.

Example 13.5 places on a formal basis the predictions made earlier when discussing standard potentials; these are seen to constitute a special case (the case $L = 1$) of the Nernst equation.

Example 13.6. What is the potential of this cell at 25°C?

$$Cu \,|\, Cu^{2+}(0.25\,M) \,\|\, Cu^{2+}(0.01\,M) \,|\, Cu$$

Obviously the two electrodes are identical except for the ion concentrations. We proceed in the usual manner:

Left electrode:	$Cu \rightleftharpoons Cu^{2+}(0.25\,M) + 2e$
Right electrode:	$2e + Cu^{2+}(0.01\,M) \rightleftharpoons Cu$
Overall reaction:	$Cu^{2+}(0.01\,M) \rightleftharpoons Cu^{2+}(0.25\,M)$

This is called a *concentration cell*. The Nernst equation applied to this cell is

$$E_{cell} = E^\circ_{cell} - \frac{0.059}{2} \log \frac{0.25}{0.01}$$

where $E^\circ_{cell} = E^\circ_{Cu,Cu^{2+}} + E^\circ_{Cu^{2+},Cu} = 0$. Thus we find $E_{cell} = -0.041\,V$. The cell reaction is nonspontaneous, which accords with expectation; the spontaneous direction of diffusion is from higher to lower concentration (actually chemical potential).

The experimental measurement of electric potential is called *potentiometry.* When a redox titration is carried out with measurement of the potential as a function of titrant volume, the plot of potential E against titrant volume has the appearance of the acid–base titration curves that we studied in Chapter 12, and the endpoint is determined from the break in this potentiometric titration curve. By applying the Nernst equation at successive stages in the titration, it is possible to calculate such a curve.

13.4. pH MEASUREMENT

pH and the Hydrogen Electrode. The potential of certain electrochemical cells depends on the pH of the cell solution, and this dependence offers a means for the potentiometric measurement of pH. The hydrogen electrode is the classic type of a pH responsive electrode. Let us consider the following electrochemical cell

$$Pt, H_2(p = 1 \text{ atm}) \,|\, H^+(a_{H^+}) \,|\, \text{reference electrode}$$

where the reference electrode need not be specified at present except to require that its potential not be affected by the pH of the cell solution. The hydrogen electrode consists of hydrogen gas bubbled through the aqueous solution; electrical contact is made through platinum metal, which is unreactive. Proceeding to describe this cell quantitatively, we write

$$E_{cell} = E_{H_2,H^+} + E_{ref}$$

The potential of the hydrogen electrode is expanded by means of the Nernst equation; the electrode reaction is

$$H_2 \rightleftharpoons 2H^+ + 2e$$

The result is (at 25°C)

$$E_{cell} = E^\circ_{H_2,H^+} - \frac{0.059}{2} \log \frac{a^2_{H^+}}{p_{H_2}} + E_{ref}$$

We combine this equation with the convention $E^\circ_{H_2,H^+} = 0$ and the definition $pH = -\log a_{H^+}$, obtaining

$$E_{cell} = 0.059\,pH + E_{ref} \tag{13.15}$$

This last equation says that the cell potential is linearly related to the pH of the cell solution. The slope of the line is $dE_{cell}/dpH = 0.059$ V, or 59 mV per pH unit. This is the theoretical response of a pH responsive electrode at 25°C. (In general, the response is 2.303 RT/F V per pH unit.) This means that in order to measure pH to within 0.01 pH unit, we must be able to measure the cell emf to within 0.00059 V.

Practical Electrodes for pH Measurement. First we consider the reference electrode whose potential appears in Eq. (13.15). The most widely used reference electrode for practical pH measurements is the *saturated calomel electrode* (SCE). The SCE is composed of a saturated solution of potassium chloride that is also saturated with mercurous chloride (calomel). The solution is in contact with mercury metal, through which electrical contact is made with the external circuit. The SCE half-reaction is

$$Hg_2Cl_2 + 2e \rightleftharpoons 2Hg + 2Cl^-$$

and its potential, which is unaffected by pH, is +0.244 V. A salt bridge must be placed between the SCE and the "test solution" whose pH is to be measured so that the SCE saturated solution is not diluted. Then a complete cell consisting of a hydrogen electrode and the SCE looks like this:

$$Pt, H_2(p = 1\ atm)\,|\,H^+(a_{H^+})\,\|\,KCl(sat), Hg_2Cl_2(sat)\,|\,Hg$$

Its cell potential is given as follows, by an argument identical to the preceding one:

$$E_{cell} = 0.059\,pH + (E_{SCE} + E_{lj}) \tag{13.16}$$

where E_{lj} is the liquid junction potential.

Since E_{lj} is unknown, we are unable to apply Eq. (13.16) directly to calculate pH from a measured value of E_{cell}. We therefore proceed by, in effect, measuring differences in pH between two solutions. Let E represent the cell potential when the cell solution has a certain pH, and similarly let E_S be the cell potential when the cell solution has the value pH_S. Then writing Eq. (13.16) for both solutions and subtracting one equation from the other gives

$$pH = pH_S + \frac{E - E_S}{0.059} \tag{13.17}$$

at 25°C, or, in general

$$pH = pH_S + \frac{E - E_S}{2.303\,RT/F} \tag{13.18}$$

The success of this procedure depends on the liquid junction potential remaining essentially constant as the pH is changed from pH to pH_S. This assumption is reasonable if pH and pH_S are not greatly different. Although Eq. (13.18) is not thermodynamically exact because of this assumption of the constancy of E_{lj}, it constitutes the operational definition of pH for practical laboratory work. If we know the value pH_S of a standard solution and measure its corresponding E_S, then replacement of the standard solution by the unknown test solution and measurement of E permits us to calculate the unknown pH by Eq. (13.18). Actually the calculation is automatically carried out by the electronic potentiometer (called a *pH meter*) used to measure the cell potential. The cell is "calibrated" by setting the pH meter to the known pH_S value with the standard solution in the cell. Then the standard solution is replaced with the test solution and the meter gives the unknown pH value. An adjustment on the meter calculates the value of $2.303\,RT/F$ for the experimental temperature.

Obviously the accuracy of this pH measurement procedure depends on the accuracy with which pH_S values are known. For all pH measurement in aqueous solutions the pH_S values given in Table 13.2 will suffice. These pH_S values were determined on cells without liquid junctions by Bates and coworkers (Bates 1962; Staples and Bates 1969). (Ordinary laboratory work yields pH measurements accurate at best to ±0.01pH unit.) Table 13.3 gives the compositions of these standard pH buffer solutions.

We have seen that the cell should be standardized with a standard buffer whose pH_S is close to the anticipated pH of the test solution in order to minimize variation in the liquid junction potential. It is also good experimental practice to measure the pH of a second standard buffer after standardization against the first one; this

Table 13.2. Standard pH$_s$ values

t (°C)	Tartrate	Citrate	Phthalate	Phosphate (1 : 1)	Phosphate (1 : 3.5)	Borax	Carbonate
0	—	3.864	4.003	6.984	7.534	9.464	10.321
5	—	3.839	3.999	6.951	7.500	9.395	10.243
10	—	3.819	3.998	6.923	7.472	9.332	10.178
15	—	3.802	3.999	6.900	7.448	9.276	10.116
20	—	3.788	4.002	6.881	7.429	9.225	10.060
25	3.557	3.776	4.008	6.865	7.413	9.180	10.012
30	3.552	3.767	4.015	6.853	7.400	9.139	9.968
35	3.549	3.759	4.024	6.844	7.389	9.102	9.928
38	3.548	—	4.030	6.840	7.384	9.081	—
40	3.547	3.754	4.035	6.838	7.380	9.068	9.892
45	3.547	3.750	4.047	6.834	7.373	9.038	9.856
50	3.549	3.749	4.060	6.833	7.367	9.011	9.825
55	3.554	—	4.075	6.834	—	8.985	—
60	3.560	—	4.091	6.836	—	8.962	—
70	3.580	—	4.126	6.845	—	8.921	—
80	3.609	—	4.164	6.859	—	8.885	—
90	3.650	—	4.205	6.877	—	8.850	—
95	3.674	—	4.227	6.886	—	8.833	—

Table 13.3. Compositions of standard buffer solutions [a]

Solution	m	Substance	Weight (g) [b]	pH$_s$ at 25°C
Tartrate	~0.034	KHC$_4$H$_4$O$_6$	Saturated at 25°C	3.557
Citrate	0.05	KH$_2$C$_6$H$_5$O$_7$	11.41	3.776
Phthalate	0.05	KHC$_8$H$_4$O$_4$	10.12	4.008
Phosphate (1 : 1)	$\begin{cases} 0.025 \\ 0.025 \end{cases}$	KH$_2$PO$_4$ Na$_2$HPO$_4$	$\left.\begin{array}{r} 3.39 \\ 3.53 \end{array}\right\}$	6.865
Phosphate (1 : 3.5)	$\begin{cases} 0.008695 \\ 0.03043 \end{cases}$	KH$_2$PO$_4$ Na$_2$HPO$_4$	$\left.\begin{array}{r} 1.179 \\ 4.30 \end{array}\right\}$	7.413
Borax	0.01	Na$_2$B$_4$O$_7 \cdot 10$H$_2$O	3.80	9.180
Carbonate	$\begin{cases} 0.025 \\ 0.025 \end{cases}$	NaHCO$_3$ Na$_2$CO$_3$	$\left.\begin{array}{r} 2.092 \\ 2.640 \end{array}\right\}$	10.012

[a] Bates 1962; Staples and Bates 1969.
[b] Weight of substance (in air near sea level) per liter of solution, prepared with carbonate-free distilled water.

step checks the correct operation of the electrode system, the pH meter, and the standardization of the cell.

To this point we have treated the hydrogen electrode as the pH responsive electrode. The hydrogen electrode, though thermodynamically well defined, is not very practical for routine use, so alternatives have been sought, and in all practical laboratory and field measurements the pH responsive electrode is a device known as the *glass electrode*. This electrode possesses a very thin glass membrane separating the test solution from a solution of fixed pH. A potential is developed across this glass membrane that is related to the pH difference on the two sides of the glass. (This is an ion-transfer effect, not a redox phenomenon; it is treated in Section 13.5.) A practical cell for pH measurement then has this form:

$$\text{Ag} \mid \text{Ag Cl(sat)}, \text{HCl} \mid \text{glass} \mid \text{test solution} \parallel \text{SCE}$$

The silver–silver chloride electrode serves to make electrical connection between the glass membrane and the external circuit. The pH response of this electrode is Nernstian, so the measurement of pH with a glass–SCE cell follows Eq. (13.16).

pK_a Determination. Accurate values of pK_a can be measured with a glass–SCE cell if appropriate attention is paid to temperature control and standardization of the electrodes. For weak acid HA the thermodynamic constant K_a is defined as

$$K_a = \frac{a_{H^+} a_{A^-}}{a_{HA}} \tag{13.19}$$

The quantity we actually measure in the laboratory, however, is called the apparent constant, K_a', defined by

$$K_a' = \frac{a_{H^+} [A^-]}{[HA]} \tag{13.20}$$

This is because the glass–SCE cell gives a pH value defined by

$$pH = -\log a_{H^+} \tag{13.21}$$

and because we prepare solutions to have known *concentrations* of A^- and HA.[4] Our first problem is to measure pK_a'; next we must correct pK_a' to pK_a.

From Eq. (13.20), we obtain

$$pK_a' = pH - \log \frac{[A^-]}{[HA]} \tag{13.22}$$

and from Eqs. (12.33) and (12.34), we have

$$pK_a' = pH - \log \frac{b + [H^+] - [OH^-]}{a - [H^+] + [OH^-]} \tag{13.23}$$

where b is the concentration of the counterion to A^- and $a + b$ is the total solute concentration: $a + b = [HA] + [A^-]$. Since we know a and b from the manner in which the solution was prepared, and we measure pH, we can calculate pK_a'.[5] A series of solutions can efficiently be prepared, each solution having varied values of b such that the pH of all solutions will be within about 1 unit of pK_a' (so as to ensure good buffer capacity). The pH values of the solutions are measured, and pK_a' is calculated for each solution. If pH is in the approximate range of 4–10, the $[H^+]$ and $[OH^-]$ quantities in Eq. (13.23) will usually be negligible.

It will be seen that this procedure is essentially a titration of the weak acid HA with the strong base MOH, where $b = [M^+]$. If the pK_a of a weak base B is to be measured, the usual procedure is to titrate B with strong acid HX in an analogous manner. Now $a + b = [BH^+] + [B]$ and $a = [X^-]$. Equation (13.23) is again applicable.

The same value for pK_a' should be obtained whether we start with the conjugate acid (e.g., acetic acid) and titrate with strong base, or start with its conjugate base (e.g., sodium acetate) and titrate with strong acid, provided the ionic strength is substantially identical in the two titrations.

With the apparent constant pK_a' at hand, we turn to the problem of finding the thermodynamic constant pK_a. For reasons discussed in Chapter 8, pK_a' varies with the ionic strength of the solution, so it is not a true constant. On the other hand, pK_a is defined to be a constant (at fixed temperature and pressure); in other words, pK_a is that unique value of pK_a' in the reference state of the solute, where activity coefficients are unity. We can correct a pK_a' value for nonideal behavior by applying the Debye–Hückel theory (Section 8.3).

Consider the uncharged acid HA, whose apparent constant K_a' is defined in Eq. (13.20). We may take it that at low to moderate values of ionic strength the activity of the uncharged form HA is equal to its concentration. The activity of the ion A^-, however, is given by

$$a_{A^-} = \gamma_{A^-} [A^-]$$

where γ_{A^-} is the mean ionic activity coefficient. With these identities, Eqs. (13.19) and (13.20) become

$$K_a = \frac{a_{H^+} \gamma_{A^-} [A^-]}{a_{HA}}$$

and

$$K_a' = \frac{a_{H^+} [A^-]}{a_{HA}}$$

or, combining these equations

$$K_a = \gamma_{A^-} K_a'$$

which in logarithmic form becomes

$$pK_a = pK_a' - \log \gamma_{A^-} \qquad (13.24)$$

Now we use the Debye–Hückel equation, Eq. (8.26), in Eq. (13.24):

$$pK_a = pK_a' + \frac{0.509\sqrt{I}}{1 + \sqrt{I}} \qquad (13.25)$$

The ionic strength I is calculated with

$$I = \frac{1}{2} \sum c_i z_i^2 \qquad (13.26)$$

where c represents the concentration of species i and z_i is its charge; the summation includes all the ions in the solution. Equation (13.25) corrects pK_a' to pK_a for uncharged acids.

For a positively charged acid such as BH^+, the ionic activity coefficient appears in the denominator of K_a, with the result that Eq. (13.24) takes the form

$$pK_a = pK_a' + \log \gamma_{BH^+} \qquad (13.27)$$

leading to

$$pK_a = pK_a' - \frac{0.509\sqrt{I}}{1 + \sqrt{I}} \qquad (13.28)$$

Equations (13.25) and (13.28) apply at 25°C.

Example 13.7. Suppose that 10.0 mL of a solution 0.10 M with respect to both acetic acid and sodium chloride was mixed with 10.0 mL of 0.05 M sodium hydroxide at 25°C. The pH of this solution was 4.64. What is the thermodynamic pK_a of acetic acid?

The total solute concentration (i.e., acetic acid plus acetate ion) is 0.05 M; this is equal to $a + b$ in the symbolism of Eq. (13.23). The quantity b is given by $(10.0)(0.05)/20.0 = 0.025$ M. From Eq. (13.23), we obtain $pK'_a = 4.64$, because the quantity $[H^+]$ is negligible.

The ionic strength receives contributions from both the sodium chloride (0.05 M) and the sodium acetate (0.025 M); from Eq. (13.26), $I = 0.075$ M. Finally, Eq. (13.25) gives

$$pK_a = 4.64 + \frac{(0.509)(0.274)}{1.274} = 4.75$$

Example 13.8. Given: 0.0541 g of 4-cresol (MW 108.1) dissolved in 47.5 mL of water at 20°C. After 1.0 mL of 0.10 M KOH was added, the pH was 9.55; after the addition of 3.0 mL of 0.10 M KOH, the pH was 10.29. Calculate the apparent constant and the thermodynamic constant.

Calculate that $0.0541/108.1 = 5.00 \times 10^{-4}$ mol of solute, or 0.5 mmol, was taken. When 1.0 mL of strong base titrant had been added, the volume was 48.5 mL, so the total solute concentration was $0.5/48.5 = 0.01031$ M; this is the quantity $a + b$. The value of b is $(1.0)(0.10)/48.5 = 0.002062$. Since the pH is quite high, let us apply the correction for $[OH^-]$. At 20°C, $pK_w = 14.17$ (Table 12.1), so $pOH = 4.62$ and $[OH^-] = 2.4 \times 10^{-5}$. Equation (13.23) gives

$$pK'_a = 9.55 - \log \frac{0.002062 - 0.000024}{0.00825 + 0.000024}$$
$$= 10.16$$

The ionic strength of this solution is (neglecting the hydroxide) equal to b, or 0.00206 M. Applying Eq. (13.25) gives $pK_a = 10.16 + 0.02 = 10.18$.

After the addition of 3.0 mL of titrant, we calculate these quantities: $a + b = 0.00990$ M; $b = 0.00594$ M; $[OH^-] = 1.3 \times 10^{-4}$, and Eq. (13.23) gives

$$pK'_a = 10.29 - \log \frac{0.00594 - 0.00013}{0.00396 + 0.00013}$$
$$= 10.14$$

The ionic strength is now 0.00607 M, and Eq. (13.25) gives $pK_a = 10.14 + 0.04 = 10.18$.

The data in Example 13.8 are from Albert and Serjeant (1984), who give much useful information on pK_a determination. These numerical examples are helpful

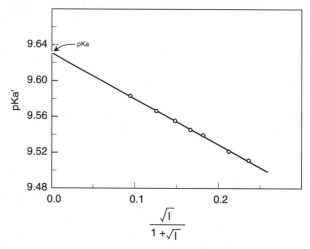

Figure 13.2. Plot according to Eq. (13.29) for β-naphthol at 20°C (Albert and Serjeant 1984).

in showing typical magnitudes of the activity coefficient corrections, which in Example 13.8 appear to be only slightly greater than the usual experimental uncertainty in the pH measurement.

An alternative approach to estimating pK_a from measurements of pK_a' is to note that Eq. (13.25) can be written in the form

$$pK_a' = pK_a - \frac{0.509\sqrt{I}}{1 + \sqrt{I}} \tag{13.29}$$

which suggests that if pK_a' is measured as a function of ionic strength, a plot of pK_a' against $\sqrt{I}/(1 + \sqrt{I})$ will be a straight line, which can be extrapolated to yield pK_a as the intercept. Figure 13.2 is a plot of Eq. (13.29) for β-naphthol (Albert and Serjeant 1984). The line extrapolates to $pK_a = 9.63$; its slope is -0.505.

13.5. ION-SELECTIVE MEMBRANE ELECTRODES

Except for our brief discussion of the pH-sensitive glass electrode, all the preceding treatment of electrical phenomena has been based on electron transfer across the electrode–solution interface. We now turn to the ion transfer mechanism as the basis of an electrochemical cell.

Theory of the Electrode Response.   Before we examine the physical nature of the electrode substance, we will simply designate it as a "membrane"; it is the site of ion-exchange with the electrolyte solution. A schematic representation of an electrochemical cell incorporating such a membrane electrode is

Internal reference electrode | a_{int} | membrane | a_{ext} ‖ external reference electrode

The activities refer to the ion for which the membrane serves as an ion exchanger; a_{int} is the internal (fixed) ion activity and a_{ext} is the sample solution ion activity. The reference electrodes are connected to the external circuit. The potential of this cell is given by

$$E_{cell} = E_{int\ ref} + E_{ext\ ref} + E_{lj} + E_{membrane} \tag{13.30}$$

Although we anticipate that the membrane response is a consequence of ion exchange between the membrane and the solution, we can model this formally as the result of two redox half-reactions. Suppose the ion in question is the cation M^{n+}. Then

Left (oxidation):	$M_{int} \rightleftharpoons M_{int}^{n+} + n(e)$
Right (reduction):	$n(e) + M_{ext}^{n+} \rightleftharpoons M_{ext}$
Overall reaction:	$M_{ext}^{n+} \rightleftharpoons M_{int}^{n+}$

Note that, in the usual manner, we write the oxidation at the left electrode. (We do not include M_{int} and M_{ext} in the overall reaction because, as pure metal, they are in the standard state of unit activity.) Comparison of the development to this point with Example 13.6 reveals that the membrane electrode is formally part of a concentration cell. The Nernst equation gives

$$E_{membrane} = -\frac{RT}{nF} \ln \frac{a_{int}}{a_{ext}}$$

which can be combined with Eq. (13.30) to yield

$$E_{cell} = \text{constant} + \frac{RT}{nF} \ln a_{ext}$$

or, at 25°C

$$E_{cell} = \text{constant} + \frac{0.059}{n} \log a_{ext} \tag{13.31}$$

Thus we predict Nernstian behavior of this cell.

Suppose that the exchangeable ion is an anion. Then the development is based on these redox reactions:

Left (oxidation): $2X_{int}^{-} \rightleftharpoons (X_2)_{int} + 2e$
Right (reduction): $2e + (X_2)_{ext} \rightleftharpoons 2X_{ext}^{-}$

Overall reaction: $X_{int}^{-} \rightleftharpoons X_{ext}^{-}$

The membrane potential is given by

$$E_{membrane} = -\frac{RT}{nF} \ln \frac{a_{ext}}{a_{int}}$$

and the analog to Eq. (13.31) becomes

$$E_{cell} = \text{constant} - \frac{0.059}{n} \log a_{ext} \qquad (13.32)$$

Summing this up, we anticipate an electrode response following the form

$$E_{cell} = \text{constant} \pm \frac{0.059}{n} \log a_{ext} \qquad (13.33)$$

with the $+$ sign applying to cations and the $-$ sign to anions.

We next turn to the mechanisms for ion-exchange between the membrane and the solution.

Glass Electrodes. A typical glass is composed of Na_2O and SiO_2, and its surface layers possess exchangeable cations. An ion exchange equilibrium is set up between the glass surface and an electrolyte solution according to

$$-SiO^-Na^- \; + \; H^+ \; \rightleftharpoons \; -SiO^-H^+ \; + \; Na^+$$
$$\text{(glass)} \qquad \text{(solution)} \qquad \text{(glass)} \qquad \text{(solution)}$$

When a pH-responsive glass electrode is first placed in water this process occurs, and when equilibrium has been reached the electrode is said to be hydrated and is ready for use. The full thickness of a glass membrane is typically 0.03–0.1 mm, and the thickness of the hydrated layers (internal and external) is only about 10^{-4} mm (Evans 1987).

Now, when this hydrated glass electrode is placed in a sample solution, in general the hydrogen ion activities in the external hydrated glass layer and in the sample solution will be different. This difference gives rise to the potential described by Eq. (13.31). In practice there can be some complicating factors. The hydrogen ion activities of the internal and external hydrated layers are seldom exactly equal, and this difference gives rise to an *asymmetry potential*, which is compensated for in the calibration process. Another complication occurs when the pH is being measured in solutions containing high sodium ion concentrations. In this case a potential difference may develop based on the different activities of sodium ion in the glass and in the solution; in effect, the electrode (or the experimentalist) is fooled into thinking that the sample solution hydrogen ion activity is higher than it really is. Since the usual source of high sodium ion concentrations is NaOH, this experimental artifact is called the *glass electrode alkaline error.* Newer glasses replace some of the sodium content with lithium and so are less susceptible to the alkaline error.

The foregoing description of the sodium ion error of the glass electrode is suggestive of an opportunity to modify the glass composition and in this way to develop glass electrodes with enhanced selectivity for ions other than H^+. This approach has been successful. Glasses are described in a shorthand manner by the symbol NAS X–Y, meaning that this glass contains X% of Na_2O, Y% of Al_2O_3, and $100 - (X + Y)\%$ of SiO_2. The conventional pH glass electrode has little Al_2O_3, and its sensitivity pattern is

$$H^+ \ggg Na^+ > K^+, Rb^+, Cs^+, \gg Ca^{2+}$$

NAS 11–18 glass has this sensitivity sequence:

$$Ag^+ > H^+ > Na^+ \gg K^+, Li^+, > Ca^{2+}$$

This glass has been used as a sodium ion-selective electrode. Obviously Ag^+ must be absent and H^+ must be fixed, but its advantage is its high sensitivity to Na^+ relative to K^+ or Li^+. Many of the newer glasses, especially the lithium glasses, possess analytically useful selectivity profiles. Glass membrane electrodes are particularly valuable because, although they are physically delicate, they are chemically quite robust.

Solid Membrane Electrodes. A sparingly soluble crystalline solid can serve as an ion-exchange electrode. Usually crystals of the substance are dispersed in a polymer matrix. Suppose we wish to design a halide ion (X^-)-sensitive electrode. We can form such an electrode with the slightly soluble AgX salt. The membrane sets up this solubility equilibrium with the solution:

$$AgX_{membrane} \overset{K_{sp}}{\rightleftharpoons} Ag^+_{soln} + X^-_{soln}$$

where K_{sp} is the solubility product (Chapter 10).

Presuming that the sample solution (into which the electrode is introduced) initially contains no Ag^+ but a relatively high concentration of X^-, the common ion effect of X^- will depress the solubility of AgX, and the concentration (activity) of the silver ion will be determined by that of X^-:

$$a_{Ag^+} = \frac{K_{sp}}{a_{X^-}} \tag{13.34}$$

From Eq. (13.31), therefore

$$E_{cell} = constant + 0.059 \log a_{Ag^+} \tag{13.35}$$

or, making use of Eq. (13.34)

$$E_{cell} = (constant)' - 0.059 \log a_{X^-} \tag{13.36}$$

where a_{X^-} refers to the total activity of X^- in the solution. This has an interesting consequence. Reverting to concentrations for convenience, we can write

$$[X^-]_{total} = [X^-]_{initial} + [X^-]_{dissolved}$$

where $[X^-]_{initial}$ is the quantity sought from the measurement and $[X^-]_{dissolved}$ is the concentration contributed by dissolution of the electrode substance. Because of the stoichiometry of the dissolution process, $[X^-]_{dissolved} = [Ag^+]$, so we find

$$[Ag^+] = [X^-]_{total} - [X^-]_{initial}$$

Restating Eq. (13.34), we also have

$$[Ag^+] = \frac{K_{sp}}{[X^-]_{total}}$$

Combining these gives a quadratic in $[X^-]_{total}$ whose solution is

$$[X^-]_{total} = \frac{[X^-]_{initial} \pm ([X^-]_{initial}^2 + 4K_{sp})^{1/2}}{2} \tag{13.37}$$

There are two extreme cases to consider. If $[X^-]_{initial}^2 \ggg 4K_{sp}$, then we find that $[X^-]_{total} = [X^-]_{initial}$. This means that the dissolved anion makes a negligible contribution to the total, and that in this region of behavior a tenfold increase in $[X^-]_{initial}$ results in a 59 mV change in cell potential [Eq. (13.36)]. At the other extreme of behavior, where $[X^-]_{initial} \lll 4K_{sp}$, Eq. (13.37) yields $[X^-]_{total} = \sqrt{K_{sp}} = [X^-]_{dissolved}$; here the initial concentration of anion is so low that it makes no sensible contribution, and from Eq. (13.36) we find that the potential is independent of $[X^-]_{initial}$. At intermediate conditions the dependence is more complicated, as shown in Fig. 13.3. The sensitivity of the system may be defined as the slope of the response curve in Fig. 13.3; thus the electrode is considered to lose useful sensitivity below the lower limit of detection.

Solid-state electrodes are quite rugged. Their sensitivity limits are, as we have seen, controlled by the K_{sp} value of the solid. Mixed solids also have been used. For example, an electrode composed of CuS and Ag_2S can respond to Ag^+, S^{2-}, or Cu^{2+}; the solubility products of both salts must be simultaneously satisfied.

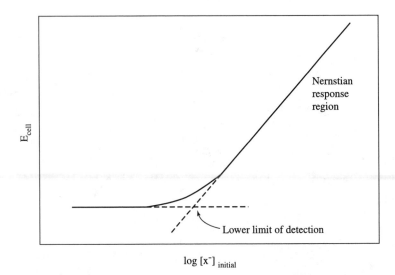

Figure 13.3. Electrode response curve of a solid membrane electrode.

Some lower limits of detection of solid-state electrodes are, for Cl^-, 10^{-5} M, for I^-, 10^{-8} M, for Cu^{2+}, 10^{-9} M, for Bi^{3+}, 10^{-11} M. These are very high sensitivities.

Liquid Membrane Electrodes. We are not accustomed to picturing liquid membranes, but the term simply implies a thin liquid phase. As the sample solution is aqueous, the liquid membrane phase will be an organic liquid that is immiscible with water. Hence the liquid membrane is very hydrophobic. By making the membrane phase quite thin, a faster response is achieved. Figure 13.4 shows some simple designs of liquid membrane electrodes. The electrode design of Fig. 13.4a will produce a slow response because of the considerable distance between the inner and outer interfaces, whereas Fig. 13.4b shows a faster responding electrode.

The basic idea is that an equilibrium is established within the membrane phase between the sample ion of interest and some hydrophobic molecule with which the ion forms a noncovalently bound complex. The sample ion thus is capable of exchanging between the membrane phase and the external aqueous sample solution. This ion exchange process is responsible for developing the potential at the interface as we have described earlier.

In one general type of electrode, a hydrophobic anion is dissolved in a hydrophobic solvent. The anion is selected so that it will form a strong complex with the exchangeable cation of interest. Since the anion is hydrophobic, it is constrained to remain in the membrane phase, but the cation can exchange between the membrane and the aqueous sample solution. A calcium-selective electrode is based on this principle. The complexing agent is bis(di-n-decyl)phosphate, and

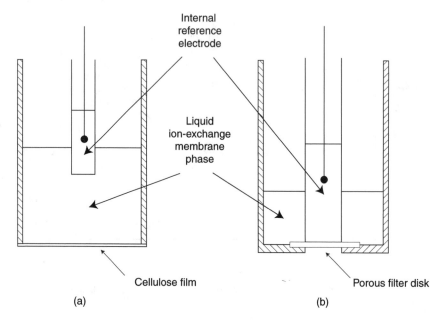

Figure 13.4. Schematic diagrams of liquid ion-selective membrane electrodes. [Reproduced by permission from Connors (1982).]

this is the equilibrium within the membrane phase

$$Ca^{2+} \; + \; 2R_2P\overset{OH}{\underset{O}{\|}} \;\; \rightleftharpoons \;\; (R_2PO_2)_2Ca \; + \; 2H^+$$

where R is $CH_3(CH_2)_9$. Clearly this electrode will suffer interference from hydrogen ions, and it is found to be usable in the pH range 5.5–11. (Above pH 11 calcium hydroxide precipitates.)

The alternative version of this electrode design makes use of a hydrophobic cation, chosen to form a complex with an exchangeable anion. Thus a nitrate ion-selective electrode is based on the ion pair formation of NO_3^- with the tridodecylhexadecylammonium ion; we can represent this equilibrium as

$$NO_3^- + R_4N^+ \rightleftharpoons R_4N^+NO_3^-$$

The second general type of liquid membrane electrode is based on an uncharged complexing agent. A potassium ion electrode uses the antibiotic valinomycin as a selective complexing agent. Much synthetic organic research is leading to the availability of macrocyclic compounds capable of complex formation with a wide variety of smaller species, and many of these compounds may be suitable as complexes in liquid membrane electrodes. An especially attractive possibility is to develop electrodes specific for drug molecules. Since most drugs are acids or bases, they are easily transformed into ions by pH control, and then their electrochemical detection becomes possible if a complexing agent can be identified that will selectively bind the ionic drug. Many such electrodes have been developed.

PROBLEMS

13.1. Balance these equations:

(a) $ClO_3^- + Sn^{2+} = Cl^- + Sn^{4+}$

(b) $PbO_2 + I^- = I_2 + Pb^{2+}$

(c) $OCl^- + NH_3 = Cl^- + N_2$

(d) $MnO_4^- + H_2O_2 = Mn^{2+} + O_2$

(e) $MnO_4^- + CuI = MnO_2 + Cu^{2+}$

(f) $S_2O_8^{2-} + 2Fe^{2+} = 2SO_4^{2-} + 2Fe^{3+}$

(g) $NH_2OH + Ce^{4+} = N_2O + Ce^{3+}$

(h) $RSH + I_2 = RSSR + I^-$

13.2. Calculate the ionic strength of a phosphate buffer prepared to be 0.025 M in NaH_2PO_4, 0.025 M in K_2HPO_4, and 0.050 M in NaCl.

13.3. Calculate the change in cell potential when a glass electrode-SCE pair is moved from 0.010 M HCl to 0.010 M KOH. (Assume that activities are equal to concentrations.)

13.4. Given this electrochemical cell, where "tris" is tris(hydroxymethyl)amino-methane, and trisH$^+$ is protonated tris:

$$Pt, H_2(p = 1 \text{ atm}) \,|\, tris(0.05 \text{ M}), trisH(0.05 \text{ M}) \,\|\, SCE$$

The potential of the SCE is $+0.244$ V and the measured cell potential was $+0.717$ V at 25°C. What is the pK_a' of trisH$^+$?

13.5. A cell consisting of a calcium ion-sensitive membrane electrode and a reference electrode gave the following cell potentials at 25°C with solutions having the listed Ca^{2+} activities:

Ca^{2+} Activity	E_{cell} (V)
0.000135	+0.136
0.00541	+0.183
0.0382	+0.208

(a) Determine whether the cell response is Nernstian.

(b) Predict the cell potential if the Ca^{2+} activity is 1.00×10^{-3}.

13.6. (a) What is the ionic strength of a solution 0.01 M in KCl and 0.01 M in Na_2SO_4?

(b) Calculate the mean ionic activity coefficient of sulfate ion in this solution.

13.7. (a) Calculate the cell potential at 25°C of this electrochemical cell:

$$Pt \,|\, Fe^{2+}(0.001\ M), Fe^{3+}(0.01\ M) \,\|\, Cu^{2+}(0.01\ M) \,|\, Cu$$

(b) Will copper metal be plated out or will it be dissolved in this cell?

13.8. (a) Calculate the potential of this cell at 25°C:

$$Zn \,|\, Zn(NO_3)_2(0.01\ M), AgNO_3(0.001\ M) \,|\, Ag$$

(b) Will this cell produce zinc-plated silver or silver-plated zinc?

13.9. What is the equilibrium constant of this reaction at 25°C?

$$AgCl + Br^- \rightleftharpoons AgBr + Cl^-$$

13.10. Standard potentials are given in parentheses for the following reactions:

$$Mg(OH)_2 + 2e \rightleftharpoons Mg + 2OH^- \qquad (E^\circ_{Mg(OH)_2,Mg} = -2.69\ V)$$
$$Mg^{2+} + 2e \rightleftharpoons Mg \qquad (E^\circ_{Mg^{2+},Mg} = -2.37\ V)$$

Calculate the solubility product of magnesium hydroxide.

NOTES

1. This concept is really the genesis of the term *oxidation* as it is also applied to inorganic reactions. Compare FeO (ferrous oxide) and Fe_2O_3 (ferric oxide). The conceptual transformation from oxygen gain to electron loss is very broadening, but it obscures the historical basis. The term *reduction* originally arose in the processing of ores, when it can be said that an ore is reduced to the pure metal, the term referring to both a typical process (also historically called *revivification*) and a diminution in volume.

2. One joule = 1 volt coulomb, so $R = 8.314\ J\ K^{-1}\ mol^{-1} = 8.314\ V \cdot C\ K^{-1}\ mol^{-1}$. This provides E with the unit V.

3. Some authors represent all electrode potentials as reductions, and then Eq. (13.11) will appear as

$$E_{cell} = E_{Cu^{2+},Cu} - E_{Zn^{2+},Zn}$$

This sign change is discussed later in the text.

4. For any practical purpose Eq. (13.21) is an adequate interpretation, but we must recall that this cell possesses a liquid junction. Moreover, Eq. (13.21) implies that we can measure the activity of a single ionic species, whereas we have seen in Chapter 8 that we can measure only a mean ionic activity.

5. There is a subtlety here. From the pH measurement we know the *activity* of H^+, but Eq. (13.23) calls for the *concentrations* of H^+ and OH^-. Activity coefficient corrections can be applied, but this will seldom be necessary.

14

NONCOVALENT
BINDING EQUILIBRIA

14.1. INTRODUCTION

The principles of thermodynamics apply to all physical and chemical equilibria, and the purpose of the present section is to concentrate attention on yet another class of chemical equilibria, namely, those processes in which the noncovalent forces of interaction are operative. The distinction between covalent ("chemical") bonds and noncovalent ("physical") interactions is not clearcut, and is based in part on theory and in part on an empirical criterion. Theoretically, using the language of molecular orbital theory, a covalent bond is a consequence of the formation of molecular orbitals from atomic orbitals; the bond usually consists of one or more electron pairs shared between the bound atoms, and is highly directional in character. Noncovalent interactions, on the other hand, are electrostatic in nature and are not highly directional. The empirical criterion is energetic; covalent bonds tend to be strong whereas noncovalent interactions are weak. Obviously this is not an absolute criterion. The single, double, and triple bonds familiar from organic chemistry are perfect examples of covalent bonds. The interactions that are responsible for the existence of condensed phases (solids and liquids) are noncovalent. Notice that we refrain from speaking of noncovalent "bonds"; this restraint is a reflection of the weakness of these interactions as well as their nondirectional nature. Most noncovalent interactions exhibit energies of $\sim 10\,\text{kcal}\,\text{mol}^{-1}$ or less (ΔH° values), whereas covalent bond energies largely lie in the range 20–200 kcal mol^{-1}.[1]

The noncovalent interactions occur between two or more molecules or ions. The manner in which we designate these interactants is arbitrary and may be determined for our convenience. We choose to call one of the interactants the *substrate* S and the other interactant the *ligand* L. Usually some chemical or physical property of the substrate, a property that is altered on interaction with the ligand, is observed by the experimenter. The product of the interaction between the substrate and the ligand is generally called a *complex*. Complexes may form between two (or more) small molecules or ions; or small molecules may bind to a macromolecule, as when a drug–protein complex is formed. Noncovalent complex formation is an essential step in many biological processes, such as antigen–antibody interaction, transport of ions across membranes, control of metabolic pathways, signal transduction, oxygen transport, and the regulation of gene expression.

14.2. THE NONCOVALENT INTERACTIONS

Potential Energy Functions. The detailed nature of the noncovalent interaction forces is not the concern of thermodynamics, but some understanding of these phenomena will be helpful in picturing the molecular processes being studied. Although we commonly speak of the forces of interaction, it is actually the energies of interaction that are of primary interest. The force F is related to the potential energy V by

$$F = -\frac{dV}{dr}$$

where r is the distance between two interacting particles. Physical theory has elucidated the potential energy functions of the noncovalent interactions (Hirschfelder et al. 1954; Israelachvili 1985). The interacting species may be ions or molecules, and the molecules may be nonpolar or may possess permanent dipole moments.

Table 14.1 gives the noncovalent potential energy functions, which are seen to fall into three classes. The Table 14.1 functions are written for interactions between species S and L in vacuo, that is, in the absence of a solvent. These are the three classes of noncovalent interactions:

1. *Electrostatic Interactions.* These take place between ions (C) or dipoles (μ). The magnitude of a charge is to be accompanied by its sign, and a negative value of energy is attractive, a positive value repulsive. (The charge–charge interaction term is Coulomb's law, which we encountered in Chapter 8.) Observe that charges and dipole moments appear as squared quantities.

2. *Induction (Polarization) Interactions.* These are a result of an ion or a dipole inducing a temporary dipole in an adjacent molecule. The interaction then consists of the electrostatic interaction between the temporary dipole and the permanent dipole or the ion. The quantity α in the expressions is the polarizability of the molecule, a measure of the ease with which the molecule's electron cloud can be deformed in the presence of an electric field.

3. *Dispersion (London) Interaction.* This is a quantum-mechanical phenomenon, although we can give a reasonable classical interpretation. Any

Table 14.1 Potential energy functions for noncovalent interactions[a]

Type of Interaction	Potential Energy Function
Electrostatic	
Charge–charge	$+\dfrac{C_S C_L}{r}$
Charge–dipole	$-\dfrac{1}{3kT} \cdot \dfrac{C_S^2 \cdot \mu_L^2}{r^4}$
Dipole–dipole	$-\dfrac{2}{3kT} \cdot \dfrac{\mu_S^2 \cdot \mu_L^2}{r^6}$
Induction	
Charge-induced dipole	$-\dfrac{C_S^2 \cdot \alpha_L}{2r^4}$
Dipole-induced dipole	$-\dfrac{\mu_S^2 \cdot \alpha_L}{r^6}$
Dispersion	
Induced dipole–induced dipole	$-\dfrac{3}{4}\left[\dfrac{\epsilon_S \cdot \epsilon_L}{\epsilon_S + \epsilon_L}\right]\dfrac{\alpha_S \cdot \alpha_L}{r^6}$

[a] C is the charge on an ion, μ is permanent dipole moment, α is polarizability, r is intermolecular distance, ϵ is a specific energy term, T is absolute temperature, and k is Boltzmann's constant, where $k = R/N_A$.

molecule, including a nonpolar molecule, may develop a momentary dipole as a result of transitory electron density displacements. This momentary dipole can induce a dipole in a neighboring molecule, and these two temporary dipoles then interact. The dispersion interaction takes place between all species; its effectiveness is dependent on their polarizabilities.

Note that, for uncharged molecules, each class of interaction includes an r^{-6} dependence on the internuclear separation distance r. For such interacting species the combined effect of these r^{-6} terms constitutes the noncovalent interactions.[2] Under the attractive influence of these terms two molecules approach until they experience an opposing repulsive force, which initially is a result of electron–electron repulsion and, at even closer distances, of nucleus–nucleus repulsion. The net effect of these forces of attraction and repulsion is reasonably expressed in Eq. (14.1), an empirical function called the Lennard-Jones 6–12 potential.

$$V = 4\,V_{\min}\left[\left(\frac{r_0}{r}\right)^{12} - \left(\frac{r_0}{r}\right)^{6}\right] \tag{14.1}$$

In Eq. (14.1), which is shown graphically as Fig. 14.1, V is the potential energy of interaction between two uncharged particles separated by distance r. $V_{\min}$ is the value of V at the equilibrium separation r_{eq}, which is the value of r when the attractive and repulsive forces exactly balance each other; r_0 is the value of r when

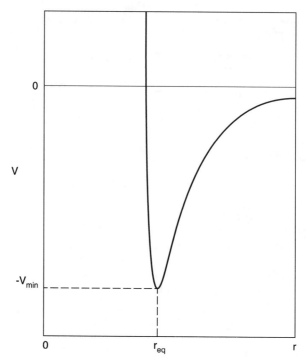

Figure 14.1. Potential energy dependence on intermolecular distance according to the Lennard-Jones potential function.

$V = 0$. The r^{-12} term empirically expresses the repulsive energy. Observe the r^{-6} term, which is attractive and embodies the r^{-6} terms in Table 14.1.

The potential energy functions in Table 14.1 are written for interactions in vacuo, that is, without a solvent present. But we are interested in condensed phase systems, most commonly consisting of substrate S and ligand L dissolved in a solvent. In such real systems the noncovalent interactions will be moderated to a degree expressed by the dielectric constant of the solvent, in the manner made explicit in our treatment of the Coulomb interaction (Chapter 8).

Chemical Interpretations. The noncovalent interactions of Table 14.1 constitute all of the forces that we need to consider[3], yet we are accustomed to invoke phenomena that may appear to be additional forces. But these phenomena are really just the noncovalent forces (perhaps with some covalent bonding mixed in) masquerading in chemically useful forms. One of these forms is *hydrogen-bonding*. A hydrogen bond (H bond) is represented by the dots in the reaction

$$A\text{--}H + B \rightleftharpoons A\text{--}H \cdots B$$

The A—H bond in the H-bond donor AH is largely covalent; the H$\cdots$B bond to the H-bond acceptor B is largely a dipole–dipole interaction. Though exceptions to the following are known, H bonding is most effective when the A—H$\cdots$B angle is 180° and when the atoms A and B are nitrogen or oxygen. The protein α-helix and the folded conformations of proteins are largely maintained by H-bonding, as is the DNA double helix. Carboxylic acids in the vapor state and in nonpolar solvents form H-bonded dimers as in

$$R-C \underset{O-H\cdots O}{\overset{O\cdots H-O}{\big\langle\big\rangle}} C-R$$

27

The rather surprising pK_a values of salicylic acid (p$K_1 = 2.98$, p$K_2 = 13.00$; for 4-hydroxybenzoic acid p$K_1 = 4.58$, p$K_2 = 9.39$) are ascribed to stabilization of the monoanion by H bonding:

28

It is interesting that intramolecular H bonding can be effective in aqueous solution, whereas intermolecular H bonding is relatively ineffective because of the overwhelming competition from the solvent, itself a good H bond donor and acceptor. The structure of water as a medium is a result of its H-bonding properties.

Another chemical phenomenon is *charge transfer* (CT) complexing, also known as electron donor–acceptor (EDA) complexing. This seems to be a combination of covalent and noncovalent effects. Apparently an electron is partly or wholly transferred from an orbital on the donor molecule to one on the acceptor molecule, so the interaction has some covalent character and it results in definite and detectable changes in electron configuration; however, the noncovalent forces also are involved. Although some covalent electron-sharing takes place, CT complexes often are very weak.

Finally we must take notice of the solvent. We can do this by treating the solvent as a structureless continuum, as when we introduce the dielectric constant as a measure of the ability of the solvent to separate charges; or more realistically we can recognize that the solvent is itself composed of molecules, which undergo the same kinds of intermolecular interactions as do the solute species. We are then led to the view that the formation of a complex SL through the reaction of S with L in the presence of solvent (medium) M is a competition among three pairwise types of interactions: solute–solute (SL), solute–solvent (SM, LM, and SL-M), and solvent–solvent (MM). Thus we can write

$$\Delta G^\circ_{net} = \Delta G^\circ_{solute-solute} + \Delta G^\circ_{solvation} + \Delta G^\circ_{solvent-solvent}$$

Each term on the right is the result of noncovalent interactions. The solute–solute interaction term is complex-stabilizing. The solvation term could be complex-stabilizing if the SL-M interaction (solvation of the complex) is stronger than the sum of the substrate-solvent plus the ligand–solvent terms, but this is unlikely, so solvation usually destabilizes the complex. The role of the solvent–solvent interaction term depends greatly on the nature of the solvent and the solute species.

Suppose, for example, that we wish to study H bonding between phenol (H-bond donor) and pyridine (H-bond acceptor). If we attempt this in water as the solvent we are unlikely to be successful because the solvation term (arising from the phenol–water and pyridine–water solvation interaction) will be complex-destabilizing. On the other hand, if carbon tetrachloride, with no H-bonding capability of its own, is the solvent we will be able to detect the phenol–pyridine interaction.

There is a particularly important kind of solvent effect observed with nonpolar solutes in aqueous solution. Since water is both an H-bond donor and an H-bond acceptor, the solvent–solvent interaction term ΔG°_{MM} is appreciable and may even be overwhelming. Water molecules form an H-bonded network having definite structural features. Now, when a nonpolar solute molecule (such as a saturated hydrocarbon) dissolves in water, no H bonds from the solute to the surrounding water molecules will form, because the solute is neither a donor nor an acceptor. The water structure in the immediate vicinity of the solute re-forms to compensate for the broken water–water H-bonds. The result is that the number of possible orientations of water molecules is reduced by the presence of the nonpolar solute; this means that the configurational entropy of the system is reduced. From this point of view, the very low aqueous solubility of nonpolar substances is caused by this unfavorable entropy change in the dissolution process. This is called the *hydrophobic effect*.

Now if two such dissolved nonpolar solute molecules come into contact, some of the "structured water" in their vicinity is released, increasing the system entropy, and resulting in a negative free-energy change. This is the driving force for association of nonpolar species in aqueous solution. This phenomenon is termed *hydrophobic interaction*. Observe that complex formation driven by this hydrophobic phenomenon owes little or nothing to solute–solute interaction (which is simply a result of the ever-present dispersion force); rather, it is essentially completely driven by solvent–solvent interaction. In a sense the solute is "squeezed out" of the water. This water-structure interpretation of the hydrophobic interaction applies strictly only to nonpolar solutes. Many solutes, however, including most drug molecules, possess both nonpolar and polar groups (we can call such molecules "semipolar"), and although the hydrophobic interaction may play a role in their complex formation, the driving force may appear as either a favorable entropy change or a favorable enthalpy change.

An alternative description of the hydrophobic effect and hydrophobic interaction adopts a thermodynamic viewpoint. The solvent is pictured as a structureless continuum. In order to dissolve a molecule in this medium, a molecule-sized cavity must be created; then the solute molecule is inserted into the cavity, and finally solute–solvent interaction take place. Creation of a cavity having surface area A

requires an expenditure of free energy equal to $A\gamma$, where γ is the solvent surface tension. We have seen (Chapter 11) that the surface tension of water is unusually high (this itself is a result of the strong water–water interaction).

On this basis alone all solutes might be expected to show low aqueous solubilities. However, recall the step in the dissolution process in which solute–solvent interactions may occur. In this step the energy expended in creating the cavity may be recovered provided the solute structure is such as to permit strong solute–solvent interactions. Semipolar solutes do lead to such interactions, but nonpolar solutes do not. Hence this thermodynamic approach accounts for the hydrophobic effect.

When two dissolved solute molecules come into contact, the total cavity surface area is reduced as the two separate cavities coalesce into a single cavity. The free energy change for this process is therefore $\gamma\Delta A$, where ΔA, a negative quantity, is the change in cavity surface area. This is the driving force for the hydrophobic interaction. Quantitative theories of this phenomenon have been developed.

If the hydrophobic interaction is substantially responsible for the strength of a given complex in aqueous solution, we can predict that incorporation of an organic solvent into the aqueous medium will result in a weakening of the complex (observed as a decrease in the equilibrium constant for its formation). We often turn the argument around, and use the complex-weakening effect of organic solvents as a diagnostic criterion for the operation of the hydrophobic interaction.

14.3. BINDING MODELS

General. We can write any complex formation equilibrium as

$$mS + nL \rightleftharpoons S_m L_n$$

and define the *overall binding constant*

$$\beta_{mn} = \frac{[S_m L_n]}{[S]^m [L]^n} \tag{14.2}$$

where we assume that activities are equal to concentrations. The simultaneous collision of m molecules of S and n molecules of L to produce the complex $S_m L_n$ is so improbable (unless $m = 1$ and $n = 1$) that it can be neglected, and so a more realistic view of what happens is that complex $S_m L_n$ is built up by successive bimolecular collisions. For example, the complex SL_2 forms in these successive steps:

$$S + L \rightleftharpoons SL$$
$$SL + L \rightleftharpoons SL_2$$

For each such step we define a *stepwise binding constant*:

$$K_{11} = \frac{[SL]}{[S][L]} \tag{14.3}$$

$$K_{12} = \frac{[SL_2]}{[SL][L]} \tag{14.4}$$

Algebraic substitution shows that $\beta_{12} = K_{11}K_{12}$. Observe how the subscripts denote the stoichiometry of the complex.

Usually reactant concentrations are expressed in mol L^{-1} (molarity, M); consequently, all stepwise binding constants have the unit M^{-1}. Binding constants are also known as stability constants, association constants, or formation constants. In some fields of study it is traditional to write the reaction in the opposite direction, and then the corresponding equilibrium constant is the reciprocal of the binding constant and is called a dissociation constant.

The experimental recognition of the existence of a complex requires that some property of the complex be quantitatively different from that property as possessed by the two interactants giving rise to the complex; in the following section we will see examples of such properties. Our first experimental goal is to establish the stoichiometry of the complex or complexes; our second goal is to evaluate the stepwise binding constants. The most general way to accomplish both goals is to postulate a reasonable stoichiometry, to derive a quantitative description of the expected experimental outcomes based on this stoichiometry, and then to test this model (hypothesis) with experimental data. The usual criterion is that the binding constant evaluated in such a test should be constant over a wide range of system concentrations. This somewhat abstract account will be made more explicit by considering several important stoichiometric models. More extensive treatments are available (Connors 1987; Wyman and Gill 1990).

The 1:1 Stoichiometric Model. This, the simplest of stoichiometric models, also happens to be applicable to many real systems, and its description is fundamental for understanding chemical equilibria. The complex formation reaction is

$$S + L \overset{K_{11}}{\rightleftharpoons} SL$$

with K_{11} defined by Eq. (14.3). Let us define f_{11} as the fraction of substrate present in the complexed (bound) form, or

$$f_{11} = \frac{[SL]}{S_t} \tag{14.5}$$

where S_t is the total substrate concentration:

$$S_t = [S] + [SL] \tag{14.6}$$

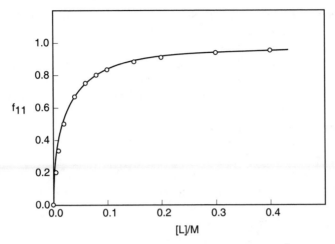

Figure 14.2. Plot of Eq. (14.7), the 1 : 1 binding isotherm, for $K_{11} = 50\,\mathrm{M}^{-1}$ (see Table 14.2).

Algebraic substitution of Eqs. (14.3) and (14.5) into Eq. (14.6) gives the quantitative 1 : 1 stoichiometric model:

$$f_{11} = \frac{K_{11}[L]}{1 + K_{11}[L]} \tag{14.7}$$

This equation is the 1 : 1 *binding isotherm*. Its functional form is known as a rectangular hyperbola. We can easily gain a sense of how f_{11} depends on [L] by making a calculation for a hypothetical system; this has been done in Table 14.2 by assuming that $K_{11} = 50\,\mathrm{M}^{-1}$ and using Eq. (14.7) to calculate f_{11} for assigned values of [L]. The results are plotted in Fig. 14.2. The shape of this curve is very

**Table 14.2 Hypothetical 1 : 1 binding isotherm
calculated with Eq. (14.7) and the value $K_{11} = 50\,\mathrm{M}^{-1}$**

[L] (M)	f_{11}
0	0
0.005	0.200
0.01	0.333
0.02	0.500
0.04	0.667
0.06	0.750
0.08	0.800
0.10	0.833
0.15	0.882
0.20	0.909
0.30	0.938
0.40	0.952

characteristic; at low values of [L], where $K_{11}[L] \ll 1$, f_{11} is nearly a linear function of [L], as can be seen from Eq. (14.7), whereas at high values of [L], where $K_{11}[L] \gg 1$, f_{11} becomes nearly independent of [L]. This region in which f_{11} shows little dependence on [L] is called the *saturation effect*; the physical interpretation is that nearly all the S molecules are already bound to L, so the addition of more L has little effect on increasing f_{11}, which increases asymptotically to a value of unity. Notice that $K = 1/[L]$ when $f_{11} = 0.5$.[4]

The chemical interpretation of 1 : 1 binding is that the substrate S possesses a single "binding site," as does the ligand L, and when the complex SL forms no further sites are available for the binding of additional species.

A quantitative test of the 1 : 1 model may be made by rearranging Eq. (14.7) into a linear plotting form. Several linear plots have been used. Since f_{11} is the fraction complexed (also known as the *fraction bound*), then $1 - f_{11}$ is the fraction uncomplexed (fraction free), or $1 - f_{11} = 1/(1 + K_{11}[L])$. Thus $f_{11}/(1 - f_{11}) = K_{11}[L]$, or

$$\log\left(\frac{f_{11}}{1 - f_{11}}\right) = \log[L] - \log K_{11} \tag{14.8}$$

A log–log plot should be linear with a slope of unity if the stoichiometry is 1 : 1. This is called a *Hill plot*. More simply, Eq. (14.7) can be rearranged to three non-logarithmic linear plotting forms. The following equation (14.9) is used by plotting $1/f_{11}$ against $1/[L]$, so it is called the *double-reciprocal plot*:

$$\frac{1}{f_{11}} = \frac{1}{K_{11}[L]} + 1 \tag{14.9}$$

When spectrophotometry is the experimental method of study, the double-reciprocal plot is called the *Benesi–Hildebrand plot*.

Equation (14.10) is another plotting form of Eq. (14.7); a plot of $[L]/f_{11}$ against [L] is expected to be linear:

$$\frac{[L]}{f_{11}} = [L] + \frac{1}{K_{11}} \tag{14.10}$$

Finally Eq. (14.11) is a third plotting form:

$$\frac{f_{11}}{[L]} = -K_{11}f_{11} + K_{11} \tag{14.11}$$

This plot of $f_{11}/[L]$ against f_{11} is sometimes called a *Scatchard plot*.

Linearity in these plots is a necessary condition if the 1 : 1 model is valid, and from the parameters of the equation K_{11} can be evaluated. Actually we seldom measure f_{11} directly, but rather some experimental quantity that is related to f_{11}, so the interpretation of the plots depends on the particular experimental method, as will be shown in Section 14.4.

A very interesting version of the $1:1$ model arises in the study of many small molecule–protein binding systems. In these systems we may consider that n small molecules, which will play the role of ligand L, may bind to a single protein molecule, which we will call the substrate S. As a measure of the extent of binding we define the quantity

$$\bar{i} = \frac{L_t - [L]}{S_t} \tag{14.12}$$

where L_t and S_t refer respectively to the total ligand and substrate concentrations; $\bar{i}$ can be interpreted as the average number of ligand molecules bound per molecule of substrate.

Now, if we impose the rather stringent conditions that all n binding sites on the protein are identical and independent, it is possible to derive the following isotherm

$$\bar{i} = \frac{nk[L]}{1 + k[L]} \tag{14.13}$$

where k is the constant for binding to a single site. According to this equation, this rather complicated system follows the hyperbolic function characteristic of simple $1:1$ binding. Usually n and k are evaluated from a Scatchard plot.

The 1 : 1+1 : 2 Model. This stoichiometric model will serve as an example of the treatment of multiple complexes. The complex stoichiometries are SL and SL_2, and the stepwise binding constants are defined in Eqs. (14.3) and (14.4). Obviously both of these equations must be simultaneously satisfied.

The existence of the SL_2 complex means that there must be two binding sites on S. If these two sites are chemically different, there may exist two different $1:1$ complexes. All of these possibilities can be related by the scheme

where XY represents the uncomplexed substrate, and X and Y are the two different binding sites. A superscript prime indicates that the site is complexed to an L molecule, so X'Y and XY' are the two possible isomeric $1:1$ complexes and X'Y' is the $1:2$ complex. The equilibrium constants shown are microscopic binding constants.

We experimentally measure K_{11} and K_{12}. These are related (Connors 1987) to the microscopic constants by

$$K_{11} = K_{X'Y} + K_{XY'} \tag{14.14}$$

$$K_{11}K_{12} = a_{XY}K_{X'Y}K_{XY'} \tag{14.15}$$

where $a_{XY} = K^*_{X'Y'}/K_{XY'} = K^{**}_{X'Y'}/K_{X'Y}$. Since these two equations constitute two independent equations with three unknowns, we are in general unable to evaluate the microscopic constants. Two special cases are of interest, however. First, suppose that the two binding sites are identical. This means that $K_{X'Y} = K_{XY'}$, so $K_{11} = 2K_{X'Y}$, and Eq. (14.15) becomes $K_{11} = 4K_{12}/a_{XY}$. The second special case occurs if the two sites are identical and are also independent. This last condition means that $a_{XY} = 1$, and we then find that $K_{11} = 4K_{12}$.

Perhaps this treatment of the $1:1+1:2$ model has seemed somewhat familiar. In fact, it is merely a rephrasing of the arguments used in Section 12.7 when discussing the assignment of pK_a values of diprotic acids. The only difference in the treatments is that for acids we defined K_a values as dissociation constants whereas for complex formation our equilibrium constants are association constants. In the acid–base system the proton plays the role of the ligand.

14.4. MEASUREMENT OF BINDING CONSTANTS

In this section we describe a few experimental techniques for the determination of complex binding constants; many more techniques are available (Connors 1987). It is obviously essential that the temperature be controlled and that the system be at equilibrium; this latter condition is easy to achieve because most noncovalent interactions take place very rapidly.

Spectrophotometry. A basic knowledge of absorption spectroscopy is assumed. We will treat the $1:1$ stoichiometric model, assuming that Beer's law is obeyed by all species. The method requires that the free substrate S and the complex SL possess significantly different absorption spectra. A wavelength is chosen at which ϵ_S and ϵ_{11} are different. (Subscripts refer to the species; 11 indicates the complex SL.) S_t and L_t represent total substrate and ligand concentrations.

In the absence of ligand we can write

$$A_0 = \epsilon_S b S_t \tag{14.16}$$

In the presence of ligand at fixed S_t value, the solution absorbance is given by

$$A_L = \epsilon_S b[S] + \epsilon_L b[L] + \epsilon_{11} b[SL]$$

which is combined with the mass balances $L_t = [L] + [SL]$ and $S_t = [S] + [SL]$ to give

$$A_L = \epsilon_S b S_t + \epsilon_L b L_t + \Delta\epsilon_{11} b[SL]$$

where $\Delta\epsilon_{11} = \epsilon_{11} - \epsilon_S - \epsilon_L$. If the solution absorbance is measured against a reference containing L_t mol L^{-1} of ligand, the absorbance actually measured is

$$A = \epsilon_S b S_t + \Delta\epsilon_{11} b[SL] \tag{14.17}$$

Now subtract Eq. (14.16) from (14.17) and incorporate the definition of K_{11} [Eq. (14.3)], obtaining

$$\Delta A = K_{11}\Delta\epsilon_{11}b[S][L] \tag{14.18}$$

where $\Delta A = A - A_0$. From the mass balance $S_t = [S] + [SL]$ and the expression for K_{11} we find $S_t = [S](1 + K_{11}[L])$, which is used in Eq. (14.18):

$$\frac{\Delta A}{b} = \frac{S_t K_{11}\Delta\epsilon_{11}[L]}{1 + K_{11}[L]} \tag{14.19}$$

This equation is the 1 : 1 binding isotherm expressed for spectrophotometric observation. Note that the functional dependence of the dependent variable $\Delta A/b$ on [L] is identical with that in Eq. (14.7).

There is a subtlety in the application of Eq. (14.19), for in this equation [L] is the free (uncomplexed) concentration of ligand, which we do not (yet) know. What we know is L_t, the total ligand concentration, for we prepare the solutions with a known constant value of S_t and varying but known values of L_t; then we measure $\Delta A/b$ in these solutions. The answer to this problem is to start with the mass balance $L_t = [L] + [SL]$, incorporating the expression for K_{11} to yield

$$L_t = [L] + \frac{S_t K_{11}[L]}{1 + K_{11}[L]} \tag{14.20}$$

Equations (14.19) and (14.20) together provide a complete description of the system. Often it is possible to design the experiment such that $L_t \gg S_t$; then Eq. (14.20) shows that $L_t \approx [L]$, and Eq. (14.19) can be analyzed with this approximation. More generally an iterative method is required; with a preliminary estimate of K_{11}, Eq. (14.20) is solved to give the [L] value corresponding to each L_t. These [L] values are used in Eq. (14.19) to obtain an improved estimate of K_{11}, and this process is repeated until the K_{11} estimates reach a constant value. The solution of Eq. (14.19) can be carried out graphically as described earlier; for example, the double-reciprocal form (the Benesi–Hildebrand plot) is

$$\frac{b}{\Delta A} = \frac{1}{S_t K_{11}\Delta\epsilon_{11}[L]} + \frac{1}{S_t\Delta\epsilon_{11}} \tag{14.21}$$

According to this equation, a plot of $b/\Delta A$ against $1/[L]$ will be linear if the stoichiometry is 1 : 1. The value of K_{11} is found from

$$K_{11} = \frac{\text{intercept on vertical axis}}{\text{slope}} \tag{14.22}$$

The parameter $\Delta\epsilon_{11}$ may be evaluated from the intercept value.

Table 14.3 Complexing of sodium cinnamate and theophylline at pH 6.5 and 25°C

$10^2\, L_t$ (M)	A^a
0.00	0.530
1.11	0.791
1.25	0.826
1.43	0.858
1.67	0.906
2.00	0.965
2.50	1.053

^{a} Pathlength $b = 1$ cm; wavelength $= 315$ nm; $S_t = 0.001$ M.

Table 14.3 lists experimental data from a study of the complex between cinnamic acid anion (the substrate S) and theophylline (the ligand L) (Kramer and Connors 1969). Figure 14.3 is the plot of these data according to Eq. (14.21). From this plot the value $K_{11} = 10.5\,\text{M}^{-1}$ was evaluated.

This absorption spectrophotometric method can be applied throughout the ultraviolet, visible, and infrared regions of the spectrum. Moreover, the same approach is applicable to fluorescence data and to nuclear magnetic resonance chemical shifts.

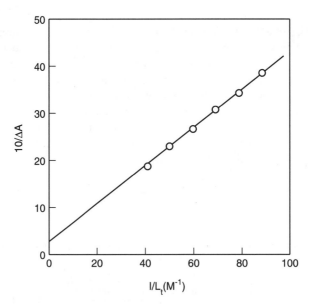

Figure 14.3. Plot of spectral data for the sodium cinnamate (S)-theophylline (L) system; pH 6.5; at 25°C; $K_{11} = 10.5\,\text{M}^{-1}$. Values of ordinates are an arithmetic average of five determinations. [Reproduced by permission from Kramer and Connors (1969).]

Solubility. When a complex is formed, the total (apparent) solubility of an inter-actant is increased, and this change in apparent solubility can be analyzed to derive the binding constant. The experiment consists of the addition of an identical weight (in considerable excess of its intrinsic solubility) of substrate S to each of numerous vials. Increasing amounts of soluble ligand L are added to successive vials, and solvent is added to make an identical volume of solution in each vial. Now the vials are agitated at constant temperature until solubility equilibrium is achieved (typically about 24 h). Then the solution phase of each vial is analyzed for its total dissolved concentration of substrate, S_t. A solubility phase diagram is constructed by plotting S_t (vertical axis) against L_t.

We will carry out the interpretation of the phase diagram for the case of $1:1$ stoichiometry. The mass balance expressions are

$$S_t = [S] + [SL]$$
$$L_t = [L] + [SL]$$

as we have often written. The manner in which the experiment was carried out ensured that pure solid S remained in each vial at equilibrium, which means that the chemical potential, and therefore the activity, of uncomplexed substrate S was the same in each vial; we can therefore reasonably conclude that the concentration of free S, namely $[S]$, was the same in each vial, including the vial containing no ligand at all. This quantity is therefore the intrinsic solubility s_0 of substrate. The mass balance on substrate can therefore be written

$$S_t = s_0 + [SL] \tag{14.23}$$

Combining Eq. (14.23) with the mass balance on ligand and the definition of K_{11} gives

$$S_t = s_0 + \frac{K_{11} s_0 L_t}{1 + K_{11} s_0} \tag{14.24}$$

as the solubility binding isotherm. Equation (14.24) predicts that S_t will be a linear function of L_t; the intercept will be s_0, and the binding constant can be calculated from

$$K_{11} = \frac{\text{slope}}{s_0(1 - \text{slope})} \tag{14.25}$$

Table 14.4 gives solubility data for a study of the complexing between theophylline (the substrate) and sodium salicylate (the ligand) (Cohen and Connors 1967). Figure 14.4 is the plot according to Eq. (14.25). From this phase diagram the value $K_{11} = 21.5\,M^{-1}$ was evaluated.[5]

The solubility method can be extended to the study of multiple complexes.

Table 14.4   Solubility data for the theophylline (S)-sodium salicylate (L) system[a]

$10^2 L_t$ (M)	$10^2 S_t$ (M)
0	3.87
2.52	5.17
5.04	6.22
10.09	8.60
12.61	9.46
15.14	10.94
20.18	12.88

[a] At 25°C in pH 6.5 phosphate buffer.

Potentiometry. We saw in Chapter 13 that it may be possible to design an electrochemical cell such that an ion activity is related to cell potential by the Nernst equation:

$$E = \text{constant} \pm \frac{RT}{nF} \ln a$$

If the activity of this ion changes in the process of complex formation, then potentiometry offers a means for studying the complex. This is what we do when we measure pK_a values of weak acids. The principle can be extended to study the formation of complexes between metal ions and bases. These complexes, which can be exceedingly strong, are the result of covalent bonding and lie somewhat outside our present concern, but they can be studied in the same way (Connors 2000).

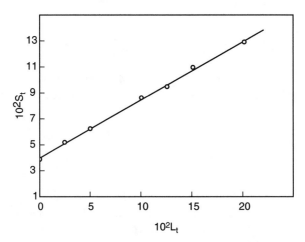

Figure 14.4. Phase solubility diagram for the theophylline (S)-sodium salicylate (L) system at 25°C. [Reproduced by permission from Cohen and Connors (1967).]

We will develop the potentiometric method for the formation of complexes between a weak acid–base conjugate pair (the substrate) and a neutral ligand. The hydrogen ion activity changes as the ligand concentration is altered, so that the ion we monitor, H^+, is a measure of the extent of complex formation but is not itself the substrate or ligand. In general both the acid form of the substrate, HA, and its conjugate base A^-, can complex with the ligand L, so we write

$$HA + L \overset{K_{11a}}{\rightleftharpoons} HAL$$

$$A^- + L \overset{K_{11b}}{\rightleftharpoons} AL^-$$

We also have the usual acid–base equilibrium

$$HA \overset{K_a}{\rightleftharpoons} H^+ + A^-$$

and there also exists this acid–base equilibrium:

$$HAL \overset{K_{a11}}{\rightleftharpoons} H^+ + AL^-$$

Defining and manipulating these four equilibrium constants gives

$$\frac{K_a}{K_{a11}} = \frac{K_{11a}}{K_{11b}} \tag{14.26}$$

Thus only three of these four quantities are independent; that is, we need measure and discuss only three of them to give a full description of this $1:1$ stoichiometric system. We will choose K_a, K_{11a}, and K_{11b}.

The experiment consists of measuring the apparent pK_a of HA as a function of added ligand. We start the analysis by defining the apparent acid dissociation constant by

$$K_a' = \frac{[HA^+]([A^-] + [AL^-])}{[HA] + [HAL]} \tag{14.27}$$

Then the expressions for K_a, K_{11a}, and K_{11b} are combined with Eq. (14.27), yielding

$$K_a' = K_a \frac{(1 + K_{11b}[L])}{(1 + K_{11a}[L])} \tag{14.28}$$

Defining $\Delta pK_a' = pK_a' - pK_a$ allows us to write Eq. (14.28) as

$$\Delta pK_a' = \log \frac{(1 + K_{11a}[L])}{(1 + K_{11b}[L])} \tag{14.29}$$

Further defining the quantity C by

$$C = \frac{1 + K_{11a}[\mathrm{L}]}{1 + K_{11b}[\mathrm{L}]} \tag{14.30}$$

we have $\Delta pK_a' = \log C$. Equation (14.30) is the 1 : 1 binding isotherm. We measure pK_a' as a function of L_t, where pK_a is the value of pK_a' when $L_t = 0$. Then C is found from $\Delta pK_a'$. A separate mass balance relates [L] to L_t. Equation (14.30) is a rectangular hyperbola, and the usual three linear plotting forms can be used to extract values of K_{11a} and K_{11b}. Equation (14.31) shows the form corresponding to Eq. (14.11), the Scatchard plot:

$$\frac{C - 1}{[\mathrm{L}]} = K_{11a} - K_{11b}C \tag{14.31}$$

Table 14.5 gives $\Delta pK_a'$ values for two complexing systems; in both of these α-cyclodextrin, a macrocyclic natural product formed of six residues of glucose, is the ligand. The substrates are benzoic acid and 4-cyanophenol (Connors et al. 1982; Lin and Connors 1983). The first interesting feature of these data is the very substantial values of $\Delta pK_a'$ that may occur. The second point is that $\Delta pK_a'$ may be either positive or negative. [If $\Delta pK_a'$ is negative, it can be redefined as

Table 14.5 $\Delta pK_a'$ values at 25°C for the complexing of benzoic acid and of 4-cyanophenol with α-cyclodextrin

L_t (M)	$\Delta pK_a'$	
	Benzoic Acid	4-Cyanophenol
0.0017	0.24	—
0.0020	—	−0.16
0.0030	—	−0.21
0.0045	—	−0.28
0.0057	0.61	—
0.0075	—	−0.38
0.01	0.84	−0.42
0.02	1.10	−0.52
0.03	1.25	−0.56
0.04	1.34	−0.58
0.05	—	−0.58
0.06	1.45	−0.59
0.07	1.48	−0.58
0.08	1.51	−0.59
0.09	1.54	−0.59
0.10	1.55	−0.58

$\Delta pK'_a = pK_a - pK'_a$ in order to generate a positive number; alternatively, define $C' = 1/C$ and use C' instead of C in Eqs. (14.30) and (14.31).] Referring to Eq. (14.30) shows that a positive $\Delta pK'_a$, which signifies that $C > 1$, means that $K_{11a} > K_{11b}$; the conjugate acid binds to the ligand more strongly than does the conjugate base. Similarly, a negative $\Delta pK'_a$ means that $K_{11b} > K_{11a}$. If $K_{11a} = K_{11b}$, $pK'_a = pK_a$ so $\Delta pK'_a = 0$, and the method is inapplicable; this circumstance is rare, however, because the conjugate acid and base differ electronically very profoundly, so their noncovalent interaction possibilities differ as a consequence.

From plots of Eq. (14.31), the values $K_{11a} = 722 \, M^{-1}$ and $K_{11b} = 11.2 \, M^{-1}$ were found for the benzoic acid–α-cyclodextrin complexes. The 4-cyanophenol complexes gave $K_{11a} = 158 \, M^{-1}$ and $K_{11b} = 662 \, M^{-1}$.

Dialysis. This interesting method is applicable to the study of the binding of small molecules to macromolecules, and it has been widely applied to drug–protein binding. The experimental method requires that two solution compartments be separated by a semipermeable membrane, that is, a membrane through which the small molecule can freely pass but the macromolecule cannot. Let us call the macromolecule the substrate S and the small molecule the ligand L. We label the compartments 1 and 2.

The substrate, at known total concentration S_t, is placed in compartment 1, where it is constrained to remain because of its size. The small ligand is placed in compartment 2. The system is allowed to come to equilibrium at constant temperature.

At equilibrium the chemical potentials of free L, the diffusible ligand, in the two compartments are equal. We may therefore (usually) infer that the concentrations of L are equal. Using subscripts to identify the compartments, we write this equality as

$$[L]_1 = [L]_2 \tag{14.32}$$

The solutions in the two compartments are analyzed to determine their total ligand concentrations, $(L_t)_1$ and $(L_t)_2$. We can now state, for compartment 1

$$(L_t)_1 = [L]_1 + [\text{bound L}]_1 \tag{14.33}$$

and for compartment 2

$$(L_t)_2 = [L]_2 \tag{14.34}$$

We therefore have all the information required to calculate the quantity $\bar{i}$ [Eq. (14.12)], rewritten here explicitly for compartment 1:

$$\bar{i} = \frac{(L_t)_1 - [L]_1}{(S_t)_1} \tag{14.35}$$

This experiment is repeated over a range of ligand concentrations, and then binding isotherm (14.13) is applied to the data to determine the parameters n and k.

Strengths of Complexes. We might express the strength of a complex in terms of either its binding constant or (what is equivalent) its standard free energy change $\Delta G°$, or as its standard enthalpy change $\Delta H°$. These may parallel each other for comparable systems, but they may diverge markedly because of the thermodynamic relationship $\Delta G° = \Delta H° - T\Delta S°$. Let us make some simple calculations to develop a sense of the magnitudes to be expected.

We recall from an earlier discussion that the net free-energy change may be divided into contributions from solute–solute (i.e., substrate–ligand) interactions, from solute–solvent (solvation) interactions, and from solvent–solvent interactions, or

$$\Delta G° = \Delta G°_{SL} + \Delta G°_{solvation} + \Delta G°_{MM} \qquad (14.36)$$

Let us first consider an H-bond complex formation reaction in vacuo or in a very nonpolar solvent, so that essentially only the solute–solute interaction makes a contribution; thus $\Delta G° = \Delta G°_{SL}$. Suppose that $\Delta H°$ for the reaction is -3 kcal mol^{-1}, a typical value for a noncovalent interaction. We also need an estimate for $\Delta S°$, which we will obtain with the following (oversimplified) argument. In the process of the two species S and L interacting to form the complex C, some modes of molecular motion are lost. Even supposing that all internal modes (vibrational and rotational) of S and L are preserved in C, three translational modes will be lost. Applying the statistical mechanical definition of entropy [Chapter 2, Eqs. (2.1) and (2.2)] to the reaction $S + L \rightleftharpoons C$, we obtain $\Delta S° = -R\ln 3 = -9.1$ J K^{-1} mol^{-1} or -2.2 cal K^{-1} mol^{-1}. For our hypothetical system we therefore calculate $\Delta G° = -3000 + (298)(2.2) = -2350$ cal mol^{-1}. With the basic equation $\Delta G° = -RT \ln K_{11}$, we calculate $K_{11} = 53$ M^{-1} at 25°C.

Now let us consider the quite different system of two nonpolar molecules in aqueous solution. The solute–solvent and solute–solute interactions will be negligible or will largely offset each other, so in this case we can write $\Delta G° = \Delta G°_{MM}$. To estimate $\Delta G°_{MM}$ we draw on the cavity theory of the hydrophobic interaction, according to which the change in free energy is equal to the product $\gamma\Delta A$, where γ is the solvent surface tension and ΔA is the change in nonpolar surface area in contact with the solvent. Suppose $\Delta A = -50$ Å^2; this is about the cross-sectional area of an aromatic ring. For water $\gamma = -71.8$ erg cm^{-2}. Thus

$$\Delta G° = \left(71.8\frac{erg}{cm^2}\right)\left(\frac{1\,J}{10^7\,erg}\right)\left(-50\,\mathring{A}^2\right)\left(\frac{10^{-8}\,cm}{1\,\mathring{A}}\right)^2 = -3.6 \times 10^{-20}\,J$$

This is the free-energy change per complex; we multiply by N_A to put it on a molar basis, finding $\Delta G° = -21.7$ kJ mol^{-1} or -5.2 kcal mol^{-1}. Converting to K_{11} gives $K_{11} = 6.5 \times 10^3$ M^{-1}.

These calculations illustrate the magnitudes of binding constants that may be expected, although the range is even larger than indicated by these numbers. Values of K_{11} smaller than 1 M^{-1} have been reported, although such results should be interpreted with caution. Very large values are not unusual. Consider the pK_a of phenol, which is 10.00 at 25°C. K_a is a dissociation constant. Its reciprocal, $1/K_a = K_{11}$, is a binding constant; this is obviously 1×10^{10} M^{-1}.

As was pointed out for acids and bases in Table 12.8, values of equilibrium constants for closely related reactants tend to fall into characteristic ranges. This behavior provides a coarse level of predictability. There is some evidence that for each identifiable "population" or class of complex equilibria the $\log K_{11}$ values are normally distributed (Connors 1995; Burnette and Connors 2000), and that the standard deviation of all such populations is about one $\log K_{11}$ unit (Connors 1997).

PROBLEMS

14.1. Define overall and stepwise binding constants for the formation of complex S_2L_3, and show how these constants are related.

14.2. Construct plots according to Eqs. (14.9)–(14.11) of the simulated data in Table 14.2.

14.3. Equation (14.19) describes the binding curve for the spectrophotometric study of 1 : 1 complex formation. What is the value of the initial slope (i.e., the slope when $[L] = 0$) of the plot of $\Delta A / b$ versus $[L]$?

14.4. (a) From Eq. (14.19) derive the Scatchard linear plotting form (corresponding to Eq. 14.11).

(b) Plot the data in Table 14.3 to evaluate K_{11} and $\Delta\epsilon_{11}$. Assume $L_t = [L]$.

14.5. What is the value of the initial slope of a plot of C against $[L]$ according to Eq. (14.30)?

NOTES

1. The classic treatment of covalent bonding is Linus Pauling's *The Nature of the Chemical Bond* (1960). Of course, more recent sources must be consulted for later theoretical and experimental findings.

2. Some authors refer collectively to these r^{-6} terms (r^{-7} in the forces) as *van der Waals* interactions, but there is some ambiguity in this term, as certain authors seem to mean only the London force by the designation van der Waals.

3. This statement is not strictly correct, as certain molecules possessing quadrupolar moments can undergo additional forces, but these can usually be neglected.

4. We have seen earlier manifestations of Eq. (14.7). The Langmuir adsorption isotherm (Chapter 11) and Eq. (12.22) have this form. The identity $K = 1/[L]$ when $f_{11} = 0.500$ is the same as the condition $pK_a = pH$ at the midpoint of an acid–base titration.

5. Earlier 1 : 1 binding isotherms [Eqs. (14.7) and (14.19)] have been hyperbolic functions of $[L]$, whereas Eq. (14.25) is a linear function of L_t. This distinction arises because of the unusual feature of the solubility experiment in which $[S]$ is maintained constant while S_t varies; in the other methods S_t is held constant and $[S]$ varies.

APPENDIXES

APPENDIX A

PHYSICAL CONSTANTS

Quantity	Symbol	Value
Avogadro's number	N_A	$6.023 \times 10^{23}\,\mathrm{mol^{-1}}$
Gas constant	R	$8.314\,\mathrm{J\,K^{-1}\,mol^{-1}}$
		$1.987\,\mathrm{cal\,K^{-1}\,mol^{-1}}$
		$0.08206\,\mathrm{L\,atm\,K^{-1}\,mol^{-1}}$
Boltzmann constant	k	$1.380 \times 10^{-23}\,\mathrm{J\,K^{-1}}$
Faraday	F	$9.6487 \times 10^{4}\,\mathrm{C\,mol^{-1}}$
Elementary charge	e	$1.602 \times 10^{-19}\,\mathrm{C}$
Planck's constant	h	$6.626 \times 10^{-34}\,\mathrm{J\,s}$
Speed of light in vacuum	c	$2.9979 \times 10^{8}\,\mathrm{m\,s^{-1}}$

APPENDIX B

REVIEW OF MATHEMATICS

B.1. INTRODUCTION

The extent of mathematics required in order to master the material in the professional pharmacy curriculum is really quite modest, comprising the basic operations of arithmetic and algebra; some fundamentals of plane geometry, analytic geometry, and calculus; and ideas from mathematical statistics. Nearly everything mathematical that you will need to know as a pharmacy student you have presumably already mastered in high school or college courses, except perhaps for the mathematical statistics content and the concept of partial differentiation (which will be treated in the following pages). You already know, or you once knew, about 95% of the material in this review (exclusive of the statistics section), which therefore should not present a difficult intellectual challenge. Although our immediate concern is to provide a basis for the mathematical needs of thermodynamics, this review goes beyond thermodynamics to include the mathematical methods useful in other parts of the curriculum.

Mathematics is treated by scientists as a tool or a language, and it is this attitude that you should adopt. Your goal in reviewing this material is to develop such a familiarity with the mathematical operations that you need not worry about them or even give much conscious thought to them. Such a capability will allow you to concentrate your attention on the new ideas being presented in your courses, whether they are physical chemical, pharmacokinetic, or biological. Not every bit of mathematics that you may encounter in your future studies will be treated here, but nearly all of it will be found here.

As a first step in developing this review of essential mathematics as the language of science, Table B.1 lists some standard mathematical symbols. As you read the following pages, keep in mind that this is a review, not a logical development

262

Table B.1. Common mathematical symbols

Symbol	Meaning
$=$	Equals; is equal to
$\equiv$	Is equivalent to
$\sim$ or $\approx$ or $\cong$	Is approximately equal to
$\neq$	Is not equal to
$\propto$	Is proportional to
$<$	Is less than
$\leq$	Is less than or equal to
$>$	Is greater than
$\geq$	Is greater than or equal to
$+$	Plus
$-$	Minus
$\times$ or $\cdot$	Times
$\div$ or $/$	Divided by
$\pm$	Plus or minus
$\sqrt{}$	The square root of
$\therefore$	Therefore
$\|$	The absolute value of

of the subject. Results are usually presented without derivation; you have already seen the derivations in your mathematics courses. Examples will draw on chemical concepts that, in many instances, will already be familiar to you, but a few ideas may appear that are new.

B.2. LOGARITHMS AND EXPONENTS

Definition and Properties. Suppose we have the power function of Eq. (B.1).

$$a = b^x \tag{B.1}$$

We define[1] the *logarithm of a to the base b* by

$$\text{Log}_b a = x \tag{B.2}$$

There are only two logarithmic bases (values of b) in common use, namely, $b = 10$ (giving *Briggsian logarithms*) and $b = e$ (giving *natural logarithms*). Briggsian logarithms are denoted *log*, whereas natural logarithms are denoted *ln*. An important property[2] of all logarithms is stated by Eq. (B.3).

$$\text{Log}_b b = 1 \tag{B.3}$$

It follows that

$$\text{Log } 10 = 1 \tag{B.4}$$
$$\ln e = 1 \tag{B.5}$$

Another property[3] is given by Eqs. (B.6) and (B.7):

$$\text{Log } 1 = 0 \tag{B.6}$$
$$\ln 1 = 0 \tag{B.7}$$

The number e is extremely important in mathematics and science. It has the value $2.718\cdots$.

At one time Briggsian logarithms were widely used to carry out arithmetic operations, but with electronic calculators and computers this use is obsolete. However, the base ten log function continues to be indispensable in the sciences, for two reasons: (1) some important physicochemical concepts (such as pH) are defined in terms of Briggsian logarithms and (2) logarithms to the base 10 have the convenient property of revealing order-of-magnitude changes or differences at a glance. For example, $\log 10^2 = 2.00$, $\log 10^3 = 3.00$, and so on.

Let us obtain a relationship by means of which we can interconvert Briggsian and natural logarithms of the same number. Let a be the number, and write

$$\ln a = c \log a \tag{B.8}$$

where we want to find the conversion factor c. Suppose for convenience (any number would do) that we set $a = 10$. From Eq. (B.8), we obtain

$$c = \frac{\ln 10}{\log 10} = \frac{2.303\cdots}{1} \tag{B.9}$$

where the numerator is found by means of an electronic calculator, and the denominator from Eq. (B.4). Therefore we can interconvert ln and log values by Eq. (B.10):

$$\ln a = 2.303 \log a \tag{B.10}$$

Operations with Logarithms. Suppose that we have both Eqs. (B.11) and (B.12):

$$a = b^x \tag{B.11}$$
$$c = b^y \tag{B.12}$$

We know from Eq. (B.2) that

$$\text{Log}_b a = x$$
$$\text{Log}_b c = y$$

But we can also write from Eqs. (B.11) and (B.12):

$$ac = b^x \cdot b^y = b^{x+y}$$

It follows that

$$\mathrm{Log}_b\, ac = \log_b a + \log_b c \tag{B.13}$$

Thus, the logarithm of a product of two numbers is equal to the sum of the logarithms of the individual numbers. This very valuable result permits several other relationships to be derived; these are stated as Eqs. (B.14)–(B.17). Although these are written in terms of log, exactly analogous equations can be given for ln:

$$\mathrm{Log}\, pq = \log p + \log q \tag{B.14}$$

$$\mathrm{Log}\, \frac{p}{q} = \log p - \log q \tag{B.15}$$

$$\mathrm{Log}\, \frac{1}{q} = -\log q \tag{B.16}$$

$$\mathrm{Log}\, p^n = n \log p \tag{B.17}$$

Example B.1. It is convenient to define, as a measure of the acidity of an aqueous solution, the pH by

$$\mathrm{pH} = -\log [\mathrm{H}^+]$$

where $[\mathrm{H}^+]$ is the hydrogen ion concentration in mol L^{-1}. This means that

$$\mathrm{pH} = \log \frac{1}{[\mathrm{H}^+]}$$

(a) Calculate the pH if $[\mathrm{H}^+] = 5.00 \times 10^{-3}$ M.

$$\begin{aligned}
\mathrm{pH} &= -\log 5.00 \times 10^{-3} \\
&= -(\log 5.00 + \log 10^{-3}) \\
&= -(0.70 - 3.00) \\
&= 2.30
\end{aligned}$$

The pH is a positive number provided that $[\mathrm{H}^+] < 1$ M. Seldom is it justifiable to express pH values beyond the second decimal place (i.e., 0.01 pH unit).

(b) What is the hydrogen ion concentration if pH $= 8.67$?

$$pH = 8.67$$
$$-\log[H^+] = 8.67$$
$$\log[H^+] = -8.67 = -9.00 + 0.33$$
$$[H^+] = 2.14 \times 10^{-9}\,M$$

This last step is called "taking the antilogarithm." It is the reverse of taking the logarithm, and is easily accomplished on the electronic calculator. A useful check on the calculation is to convert the $[H^+]$ back to pH. Another check is to be sure that the order of magnitude is reasonable; this means that the answer is as expected at least to within a factor of 10.

Operations with Exponents. The following identities follow from the properties of logarithms [actually we used Eq. (B.20) in order to derive Eq. (B.13)]:

$$a^0 = 1 \tag{B.18}$$
$$a^1 = a \tag{B.19}$$
$$a^u \cdot a^v = a^{u+v} \tag{B.20}$$
$$a^{-u} = \frac{1}{a^u} \tag{B.21}$$
$$(a^u)^v = a^{uv} \tag{B.22}$$
$$(ab)^u = a^u b^u \tag{B.23}$$

Scientific Notation. Many quantities in theoretical and experimental science are either extremely large or extremely small, so an exponential form of expressing them is convenient. Nearly always these are written as an integral power of 10, as shown in these examples:

$$51{,}000 \equiv 5.1 \times 10^4 \equiv 51 \times 10^3$$
$$0.00000417 \equiv 4.17 \times 10^{-6}$$

As seen in Example B.1, this is a very convenient way in which to express a number whose logarithm is to be taken, because [as seen in Eq. (B.13)] the logarithm of a product is equal to the sum of the logs, and because $\log 10^n = n \log 10 = n$. Thus

$$\text{Log}\,4.17 \times 10^{-6} = (\log 4.17) - 6 = -5.38$$

B.3. ALGEBRAIC AND GRAPHICAL ANALYSIS

Setting up Proportions. It often happens that we know three related items of information and seek a fourth member of the set. In order to solve for this fourth, unknown, item, we write an equation. One way to do this is to express the relationships in terms of sentences, by means of which we can more readily detect analogous patterns. Then we replace the English words with mathematical symbols.

Example B.2. How many moles of sodium chloride are contained in 5.00 g of NaCl?

The first of the following statements gives two pieces of known information; the second analogous statement contains the unknown.

$$58.45 \text{ g of NaCl corresponds to 1 mol}$$

so

$$5.00 \text{ g of NaCl corresponds to how many mol?}$$

Now we replace the words with symbols (and notice how the units cancel):

$$\frac{58.45}{5.00} = \frac{1}{x}$$

$$x = \frac{5.00}{58.45} = 0.0855$$

Generalizing this equation gives these important formulas:

$$\text{mol} = \frac{W\,(\text{g})}{\text{MW}} \qquad\qquad (\text{B.24})$$

$$\text{mmol} = \frac{W\,(\text{mg})}{\text{MW}} \qquad\qquad (\text{B.25})$$

Eq. (B.25) is obtained from Eq. (B.24) by multiplying both sides by 10^3. A millimole (mmol) is one-thousandth of a mole.

Example B.3. A sample of aspirin weighing 305 mg was found by analysis to contain 294 mg of aspirin. What is its percent purity?

If the sample contained 305 mg, it would be 100% pure. Actually it contains 294 mg, so it is $x\%$ pure. Therefore

$$\frac{305}{294} = \frac{100}{x}$$

or 96.4% pure. Generalizing this result, we obtain

$$\% \text{ purity} = \frac{W_{\text{found}}}{W_{\text{taken}}} \times 100 \qquad\qquad (\text{B.26})$$

In a later section we will treat the conversion of physical units. Here we see that setting up a proportion is one way to handle this problem.

Example B.4. Convert 75 min to hours.
   If 60 min is equivalent to 1 h, then 75 min is equivalent to x h?

$$\frac{60}{75} = \frac{1}{x}$$
$$x = 1.25 \, \text{h}.$$

Ratios and Fractions. We are going to consider this subject in the context of chemistry rather than of pure mathematics. To clarify the distinction between a ratio and a fraction, consider the dissociation of a weak acid (like a carboxylic acid) in water:

$$\text{HA} \rightleftharpoons \text{H}^+ + \text{A}^-$$

Here we let HA represent any neutral weak acid, where A^- is the anion resulting from the dissociation. We define the *ratio* of anion to neutral acid by

$$\frac{[\text{A}^-]}{[\text{HA}]} = \text{ratio of anion to acid} = R_{\text{A}^-}$$

where square brackets signify molar concentrations. Similarly we have

$$\frac{[\text{HA}]}{[\text{A}^-]} = \text{ratio of acid to anion} = R_{\text{HA}}$$

These ratios play an important role in describing chemical equilibria.
   There can also be situations in which we wish to define the *fraction* of anion in the mixture of A^- and HA. This fraction, which we will label F_{A^-}, is defined as

$$\frac{[\text{A}^-]}{[\text{HA}] + [\text{A}^-]} = F_{\text{A}^-} = \text{fraction of anion}$$

Similarly the fraction present as the neutral acid is given by

$$\frac{[\text{HA}]}{[\text{HA}] + [\text{A}^-]} = F_{\text{HA}} = \text{fraction of acid}$$

By substitution it is easily found that

$$F_{\text{A}^-} + F_{\text{HA}} = 1$$

This is a general property of fractions as defined in this way; they sum to unity. As a consequence, if the whole is divided into n fractions, only $n - 1$ of these are independent (i.e., capable of independent variation).

Example B.5. A solution made up to contain a *total* concentration (also called an *analytical concentration*) of weak acid 3.50×10^{-3} M is found to have an anion concentration of 8.95×10^{-4} M. Calculate the fractions of solute in the anion and neutral forms.

We are told that the total concentration is 3.50×10^{-3} M. This is the sum $[HA] + [A^-]$, since the solute can exist in either or both forms, and no other. Hence

$$F_{A^-} = \frac{[A^-]}{[HA] + [A^-]} = \frac{0.895 \times 10^{-3}}{3.50 \times 10^{-3}} = 0.256$$

From the identity $F_{A^-} + F_{HA} = 1$, we immediately obtain $F_{HA} = 1 - 0.256 = 0.744$.

A fraction can be converted to a percentage through multiplication by 100, Eq. (B.27); see also Eq. (B.26).

$$\text{Percent} = 100 \times \text{fraction} \tag{B.27}$$

Thus in this example 25.6% is in the form of the anion and 74.4% is in the form of the neutral acid.

Example B.6. For the system in Example B.5, calculate the ratios $[A^-]/[HA]$ and $[HA]/[A^-]$.

We know that $[A^-] = 0.895 \times 10^{-3}$ M and $[HA] + [A^-] = 3.50 \times 10^{-3}$ M, so we find that $[HA] = 2.605 \times 10^{-3}$ M. Therefore

$$\frac{[A^-]}{[HA]} = \frac{0.895}{2.605} = 0.344$$

The reciprocal gives us the other ratio:

$$\frac{[HA]}{[A^-]} = \frac{1}{0.344} = 2.91$$

Fractions must be less than (or equal to) unity, but a ratio can be greater than unity. Ratios and fractions (in this context) are dimensionless.

Students sometimes wonder why, in calculations like this (the dissociation of HA according to $HA \rightleftharpoons H^+ + A^-$) we were able to ignore the H^+ produced in the reaction. The answer is that we are counting molecules or moles, not grams; each molecule of HA that dissociates yields one H^+ ion and one A^- ion. If we counted both ions, we would be double-counting, with the result that we would appear to be creating matter, which we know is impossible.

Solving Simultaneous Equations. From algebra we know that if we have n simultaneous independent equations in n unknowns, we can solve the equations to find all n unknowns. Usually, of course, we encounter the simplest case in which we have one equation and one unknown. It is more interesting when we have two or more unknowns.

Let us continue to discuss our earlier example of the dissociation of weak acid HA to yield anion A^-. Often it happens that we know the total concentration and can measure the ratio of concentrations. From this information we seek the individual concentrations [HA] and $[A^-]$.

We have two unknowns, so we hope that we can write two independent equations. We begin by setting in equation form that which we know. We write

$$\frac{[A^-]}{[HA]} = R_{A^-} \tag{B.28}$$

$$[HA] + [A^-] = c_t \tag{B.29}$$

where we know (have numerical values for) R_{A^-} and c_t. Equations (B.28) and (B.29) are two independent equations in two unknowns.

There are several ways to solve simultaneous equations; the simplest is by algebraic substitution. Solve Eq. (B.28) for $[A^-]$ and substitute this into Eq. (B.29). From Eq. (B.28), $[A^-] = R_{A^-}[HA]$, so we get from Eq. (B.29),

$$[HA] + R_{A^-}[HA] = c_t$$

We have reduced two equations with two unknowns to one equation with one unknown, for which we solve

$$[HA] = \frac{c_t}{1 + R_{A^-}}$$

Having found [HA], we can use Eq. (B.28) or (B.29) to find $[A^-]$.

The requirement that the equations be independent means that there is no possible way to obtain (to derive) one of them from the others; that is, each equation must contribute some additional information to the problem. For example, in the preceding case suppose that we only know c_t. There is no way from this knowledge alone that we could deduce the value of R_{A^-}, so we could not calculate individual values of [HA] and $[A^-]$; we would have a single equation [Eq. (B.29)] and two unknowns.

The solution of simultaneous equations is usually easy. The difficult tasks are to analyze the problem so as to identify and write down the equations, and to collect the necessary information so they can be solved numerically.

Solution of Quadratic Equations. Everyone learns in high school algebra how to solve a quadratic equation, that is, an equation in which the unknown quantity appears to the second power. In its "standard" form a quadratic equation can be written

$$ax^2 + bx + c = 0 \qquad (B.30)$$

where x is the unknown quantity and a, b, c are known quantities; $a, b,$ and c can be viewed as constants in the particular situation. The solution of Eq. (B.30) is given by Eq. (B.31).

$$x = \frac{-b \pm \sqrt{b^2 - 4ac}}{2a} \qquad (B.31)$$

This equation should be memorized. It shows that there are two solutions to Eq. (B.30), corresponding to the use of either the plus or the minus sign in Eq. (B.31). Usually only one of these solutions has physical significance; the other solution can be ignored. By "physical significance" we mean that it makes sense in the context of the physical situation. For example, if x is a concentration, obviously a negative value has no physical significance. The capability of some theories or mathematical operations to generate solutions lacking physical significance is known as "formal surplus structure."

Example B.7. We will continue to use our example of the dissociation of weak acid HA according to

$$HA \rightleftharpoons H^+ + A^-$$

Let us define an equilibrium constant by

$$K_a = \frac{[H^+][A^-]}{[HA]} \qquad (B.32)$$

We also have the equation giving the total solute concentration:

$$c_t = [HA] + [A^-] \qquad (B.33)$$

We now observe that each molecule of HA that dissociates yields one H^+ and one A^-, suggesting (this is not quite true, but is nearly always a very good approximation) that we can write

$$[A^-] = [H^+]$$

Making this substitution in Eq. (B.32) gives

$$K_a = \frac{[H^+]^2}{c_t - [H^+]} \qquad (B.34)$$

This is a quadratic equation. First we rearrange it to place it in the standard form, obtaining

$$[H^+]^2 + K_a[H^+] - K_a c_t = 0 \tag{B.35}$$

Comparing Eqs. (B.30) and (B.35) gives these identities:

$$a = 1$$
$$b = K_a$$
$$c = -K_a c_t$$
$$x = [H^+]$$

The solution is accordingly

$$[H^+] = \frac{-K_a \pm \sqrt{K_a^2 + 4K_a c_t}}{2} \tag{B.36}$$

Example B.8. Calculate the pH in a solution that is 0.010 M with respect to a weak acid if $K_a = 1.00 \times 10^{-5}$.

We use Eq. (B.36):

$$[H^+] = \frac{-1.0 \times 10^{-5} \pm \sqrt{1.0 \times 10^{-10} + (4 \times 10^{-5})(1 \times 10^{-2})}}{2}$$

$$= \frac{-1.0 \times 10^{-5} \pm \sqrt{1 \times 10^{-10} + 4 \times 10^{-7}}}{2}$$

$$= \frac{-1.0 \times 10^{-5} \pm \sqrt{0.01 \times 10^{-8} + 40 \times 10^{-8}}}{2}$$

$$= \frac{-1.0 \times 10^{-5} \pm \sqrt{40.01 \times 10^{-8}}}{2}$$

$$= \frac{-1.0 \times 10^{-5} \pm 6.325 \times 10^{-4}}{2}$$

$$= \frac{-1.0 \times 10^{-5} \pm 63.25 \times 10^{-5}}{2}$$

$$= 31.125 \times 10^{-5} = 3.11 \times 10^{-4}$$

So pH $= -\log [H^+] = 3.51$. Note that the solution employing the negative sign has been rejected.[4]

Approximations. Scientists, unlike mathematicians, are often satisfied with approximate rather than exact solutions. The level of approximation that is acceptable is determined by practical criteria and is not completely arbitrary. If we cannot experimentally detect or measure an effect, we may feel justified in neglecting it. Or how we use the result may determine the acceptable level of approximation; for example, if we are to measure the pH of Lake Mendota water, we may be satisfied with a result accurate ±0.1 pH unit (for various practical reasons), whereas if we are measuring the equilibrium constant of a weak acid, we will surely hope for measurements accurate to ±0.01 pH unit. This kind of thinking is then extended to the equations that enable us to describe and interpret the measurements. If we make an approximation in an equation it is no longer exact in a mathematical sense,[5] but it may be acceptably accurate in a scientific sense.

Example B.9. Calculate the pH in a solution that is 0.010 M with respect to a weak acid if $K_a = 1.00 \times 10^{-5}$.

This is the same problem for which we obtained an accurate solution in Example B.8. In that calculation we used the equation

$$K_a = \frac{[H^+]^2}{c_t - [H^+]} \tag{B.37}$$

Now suppose that the hydrogen ion concentration is much smaller than is the total concentration c_t. Then we can reasonably make this approximation:

$$c_t - [H^+] \approx c_t$$

Making this substitution in Eq. (B.37) gives

$$K_a \approx \frac{[H^+]^2}{c_t}$$

or

$$[H^+] \approx \sqrt{K_a c_t} \tag{B.38}$$

Applying Eq. (B.38) to our problem, we get

$$\begin{aligned}
[H^+] &= \sqrt{(1 \times 10^{-5})(1 \times 10^{-2})} \\
&= \sqrt{1 \times 10^{-7}} \\
&= \sqrt{10 \times 10^{-8}} \\
&= 3.16 \times 10^{-4} \, M
\end{aligned}$$

or pH = 3.50. Our approximation has led to a very simple solution, and comparison with Example B.8 shows the level of error that has been introduced.

When is it acceptable to use such an approximation? This depends on those factors already mentioned. In the present example we might examine the quantity $c_t - [H^+]$ to see if $[H^+]$ is indeed much smaller than c_t (for that is the assumption on which the approximation is based). In Example B.9 we can compare these numbers:

Exact: $c_t - [H^+] = 1.00 \times 10^{-2} - 3 \times 10^{-4} = 0.97 \times 10^{-2}$

Approximate: $c_t - [H^+] \approx c_t = 1.00 \times 10^{-2}$

Therefore the approximation introduces about a 3% error into the denominator of Eq. (B.37). The error in the final answer is even smaller than this, and for most purposes the approximate result would be acceptable. This is the practical point of view that is adopted, and it can be seen that decisions of this sort depend greatly on experience with making calculations and with interpreting experimental results.

Graphical Properties of Linear Functions. Let us begin this treatment by writing this linear equation in a standard form:

$$y = mx + b \qquad (B.39)$$

We call this "linear" because y depends on x to the first power. The following terminology is used:

x, y are *variables*

m, b are *parameters* (i.e., constants of the system)

More specifically, x is often called the *independent variable* and y the *dependent variable*. This terminology signifies that the value of x is under our control, and that the value of y then depends on x.

If paired x, y data are related by Eq. (B.39), when plotted on graph paper they yield a straight line (which is another reason why we call Eq. (B.39) "linear"). Figure B.1 shows how the plot is conventionally made. It is traditional to plot the x values on the horizontal axis (the abscissa) and the y values on the vertical axis (the ordinate).

Let us set $x = 0$ in Eq. (B.39); we get $y = b$; that is, b is the value of y when $x = 0$. We call this the *intercept on the y axis*. The parameter m describes the steepness with which y increases (or decreases) as x increases; m is called the *slope*. Evidently if we know the values of m and b, we know everything there is to know about Eq. (B.39).

Now let us review the calculation of m, the slope. In Fig. B.2, two points, on the line, having coordinates (x_1, y_1) and (x_2, y_2), are identified. We write the equation of the line for each of these points (for the equation is satisfied at every point on the line):

$$y_1 = mx_1 + b$$

$$y_2 = mx_2 + b$$

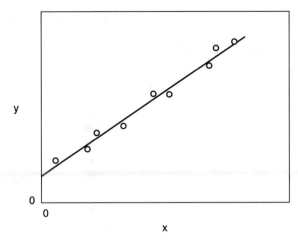

Figure B.1. A typical straight-line plot of data points.

Now subtract y_1 from y_2 and solve for m:

$$m = \frac{y_2 - y_1}{x_2 - x_1} \tag{B.40}$$

This equation allows us to calculate the slope of any straight line. The slope m can be positive (y increases as x increases), negative (y decreases as x increases), or zero (y does not depend on x). We can read b from the graph as the value of y when $x = 0$, or more accurately and sometimes more conveniently (because sometimes the plot doesn't include the $x = 0$ region), b can be calculated from Eq. (B.38),

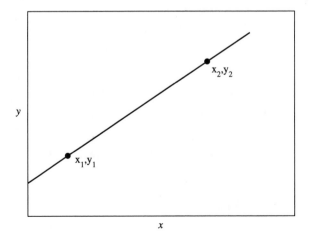

Figure B.2. Illustrating the calculation of the slope of a straight line; see text.

since we now know *m*. Simply choose any point on the line and substitute the corresponding numerical values into $b = y - mx$.

Here are two interesting special cases of Eq. (B.38).

1. $m = 0$. Then the line is horizontal, parallel to the *x* axis, since substituting this value of *m* into Eq. (B.38) gives $y = b$.
2. $b = 0$. Then Eq. (B.38) yields

$$y = mx \tag{B.41}$$

showing that the line passes through the origin at $y = 0$, $x = 0$.

Example B.10. Table B.2 lists experimental data (Cohen and Connors 1967) giving the solubility of the drug theophylline (in water at 25°C) as a function of the concentration of added sodium salicylate. Analyze the data.

The first thing to do is to plot the data. Use graph paper having fine enough divisions to preserve the accuracy of the data; 1-mm divisions usually work well, whereas $\frac{1}{4}$-in. divisions are too coarse.[6] Figure B.3 shows the plot of the data. Since the sodium salicylate concentration was set by the experimenter, we consider it to be the independent variable *x*.

The data points appear to describe a straight line. There is a theoretical reason for this, but we can view it purely experimentally as a pleasingly simple result. Note that the data points show some small but significant "scatter" about the line that has been drawn. This scatter introduces ambiguity into the question of how best to draw the line. Later, in Section B.5, we will deal with this issue of the "best straight line," but for the present it is sufficient to note that we draw a line that appears to approximately balance the deviations of the points above and below the line.

Next we calculate the slope of the line. Because of the scatter seen in the experimental points, our two points for the slope calculation will be taken from the line itself, for it is the slope of the line that we want.[7] Any two points will do, but they should be far enough apart to yield an accurate result. Points

Table B.2. Solubility of theophylline in water at 25.0°C as a function of added sodium salicylate

Sodium Salicylate Concentration (M)	Theophylline Concentration (M)
0	0.0387
0.0252	0.0517
0.0504	0.0622
0.1009	0.0860
0.1261	0.0946
0.1514	0.1094
0.2018	0.1288

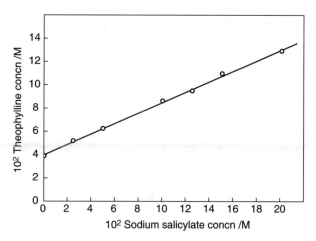

Figure B.3. Plot of the data in Example B.10.

corresponding to $x_1 = 0.060$ and $x_2 = 0.160$ were chosen. Reading directly from Fig. B.3 gives

At $x_1 = 0.060\,M$, $y_1 = 0.0669\,M$
At $x_2 = 0.160\,M$, $y_2 = 0.1122\,M$

These numbers are used in Eq. (B.40):

$$m = \frac{0.1122 - 0.0669}{0.160 - 0.060} = 0.453$$

Now we calculate b using (for convenience, because we already have the values) point x_1, y_1:

$$b = y - mx$$
$$= 0.0669 - (0.453)(0.060)$$
$$= 0.0397\,M$$

Note that b has the units of y whereas m has the units of y/x. Also observe that b as calculated from the line is slightly different from the experimental value of $0.0387\,M$ when $x = 0$. Such discrepancies are common in scientific work. They add interest to the interpretation of experimental data.

We can now state that the set of data given in Example B.10 can be described by the equation

$$y = 0.453x + 0.0397$$

where x = sodium salicylate concentration in M
    y = theophylline concentration in M

and the equation is valid over the range $x = 0$–0.20 M. The physical interpretation is that the presence of sodium salicylate increases the theophylline solubility in a linear manner. How this comes about chemically we will not pursue here (but see Chapter 14 for an interpretation).

Linearization of Nonlinear Functions. The experimental data of Example B.10 consisted of molar concentrations, and we found empirically that a plot of theophylline solubility as a function of sodium salicylate concentration gave a straight line. We could conclude that the concentrations were linearly related, and we obtained the parameters of the straight-line relationship.

It is not always this simple. Often, perhaps usually, the data are smoothly but nonlinearly related. In such circumstances we may be able to carry out a mathematical transformation that converts a nonlinear function to a linear function. This is often very desirable, because of the simplicity with which we can describe straight lines. We may have theoretical reasons to expect certain transformations to work in this way, or we may just try different plotting forms empirically, hoping that we will generate a straight line. Here are some of the most common transformations.

1. *Exponential Functions.* These have the general form

$$y = ae^{bx} \tag{B.42}$$

where, as before, x and y are variables, a and b are parameters, and e is the base of natural logarithms. We take the natural logarithm of both sides:

$$\ln y = \ln a + bx \tag{B.43}$$

This operation has converted the nonlinear function Eq. (B.42) to the linear function Eq. (B.43), which has the form of Eq. (B.39) for a straight line. In other words, if Eq. (B.42) describes the data, a plot of $\ln y$ against x should be linear with slope value b and intercept (on the vertical axis when $x = 0$) equal to $\ln a$. This is often called a *semilog plot*. It is widely used in kinetic studies.

2. *Power Functions.*

$$y = ax^b \tag{B.44}$$

Again we take the logarithm.

$$\ln y = \ln a + b \ln x \tag{B.45}$$

A plot of $\ln y$ against $\ln x$ will be linear if Eq. (B.44) describes the data. This is called a *log–log plot*.

3. *Polynomial Functions*

$$y = a + bx + cx^2 \tag{B.46}$$

This equation is a quadratic function, which can be linearized as in

$$\frac{y-a}{x} = b + cx \tag{B.47}$$

Evidently a plot of $(y - a)/x$ against x will give a straight line if Eq. (B.46) describes the data. Of course, the parameter a must be known in order to construct this plot.

4. *Rectangular Hyperbola.* Any equation having the following form is called a *rectangular hyperbola*:

$$y = \frac{ax}{1 + bx} \tag{B.48}$$

This is nonlinear when plotted as y against x. We can linearize it in several ways. Taking the reciprocals of both sides gives

$$\frac{1}{y} = \frac{1}{ax} + \frac{b}{a} \tag{B.49}$$

so a plot of $1/y$ against $1/x$ (this is called a *double-reciprocal plot*) will be linear. You may encounter this plot in your study of enzyme kinetics, where it is called the *Lineweaver–Burk* plot. Algebraic manipulation also leads to the following equation, another linear plotting form.

$$\frac{x}{y} = \frac{b}{a}x + \frac{1}{a} \tag{B.50}$$

In this version, x/y is plotted against x. A third linear transformation can be obtained; this is shown as

$$\frac{y}{x} = a - by \tag{B.51}$$

A plot of y/x against y is linear. Notice that the slope is negative. In protein binding studies a plot according to Eq. (B.51) is called a *Scatchard plot*. The rectangular hyperbola arises naturally in mathematical descriptions of chemical equilibria.

It will be evident that a facility for recognizing the standard linear form $y = mx + b$ (where the definitions of the variables and parameters depend on the particular system) is invaluable in seeking linear forms from nonlinear functions.

Example B.11. Table B.3 gives kinetic data for the decomposition of nitrogen pentoxide in carbon tetrachloride solution at 45°C.[8] Analyze the data.

The experimental data consist of the concentration of N_2O_5 (c) as a function of time (t). Figure B.4 is a direct plot of c (as the dependent variable) against t. The

Table B.3. Kinetics of N_2O_5 decomposition at 45°C in CCl_4

t (s)	c (M)	$\log [c \, (M)]$
0	2.33	0.367
184	2.08	0.318
319	1.91	0.281
526	1.67	0.223
867	1.36	0.134
1198	1.11	0.045
1877	0.72	−0.143
2315	0.55	−0.260
3144	0.34	−0.469

plot is obviously nonlinear. As it happens, we have some theoretical guidance for this reaction (and for many other processes that follow the same functional dependence on time). We anticipate that the progress of the reaction is described by Eq. (B.52), where c_0 is the reactant concentration when $t = 0$ (the beginning of the reaction) and c is the concentration at any time t:

$$c = c_0 e^{-kt} \tag{B.52}$$

The parameter k is called the *rate constant*.

We recognize Eq. (B.52) as an exponential function, which we can linearize by taking the logarithm.

$$\ln c = \ln c_0 - kt \tag{B.53}$$

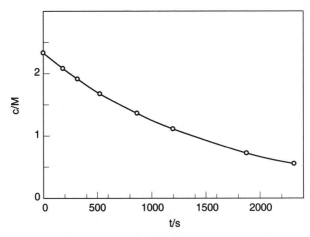

Figure B.4. Direct plot of data in Example B.11.

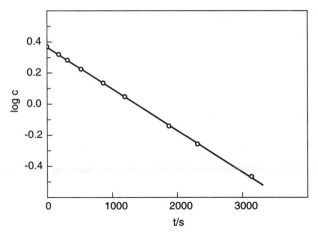

Figure B.5. Semi-log plot of data in Example B.11.

or

$$\text{Log } c = \log c_0 - \frac{kt}{2.303} \tag{B.54}$$

We can use either Eq. (B.53) or eq. (B.54). The table of data shows values of log c, and Fig. B.5 is the plot of log c against t as suggested by Eq. (B.54). Evidently we have succeeded in linearizing the data, which we interpret to mean that Eq. (B.52) describes the reaction.

From Fig. B.5 we calculate the slope as follows:

$$\text{Slope} = \frac{-0.167 - (+0.100)}{2000 - 1000}$$
$$= -2.67 \times 10^{-4} \text{s}^{-1}$$

Observe the sign and units of the slope. Now, from Eq. (B3.31) we can write

$$\text{Slope} = -\frac{k}{2.303}$$

so

$$k = 6.15 \times 10^{-4} \text{s}^{-1}$$

B.4. DEALING WITH CHANGE

Change in Physical and Chemical Processes. We are often interested in some sort of process that has happened, is happening, or is expected to happen;

Table B.4. Types of physicochemical processes

Solid	$\xrightleftharpoons[\text{crystallization}]{\text{melting (fusion)}}$	liquid
Liquid	$\xrightleftharpoons[\text{condensation}]{\text{vaporization}}$	gas (vapor)
Solid	$\xrightleftharpoons{\text{sublimation}}$	gas
Solvent + solid	$\xrightleftharpoons[\text{precipitation}]{\text{dissolution}}$	solution
Solute in solvent A	$\xrightleftharpoons{\text{partitioning}}$	solute in solvent B
Gas at volume 1	$\xrightleftharpoons[\text{expansion}]{\text{compression}}$	gas at volume 2
System at temperature 1	$\xrightleftharpoons[\text{cooling}]{\text{heating}}$	system at temperature 2
Reactants	$\xrightleftharpoons{\text{chemical reaction}}$	products

in other words, something changes. We need to be able to describe and analyze such changes. Table B.4 shows the kinds of processes that may concern us.

Suppose that we want to specify quantitatively the value of some property P that changes as the physical or chemical system passes from its initial state A to its final state Z. The process itself is symbolized $A \to Z$, and the change (or increment) in P is defined as

Change in $P = $ (value of P in final state) $-$ (value of P in initial state)

or

$$\Delta P = P_Z - P_A \tag{B.55}$$

If P increases during the process, then $P_Z > P_A$ and ΔP is positive; if P decreases, then ΔP is negative.

Incremental and Differential Change. We have defined an increment in a quantity by Eq. (B.55). Let us now revert to our study of a straight-line function

$$y = mx + b \tag{B.56}$$

and recall how we calculated the value of the slope m. We chose two points on the line (see Fig. B.2) and found that m is equal to the function in

$$m = \frac{y_2 - y_1}{x_2 - x_1} \tag{B.57}$$

If we think of larger positive values of x (values increasing toward the right on the abscissa) as "later," then we can identify the point (x_1, y_1) as an initial state and point (x_2, y_2) as a final state. Then we see that m can be written in our delta symbolism as

$$m = \frac{\Delta y}{\Delta x} \tag{B.58}$$

Carrying out the division on the right-hand side with numerical quantities yields a number equal to m. Since this result can be viewed as the number divided by 1, we interpret $m = \Delta y / \Delta x$ as *the change in y per unit change in x*. In Example B.10 we found $m = 0.453$, which we interpret to mean that as x increases by one unit, y increases by 0.453 unit. Recall also that m can be negative; this would mean that y decreases as x increases.

Now the essence of a straight line is that its slope m is a constant, so that we would obtain the same value for m no matter which two points, wherever they may be on the line, we choose for its calculation. But suppose the plot of y against x yields a curved (nonlinear) line, as in Fig. B.6? Obviously if we calculate the slope value using points (x_1, y_1) and (x_2, y_2), we will get a different value from that using points (x_2, y_2) and (x_3, y_3). In fact, we have to ask if the concept of "slope" has meaning in this circumstance. The answer is that we can expand our definition of the slope to include such circumstances. We will now define the slope of any line *at a point p* as the value of the tangent to the line at p, as shown in Fig. B.7.

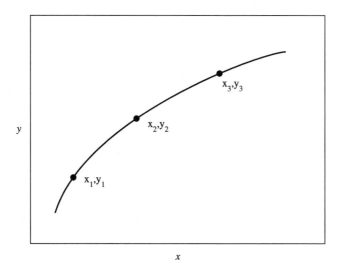

Figure B.6. A curvilinear function $y = f(x)$. The slope of the line depends on the value of x.

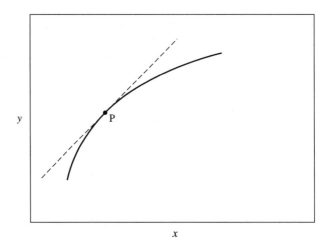

Figure B.7. The slope at point *p* is the value of the tangent to the curve at *p*.

How can we evaluate the numerical value of the slope at point *p*? We simply return to our original definition

$$m = \frac{\Delta y}{\Delta x}$$

and require that Δx (in the immediate vicinity of point *p*) be made smaller and smaller until it is so small that *m* approaches an essentially constant value; that is, making Δx still smaller doesn't sensibly alter the value of *m*. Now the ratio $\Delta y / \Delta x$ gives the slope (tangent) of the line at point *p*. We write this

$$m = \lim_{\Delta x \to 0} \frac{\Delta y}{\Delta x} \tag{B.59}$$

which is read "*m* is the limiting value of $\Delta y / \Delta x$ as Δx approaches zero." Of course, it would be cumbersome to write Eq. (B.59) repeatedly, so a new terminology is introduced, namely

$$m = \lim_{\Delta x \to 0} \frac{\Delta y}{\Delta x} = \frac{dy}{dx} \tag{B.60}$$

where *dy* and *dx* are individually referred to as *differentials* and the ratio *dy/dx* is called *the derivative of y with respect to x*.

We interpret the derivative *dy/dx* of any function $y = f(x)$ as the slope of the function (when plotted in the usual manner). If the function is a straight line, *dy/dx* is a constant (its value does not depend on *x*), whereas for curved functions the slope *dy/dx* depends on (varies with) *x*. Thus *dy/dx*, for both straight and curved lines, is a measure of change.

Formulas for Derivatives. One of the interesting properties of derivatives is that the individual differentials can be treated as algebraic quantities. Thus we can write

$$\frac{dy}{dx} \cdot dx = dy \qquad \text{(B.61)}$$

and

$$\frac{dy}{dx} = \frac{dy}{du} \cdot \frac{du}{dx} \qquad \text{(B.62)}$$

Equation (B.62) is known as the "chain rule." Evidently we also have $dx/dx = 1$.

Table B.5 collects some formulas [Eqs. (B.63)–(B.70)] for derivatives and differentials that will be found useful in scientific settings. In these formulas u and v are functions of x, c and n are constants, and e is the base of natural logarithms. The differential form is obtained from the derivative through multiplication by dx. Table B.5 is a compact way of summarizing these formulas, and a more expanded form might express the results as follows, where we take Eq. (B.65) as an example:

$$\begin{aligned}
\text{Function:} &\quad y = u + v \\
\text{Derivative:} &\quad \frac{dy}{dx} = \frac{du}{dx} + \frac{dv}{dx} \\
\text{Differential:} &\quad dy = du + dv
\end{aligned}$$

Table B.5. Some derivatives and differentials[a]

Derivative	Differential	Eq.
$\dfrac{dc}{dx} = 0$	$dc = 0$	(B.63)
$\dfrac{d(cu)}{dx} = c\dfrac{du}{dx}$	$d(cu) = c\,du$	(B.64)
$\dfrac{d(u+v)}{dx} = \dfrac{du}{dx} + \dfrac{dv}{dx}$	$d(u+v) = du + dv$	(B.65)
$\dfrac{d(uv)}{dx} = u\dfrac{dv}{dx} + v\dfrac{du}{dx}$	$d(uv) = u\,dv + v\,du$	(B.66)
$\dfrac{d(u/v)}{dx} = \dfrac{v(du/dx) - u(dv/dx)}{v^2}$	$d\dfrac{u}{v} = \dfrac{v\,du - u\,dv}{v^2}$	(B.67)
$\dfrac{du^n}{dx} = nu^{n-1}\dfrac{du}{dx}$	$d(u^n) = nu^{n-1}du$	(B.68)
$\dfrac{d\ln u}{dx} = \dfrac{1}{u}\dfrac{du}{dx}$	$d\ln u = \dfrac{du}{u}$	(B.69)
$\dfrac{de^u}{dx} = e^u\dfrac{du}{dx}$	$de^u = e^u du$	(B.70)

[a] u, v, x are variables; c, n are constants.

Observe also that some entries can be derived from others; for example, Eq. (B.64) is a special case of Eq. (B.66), and Eq. (B.67) can be obtained from Eq. (B.66) by writing the quotient u/v as the product uv^{-1}.

All the derivatives in Table B.5 are first derivatives. We can also define higher derivatives. Suppose that we define $u = dy/dx$; then

$$\frac{du}{dx} = \frac{d(dy/dx)}{dx} = \frac{d^2y}{dx^2}$$

is called a *second derivative*. A second derivative is a measure of change of the first derivative.

Example B.12. Find the slope of the hyperbolic function

$$y = \frac{ax}{1 + bx} \tag{B.71}$$

We want the slope dy/dx. Equation (B.71) is a quotient, so we use Eq. (B.67) combined with Eq. (B.64):

$$\frac{dy}{dx} = \frac{(1 + bx)a - (ax)b}{(1 + bx)^2}$$

$$= \frac{a}{(1 + bx)^2} \tag{B.72}$$

Thus the slope depends on x, as can be seen graphically in Fig. B.8. As $x \to 0$, $dy/dx \to a$, a constant; this is the "limiting slope" or "initial slope," that is, the

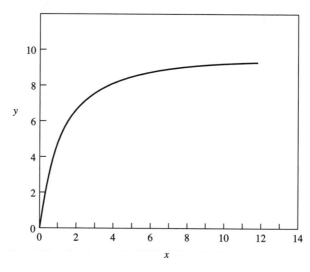

Figure B.8. The rectangular hyperbola, Eq. (B.71), for the case $a = 10$, $b = 1$.

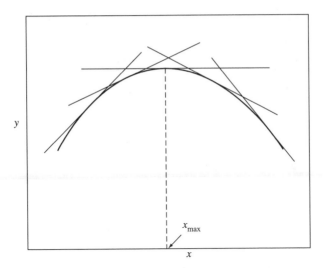

Figure B.9. The tangent lines show how dy/dx changes as y passes through a maximum.

tangent to the curve at the point $x = 0$. On the other hand, when $x \rightarrow \infty$ [x becomes so large that the denominator of Eq. (B.71) becomes much greater than the numerator], $dy/dx \rightarrow 0$; in this circumstance the value of y becomes essentially independent of x.

Maxima, Minima, and Inflection Points. Figure B.9 shows a function $y = f(x)$ that passes through a maximum.

Picture how the slope dy/dx changes as x increases from left to right. This is indicated by the tangent lines. In the vicinity of the maximum, whose location is labeled x_{max}, the slope decreases as x approaches x_{max} from the left. At $x = x_{max}$, $dy/dx = 0$; then as x leaves x_{max}, moving to the right, dy/dx becomes an increasingly large negative number.

This behavior provides a criterion for the location of a maximum in a function. At a maximum, $dy/dx = 0$, dy/dx is positive at $x < x_{max}$, and dy/dx is negative at $x > x_{max}$. (In addition, the second derivative d^2y/dx^2 is negative at a maximum.) Analogous conditions locate a minimum: $dy/dx = 0$, dy/dx is negative for $x < x_{min}$, dy/dx is positive for $x > x_{min}$, and the second derivative is positive.

An inflection point in a plot of y against x is a point where the first derivative passes through a maximum; hence it is also detectable as the point where the second derivative is equal to zero. This idea is clarified with some experimental data in Example B.13 (Connors 1967, Chapter 6).

Example B.13. Given: 0.3070 g of a weak base dissolved in glacial acetic acid was titrated with 0.1138 M acetous perchloric acid; the data in Table B.6 are the titrant volume V and the electrochemical cell potential E in the vicinity of the endpoint. Estimate the endpoint volume by the second derivative method.

Table B.6. Potentiometric titration data (Example B.13)

V (mL)	E (mV)	$\Delta E/\Delta V$ (mV/mL)	$\Delta^2 E/\Delta V^2$ (mV/mL^2)
7.50	490		
		44	
7.75	501		112
		72	
8.00	519		192
		120	
8.25	549		48
		132	
8.50	582		−176
		88	
8.75	604		−112
		60	
9.00	619		

The third column in Table B.6 shows $\Delta E/\Delta V$ (an approximation to the first derivative) as calculated from the V, E data; note how the values of $\Delta E/\Delta V$ are centered on the V, E intervals. In column 4 the "second derivative" $\Delta^2 E/\Delta V^2$ is similarly calculated from

$$\frac{\Delta^2 E}{\Delta V^2} = \frac{(\Delta E/\Delta V)_2 - (\Delta E/\Delta V)_1}{V_2 - V_1}$$

Figure B.10 shows plots of E against V, of $\Delta E/\Delta V$ against V, and of $\Delta^2 E/\Delta V^2$ against V.

The endpoint could be estimated directly from Fig. B.10a as the volume corresponding to the steepest point of the curve, but Fig. B.10b shows how this point can also be found through extrapolation from the $\Delta E/\Delta V$ values on either side of the maximum. Figure B.10c uses an interpolation from the $\Delta^2 E/\Delta V^2$ calculation to find the endpoint; the calculation, from the table, is

$$V_{endpoint} = 8.25 + 0.25 \left(\frac{48}{48 + 176}\right) = 8.30 \, \text{mL}$$

Thus, the point at which $\Delta^2 E/\Delta V^2 = 0$ is found by linear interpolation between the two data points on either side of zero. (We now have enough data to calculate the equivalent weight of the weak base.)

Integration. Integration is the opposite of differentiation; starting from the derivative, we seek to recover the original function. An equation of the form

$$\frac{dy}{dx} = f(x) \tag{B.73}$$

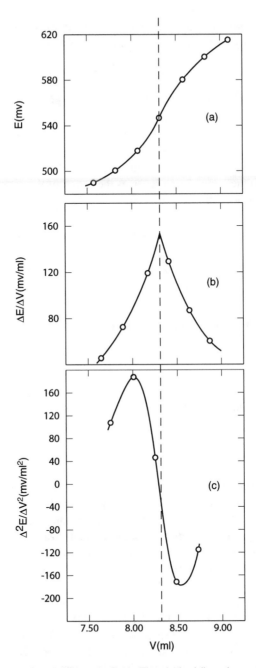

Figure B.10. Plots of the data in Example B.13. The dashed line shows the endpoint of the titration. [Reproduced by permission from Connors (1967).]

is called a *differential equation*; we have seen many examples. We wish to learn how y is related to x; our only clue is Eq. (B.73). We rearrange to the form

$$dy = f(x)\,dx \tag{B.74}$$

and integrate both sides as directed by the integral signs:

$$\int dy = \int f(x)\,dx \tag{B.75}$$

(An integral sign must always be accompanied by a differential.) On the left-hand side of Eq. (B.75) the integral sign reverses the action of the differential sign, since y is the function whose differential is dy. Hence

$$y = \int f(x)\,dx \tag{B.76}$$

To proceed, we will take some special cases.

Example B.14.

(a) Integrate $dy/dx = a$, where a is a constant. In the form of Eq. (B.76) we have

$$y = \int a\,dx \tag{B.77}$$

One rule of integration is that we can take constants outside the integral sign, so

$$y = a \int dx \tag{B.78}$$

This suggests that $y = ax$. But consider the following. Suppose that the original function was $y = ax + 2$, or $y = ax + 10^6$, or $y = ax - 15$, or the like. All of these functions (and there are an infinite number of them) have the derivative $dy/dx = a$, because the derivative of a constant is zero. So when we integrate Eq. (B.78) we must restore the constant that *might* have been there. Our final result is therefore

$$y = ax + C \tag{B.79}$$

where C is called the *constant of integration*.

(b) Integrate $dy/dx = 24x^2$. Experience with derivatives leads us to expect [see Eq. (B.68) in Table B.5] that if $dy/dx = 24x^2$, then y is some function of x^3. A bit of guessing shows us that if $y = 8x^3$, then $dy/dx = 24x^2$. We therefore have

$$y = 24 \int x^2\,dx = (24)\left(\frac{x^3}{3}\right) + C = 8x^3 + C$$

Table B.7. Some indefinite integrals

$$\int du = u + C \qquad\qquad (\text{B.80})$$

$$\int a\, du = a \int du \qquad\qquad (\text{B.81})$$

$$\int (du + dv) = \int du + \int dv \qquad\qquad (\text{B.82})$$

$$\int u^n\, du = \frac{u^{n+1}}{n+1}\,(n \neq -1) \qquad\qquad (\text{B.83})$$

$$\int \frac{du}{u} = \ln u + C \qquad\qquad (\text{B.84})$$

$$\int e^{au}\, du = \frac{e^{au}}{a} + C \qquad\qquad (\text{B.85})$$

$$\int a^u\, du = \frac{a^u}{\ln a} + C \qquad\qquad (\text{B.86})$$

$$\int (a + bu)^n\, du = \frac{(a + bu)^{n+1}}{(n+1)b} + C(n \neq -1) \qquad\qquad (\text{B.87})$$

$$\int \frac{du}{a + bu} = \frac{1}{b}\ln(a + bu) \qquad\qquad (\text{B.88})$$

Integrals of the type discussed above are called *indefinite integrals*, at least in part because the value of the constant C is unspecified. A short tabulation of indefinite integrals is given in Table B.7 [which contains Eqs. (B.80)–(B.88)]. The *CRC Handbook of Chemistry and Physics* gives a table with hundreds of integrals.

A *definite integral* has specified initial and final points over which the integral is to be evaluated. We will develop this concept with an example of great importance in many types of scientific work.

Example B.15. Let us study a chemical reaction described by the scheme $A \rightarrow Z$, where A is the reactant and Z is the product. It is often observed experimentally, for reactions fitting this scheme, that the rate of loss of reactant is directly proportional to the concentration of A at that moment. Expressed mathematically, this observation becomes

$$-\frac{dc_A}{dt} = kc_A \qquad\qquad (\text{B.89})$$

Here dc_A/dt is the *reaction rate*; the negative sign arises because c_A, the concentration of A, is decreasing as time t increases. The quantity k is the *rate constant*. Because c_A appears on the right-hand side to the first power, Eq. (B.89) is called the *first-order differential rate equation*, and k is a first-order rate constant. [In Problem B.22, Eq. (B.89) is obtained from a set of experimental kinetic data.]

Equation (B.89) expresses a rate as a function of a concentration, but it is more convenient experimentally to measure a concentration as a function of time. Integration will convert Eq. (B.89) into such a form. Let us make these definitions:

c_A^0 is the concentration of A when $t = 0$, which means "at the beginning of the reaction."

c_A is the concentration of A at any time t.

Now, to place Eq. (B.89) into an integrable form, we collect like variables; in this case we want c_A and dc_A on the same side of the equation. Algebraic rearrangement gives

$$\frac{dc_A}{c_A} = -k\,dt \tag{B.90}$$

We are going to carry out a definite integration between the limits $c_A = c_A^0$ when $t = 0$ and $c_A = c_A$ when $t = t$. This is indicated as in

$$\int_{c_A^0}^{c_A} \frac{dc_A}{c_A} = -k \int_0^t dt \tag{B.91}$$

Note that the initial state is at the lower end of the integral sign and the final state at the upper end. Next we integrate both sides, making use of Eqs. (B.80) and (B.84) (from Table B.7):

$$\ln c_A \big]_{c_A^0}^{c_A} = -kt \big]_0^t \tag{B.92}$$

This symbolism shows that we have carried out the integration but have not yet applied the integration limits, so next we do this, writing the final state first and subtracting off the initial state, exactly as in our earlier definitions of changes:

$$\ln c_A - \ln c_A^0 = -k(t - 0)$$

This is obviously equivalent to

$$\ln \frac{c_A}{c_A^0} = -kt \tag{B.93}$$

or, in Briggsian logarithms

$$\log \frac{c_A}{c_A^0} = \frac{-kt}{2.303} \tag{B.94}$$

Yet another rearranged form is shown as

$$c_A = c_A^0 e^{-kt} \tag{B.95}$$

Equations (B.93)–(B.95) are equivalent forms of the *integrated first-order rate equation* (this is sometimes called the *first-order rate law*, *first-order decay*, or the *exponential rate law*). We have seen here that it appears naturally in the field of chemical kinetics. It is also important for describing radioactive decay, pharmacokinetic processes, and other applications. Mastery of the material in Example B.15 is essential. Note also how Example B.11 and Problem B.22 are related to this treatment.

More complicated rate equations will sometimes be encountered, but a thorough treatment is not appropriate here. Sometimes the kinetic scheme and the differential rate equation can suggest the qualitative nature of the integrated equation. Consider this scheme of two first-order reactions in series:

$$A \xrightarrow{k_1} B \xrightarrow{k_2} C$$

The differential rate equations are

$$-\frac{dc_A}{dt} = k_1 c_A$$

$$\frac{dc_B}{dt} = k_1 c_A - k_2 c_B$$

$$\frac{dc_c}{dt} = k_2 c_B$$

We can therefore anticipate that the dependence of c_A on t will be given by Eq. (B.95), since the rate of loss of A depends only on rate constant k_1. Intermediate B, however, involves both k_1 and k_2, so we expect that c_B will be a biexponential function. The integrated result for c_B [which we will not derive here (Connors 1990, Chapter 3)], is

$$c_B = \frac{c_A^0 k_1}{k_2 - k_1}[e^{-k_1 t} - e^{-k_2 t}] \tag{B.96}$$

except for the special case $k_1 = k_2$. The dependence of c_C on time can be found from the conservation equation $c_A^0 = c_A + c_B + c_C$ combined with Eqs. (B.95) and (B.96) for c_A and c_B.

Partial Differentiation and the Total Differential. Up to this point in our treatment of change we have dealt with functions of a single variable. For example, if y is a function of the variable x alone, we write $y = f(x)$, and we can evaluate the derivative dy/dx. Very often, however, we encounter functions of two or more variables, and here we consider how to describe changes in such quantities. This material may not have been covered in an introductory calculus course.

Suppose that we have a function $z = f(x,y)$, meaning that the value of z depends on both of the variables x and y. We wish to describe how z changes when we alter x or y, or both x and y. We do this as follows. First take the derivative of z with respect to x *while holding y constant*. In order to make transparently clear what is going on we use a slightly different symbolism for this derivative, writing

$$\left(\frac{\partial z}{\partial x}\right)_y$$

Note the subscript y; this tells us that y is held constant while x is changing. In like manner we can take the derivative of z with respect to y while x is held constant, writing the result as

$$\left(\frac{\partial z}{\partial y}\right)_x$$

Observe the use of the symbol in these expressions. The operation just described is called partial differentiation and the quantities written above are *partial derivatives*.

Next we make use of a chain rule to define the *total differential dz* of the function $z = f(x,y)$:

$$dz = \left(\frac{\partial z}{\partial x}\right)_y dx + \left(\frac{\partial z}{\partial y}\right)_x dy \qquad (B.97)$$

These considerations may seem somewhat abstract, but it happens that many quantities of scientific interest are functions of more than one variable. Incidentally, Eq. (B.97) can be generalized to functions of more than two variables; the pattern will be evident from Eq. (B.97) (see also Problem B.31).

Example B.16. The volume V of a fixed amount of a homogenous gas depends only on its temperature T and its pressure P. Write the total differential dV.

By analogy with the foregoing we write

$$V = f(T, P)$$

so

$$dV = \left(\frac{\partial V}{\partial T}\right)_P dT + \left(\frac{\partial V}{\partial P}\right)_T dP \qquad (B.98)$$

Experimental measurements can provide numerical quantities for these partial derivatives, so Eq. (B.98) has a definite physical meaning.

Recall from our earlier definition of change in a chemical process that we defined an increment as the difference between values in final and initial states.

Taking volume V as an example of a property undergoing change we have, using the language of calculus

$$\Delta V = \int_{V_{\text{initial}}}^{V_{\text{final}}} dV = V_{\text{final}} - V_{\text{initial}} \tag{B.99}$$

Now suppose that we carry out the change in two steps, first $A \rightarrow B$ and then $B \rightarrow C$. What is the change ΔV for the overall process $A \rightarrow C$? We apply Eq. (B.99):

$$\Delta V = \int_{V_A}^{V_B} dV + \int_{V_B}^{V_C} dV = (V_B - V_A) + (V_C - V_B)$$
$$V = V_C - V_A$$

We have found that state B plays no role in determining ΔV. State B is an intermediate state on the path from A to C, and since B could have been any intermediate state, evidently the change ΔV is independent of the path or mechanism of the process.

If the change in a property or function between two *states* of a system is independent of the path taken between the states, the total differential is called an *exact differential* and the property or function is called a *state function*. Whether or not a function is a state function (path-independent) is ultimately based on experimental observations, but extensive laboratory studies have clarified the situation. The subject of thermodynamics (which describes systems at equilibrium) deals largely with state functions, including the temperature, volume, pressure, and energy.[9] On the other hand, chemical kinetics, which describes systems changing in time, largely treats path-dependent quantities; in this context, the path taken by a reaction is the reaction mechanism, and a major role of chemical kinetics studies is to investigate reaction mechanisms.

B.5. STATISTICAL TREATMENT OF DATA

The results of a quantitative experimental study often consist of a set of numbers obtained from replicate determinations made under essentially identical conditions, or a set of numbers corresponding to one quantity as a function of another quantity. These numbers may represent concentrations, weights, equilibrium constants, rate constants, pH values, and so on. The interpretation of these data by the experimentalist answers two general questions:

1. What is the *best estimate* of the quantity or function being investigated?
2. *How reliable* is this estimate as a measure of the true value?

The branch of mathematics called *statistics* deals with such issues. Our present treatment will be very brief, intended to provide an immediately usable tool for the interpretation of data obtained in laboratory coursework.

Random Errors and the Normal Distribution. Every measurement has some error associated with it. These errors may be of two types. *Systematic errors* are errors introduced by some inadequacy in the experimental technique (such as an improperly calibrated balance or an interference caused by impurities in reagents) or poor judgment or unconscious bias on the part of the experimentalist (as may happen through parallax error when reading the meniscus in a burette). Systematic errors can be tracked down and substantially eliminated (or the method may have to be abandoned); we will not consider them further.

Even after all systematic errors have been eliminated, it is a familiar observation that repeated determinations of a quantity almost never result in the same number. This variability in experimental data is a manifestation of *random error.* We usually observe that replicate observations are grouped about a most frequently observed value, and that large deviations from this value are rarer than small deviations. Random errors are the consequence of limitations inherent in the observational method. They can perhaps be reduced in magnitude by careful work, but they cannot be eliminated. Statistics helps the experimentalist to interpret the data, given this inevitable presence of random error.

The statistician adopts a point of view concerning experimental data that may seem peculiar to the experimentalist. The statistician considers an experimental observation to be a single member that has been randomly selected from an infinite population of individual observations that are characteristic of the system being investigated. Replicate observations will exhibit variation owing to the operation of random errors. If we draw a graph of the value of each experimental observation on the horizontal (x) axis against the number of times each value is observed (its frequency) on the vertical (y) axis, a symmetric figure usually is obtained, with a maximum corresponding to the most frequently observed value. As the number of observations increases toward the (unattainable) limit of infinity, the graph will assume the form of a smooth curve. This curve is called a *frequency distribution.*

In scientific practice experimental frequency distributions can usually be closely fitted to a theoretical frequency distribution that is called the *normal distribution,* the *Gaussian error curve,* or the *normal error curve.* The equation of the normal distribution is

$$f(x) = \frac{1}{\sigma\sqrt{2\pi}} e^{-(1/2)[(x-\mu)/\sigma]^2} \qquad (B.100)$$

where $f(x)$ is the frequency of occurrence of the value x of the "random variable," which is the experimental observable, and σ and μ are parameters of the population. The symbol μ signifies the *population mean,* which is the value of x corresponding to the maximum in the distribution; and σ, the *population standard deviation,* determines the "spread" or width of the bell-shaped curve. Figure B.11 shows a plot of the normal distribution. Graphically the quantity σ is the horizontal distance from the mean to either inflection point of the curve, as shown in Fig. B.11. Approximately 68% of the area under the normal curve, and therefore 68% of the members of the population, lie within one standard deviation of the mean,

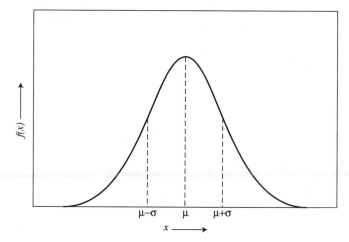

Figure B.11. The normal error curve with mean μ and standard deviation σ.

$\mu \pm \sigma$. About 95% of the population are found in the range $\mu \pm 2\sigma$, and over 99% in the range $\mu \pm 3\sigma$. Scientists usually assume that their data can be described by the normal distribution, and we will adopt this assumption in the following treatment.

Estimation of Statistical Parameters. The population parameters μ and σ are not accessible to us because we would have to sample an infinity of random variables in order to define the population frequency distribution. Nevertheless, we desire estimates of μ and σ. Because of the symmetry of the normal distribution, the best estimate of the population mean is the arithmetic average, or *mean*, $\bar{x}$, defined by

$$\bar{x} = \frac{\sum x_i}{n} \tag{B.101}$$

where x_i is the value of the ith observation $(i = 1, 2, 3, \ldots, n)$ and n is the total number of observations.

The *accuracy* of an experimental result is the closeness with which the experimental mean $\bar{x}$ approaches the population mean μ. Since we do not know μ, we cannot in general assess the accuracy. Sometimes, however, an experiment can be designed so that the experimental $\bar{x}$ can be compared with a known value that has been set by the experimentalist with a standard sample. There also exist a few quantities that have been measured by so many workers, using different methods in different laboratories, that we have developed great confidence in their accuracy. For example, the K_a value of benzoic acid at 25°C is 6.26×10^{-5}, an average of many experimental results; and so much care and effort has gone into this number that we may reasonably take it as very accurate.

The *median* is sometimes used as an estimate of the population mean, especially if the set of experimental results includes one or two widely divergent results. The median is that value that exceeds as many values as it itself is exceeded by, for *n* odd. If *n* is even, the median is the average of the two values satisfying the same criterion. The median is easily picked out if the numbers are arranged in order of increasing magnitude.

It is a valuable result of statistical theory that, even if the experimental variable is not normally distributed, the means of small sets of the variable are normally distributed. Since the mean $\bar{x}$ is our best estimate of the true value, we are assured that these $\bar{x}$ estimates follow a normal distribution.

We have next to obtain an estimate of σ, the population standard deviation, which we see from Fig. B.11 to be a measure of the width of the normal distribution. This width reflects the reproducibility of the measurements; the more reproducible, the narrower the curve, and the smaller the value of σ. *Precision* is the term usually used to describe reproducibility. Our estimate of σ is labelled *s* and is called the *experimental standard deviation*; *s* is our measure of the precision of $\bar{x}$, and sometimes *s* is said to measure the "uncertainty" of $\bar{x}$. Its calculation begins with the definition of the following equation, where s^2 is called the *variance*:

$$s^2 = \frac{\sum (x_i - \bar{x})^2}{n - 1} \tag{B.102}$$

The standard deviation is then found as the square root of the variance. Note the denominator in this equation; the quantity $n - 1$ is called the *degrees of freedom*, for it specifies the number of independently assignable quantities needed to completely determine the system. This is $n - 1$ because we already have calculated one parameter, namely, $\bar{x}$. The units of *s* are the same as those of $\bar{x}$.

At one time (before electronic calculators and computers made statistical calculations easy), the *average deviation*, expressed as follows, was often used as a measure of precision:

$$\text{Average deviation} = \frac{\sum |x_i - \bar{x}|}{n - 1} \tag{B.103}$$

The *range w* is the difference between the largest and the smallest results in a set; *w* can be a useful indicator of the spread of results when *n* is small.

The precision can be expressed in relative terms as the quotient $s/\bar{x}$, or more frequently on a percent basis by $100s/\bar{x}$, which is called the *coefficient of variation* or the *relative standard deviation* (RSD). Similarly, we might report

$$\text{Precision in parts per thousand} = \frac{10^3 s}{\bar{x}}$$

$$\text{Precision in parts per million} = \frac{10^6 s}{\bar{x}}$$

It is important to appreciate that the accuracy and precision of an experimental result are very different concepts. In the best of circumstances we may have good accuracy ($\bar{x}$ closely approximates μ) and high precision (s is small relative to $\bar{x}$), but it is also possible to encounter poor accuracy with high precision.

A more complete description of s is that it is the standard deviation of a single observation. However, it is the mean $\bar{x}$ that we take as our best estimate, so we really would like a measure of the precision of the mean. This is provided by the *standard deviation of the mean*, s_m:

$$s_m = \frac{s}{\sqrt{n}} \tag{B.104}$$

Some authors call s_m the *standard error*.

Example B.17. The following numbers are the percent recoveries in seven identical nonaqueous titrations of a urea sample: 98.4, 100.2, 99.3, 101.7, 97.4, 98.2, and 100.8. Calculate the mean, median, range, variance, standard deviation, relative standard deviation, and standard deviation of the mean.

It is best to arrange the work in tabular form. Notice that the variance is calculated according to Eq. (B.104) with the arithmetic operations carried out in the following order: (1) differences are taken, (2) differences are squared, and (3) squares are summed:

Titration, i	Percent Recovery (x_i)	$(x_i - \bar{x})$	$(x_i - \bar{x})^2$
1	98.4	−1.0	1.00
2	100.2	0.8	0.64
3	99.3	−0.1	0.01
4	101.7	2.3	5.29
5	97.4	−2.0	4.00
6	98.2	1.2	1.44
7	100.8	1.4	1.96
	696.0		14.34

Mean: $\bar{x} = 696.0\%/7 = 99.4\%$

Median: 99.3%

Range: $101.7\% - 97.4\% = 4.3\%$

Variance: $s^2 = [14.34(\%^2)]/6 = 2.39(\%^2)$

Standard deviation: $s = \sqrt{2.39} = 1.55\%$

RSD: $100(1.55/99.4) = 1.56\%$

Standard deviation of the mean: $s_m = 1.55/2.65 = 0.58\%$

Equation (B.102) for the variance can be placed in other forms that are more convenient for electronic calculation. You will undoubtedly use your electronic calculator (which should be capable of the routine statistical calculations described in this Section B.5), but make sure that the calculator uses $n - 1$ rather than n in the denominator of Eq. (B.102). Of course, if n is very large (an unusual circumstance in much experimental work), the difference between n and $n - 1$ becomes negligible.

Confidence Limits of the Mean. We have seen that the mean $\bar{x}$ can be treated as a normally distributed random variable. $\bar{x}$ is our best estimate of the quantity we seek, and now we would like some measure of the reliability of $\bar{x}$. It might seem that we could achieve this by taking note of the properties of the normal distribution. For example, we saw that 95% of the members of a normally distributed population fall within two standard deviations of the mean, so perhaps we could state that the interval $\bar{x} \pm 2s$ should include 95% of any future estimates of $\bar{x}$ for the same quantity.

This sounds plausible, but as it happens, if n is fairly small, the actual distribution of $\bar{x}$ is somewhat wider than is specified by the normal distribution. The actual distribution for small n is given by a different function called Student's t distribution,[10] which approaches the normal distribution as n becomes large. Table B.8 lists some values of Student's t. In this table the column headed "Degrees of Freedom" is to be interpreted as $n - 1$. The headings of the other columns give the value of P, which is the probability that the limits to be calculated may be exceeded by chance. The values in the table are the Student's t. Observe how t seems to be approaching 2 for the column $P = 0.05$ and recall that for the normal distribution 95% of the population lies in the interval $\bar{x} \pm 2s$; this comparison gives some meaning to the t values.

We now wish to measure the reliability of our $\bar{x}$ estimate. This measure of reliability is called the *confidence limits of the mean*, and it is calculated with the aid of Student's t distribution. We suppose that n replicate observations have been made,

Table B.8. Some values of Student's t distribution

Degrees of Freedom	$P = 0.10$	0.05	0.01
1	6.314	12.706	63.657
2	2.920	4.303	9.925
3	2.353	3.182	5.841
4	2.132	2.776	4.604
5	2.015	2.571	4.032
6	1.943	2.447	3.707
7	1.895	2.365	3.499
8	1.860	2.306	3.555
9	1.833	2.262	3.250
10	1.812	2.228	3.169

and $\bar{x}$, s, and s_m have been calculated. We then calculate the confidence limits of $\bar{x}$ by

$$\bar{x} \pm ts_m$$

where t is read from the appropriate column in Table B.8. For example, if we wish to know the limits within which 95% of further $\bar{x}$ values would fall (if we undertook to measure them), we would choose the column $P = 0.05$, where the quantity P is the fraction of results that are expected to fall *outside* the limits. Similarly the $P = 0.01$ column gives the 99% confidence limits.

Example B.18. Find 95% and 99% confidence limits of the mean calculated in Example B.17.

95% Confidence Limits. For $P = 0.05$ and 6 degrees of freedom, Table B.8 gives $t = 2.447$. The confidence limits $(P = 0.05)$ are therefore $\bar{x} \pm ts_m$ or $99.4 \pm 2.447 \,(0.58)\% = 99.4 \pm 1.4\%$. The meaning of this result is that, if many additional sets of seven observations were made, about 95% of the means of these sets would be expected to fall within the range 98.0–100.8% (the confidence interval).

99% Confidence Limits. For $P = 0.01$, $t = 3.707$. The limits $(P = 0.01)$ are $99.4 \pm 2.2\%$. The limits are wider at $P = 0.01$ than at $P = 0.05$ because we have used the same information but have required that a larger percentage of additional results will fall within specified limits; that is, we have asked for a greater level of confidence, so we must pay for this with a wider confidence interval.

Comparison of Two Means. It is often required that two experimental results are to be compared to determine whether they are different. For example, we might wish to know if a newly developed chromatographic method yields the same analytic result as a well-tested spectrophotometric method. Such problems are dealt with by *tests of significance*, meaning that a decision is sought concerning whether the difference between the two results is significant or negligible.

In statistical terms, one tentatively assumes that there is no difference between the two results—this is called the *null hypothesis*—and then tests this assumption. Usually two means are to be compared. Let us symbolize these means as $\bar{x}$ and $\bar{y}$. According to the null hypothesis, $\bar{x}$ and $\bar{y}$ describe the same population. To show the basis of the significance test, suppose that $\bar{x}$ and $\bar{y}$ have the same value s_m for the standard deviation of the mean. As we have seen, confidence intervals can be defined by

Confidence interval for $\bar{x} = \bar{x} \pm ts_m$
Confidence interval for $\bar{y} = \bar{y} \pm ts_m$

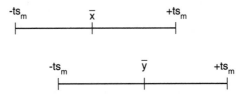

Figure B.12. The means $\bar{x}$ and $\bar{y}$ are not significantly different if their confidence intervals overlap.

We can therefore say that $\bar{x}$ and $\bar{y}$ are not significantly different (at the P level of confidence expressed by t) if $\bar{x}$ lies within the confidence interval of $\bar{y}$ (and vice versa), as indicated graphically in Fig. B.12.

Therefore $\bar{x} = \bar{y} \pm t s_\mathrm{m}$ expresses the null hypothesis, and rearranging, we obtain

$$t = \left| \frac{\bar{x} - \bar{y}}{s_\mathrm{m}} \right| \qquad (\text{B.105})$$

The approach is to calculate t by eq. (B.105). If the calculated t exceeds the tabulated t value at the chosen level of significance, the null hypothesis may be rejected; that is, $\bar{x}$ and $\bar{y}$ are significantly different.

This demonstrates the principle. Some subtleties enter when, as may happen, the numbers of observations contributing to $\bar{x}$ and $\bar{y}$ are different, and when s_m for $\bar{x}$ is different from s_m for $\bar{y}$. We will not pursue these matters here, except as seen in the following example.

Example B.19. These are analytical results for the analysis of two lots of aspirin tablets, given in milligrams of aspirin per tablet. Are the aspirin contents of the two lots different at the 95% significance level?

x_i	y_i
295.4	300.5
301.1	310.9
297.8	307.1
305.0	302.6
297.5	305.9

For lot x we find $\bar{x} = 299.4$, $s = 3.755$, $s_\mathrm{m}^x = 1.679$.
For lot y we find $\bar{y} = 305.4$, $s = 4.039$, $s_\mathrm{m}^y = 1.806$.

We now introduce this modification. Somewhat later in this section we will discover that variances of both sums and differences are additive. Since the numerator of Eq. (B.105) is a difference, we really want the standard deviation of the mean of this difference in the denominator. We therefore take the square root (to get the standard deviation) of the sum of the variances:

$$s_m = \sqrt{(s_m^x)^2 + (s_m^y)^2} = 2.466$$

Now we calculate t with Eq. (B.105):

$$t = \frac{305.4 - 299.4}{2.466} = 2.433$$

Consulting Table B.8, we find that the tabulated $t[P = 0.05; (n_x - 1) + (n_y - 1) = 8$ degrees of freedom] is 2.306. The calculated t exceeds the tabulated t, so the null hypothesis may be rejected, and we conclude that the two batches are different at the 95% significance level.

It is interesting that at the 99% significance level the tabulated $t = 3.555$, so the null hypothesis may not be rejected; the two batches are not different at this significance level. This result shows that statistics alone cannot make decisions; the experimentalist must exercise judgment. When reporting statistical results of this type it is essential to specify the chosen level of significance.

Linear Correlation. In Section B.3 we discussed linear relationships in detail. Our general formula for a *linear correlation* is

$$y = mx + b \tag{B.106}$$

where m is the slope and b is the intercept on the y axis. When confronted with a set of x, y data, we constructed a plot of y against x, determined by inspection whether it was linear, and drew our best straight line using a straightedge (ruler) and our intuition. We now wish to learn how statistics can assist us in such an analysis.

Our first task is to decide whether the correlation between x and y is linear. Visual inspection is usually adequate, but many scientists like to calculate a quantity r called the *correlation coefficient*:

$$r = \frac{s_{xy}}{s_x s_y} \tag{B.107}$$

where s_x is the standard deviation of all the x values, calculated in the usual way, and similarly s_y is the standard deviation of the y values. The quantity s_{xy} is called the *covariance* and is given by

$$s_{xy} = \frac{\sum (x_i - \bar{x})(y_i - \bar{y})}{n - 1} \tag{B.108}$$

Electronic calculators yield r directly without requiring the user to proceed through Eqs. (B.107) and (B.108).

The numerator of Eq. (B.107) is a measure of how strongly correlated the x and y values are, and the denominator "normalizes" r so that it must lie in the interval 0 to 1 (for positive slope) or 0 to -1 (for negative slope). The closer r is to 1 (or -1), the more linear the correlation. That, at least, is the conventional interpretation, but it must be treated with caution. This is because r depends not only on the linearity of the relationship but also on the slope of the line (a steeper slope giving a larger r value) and on the scatter of the points (more scatter giving a smaller r value).

Figures B.13 and B.14 illustrate these points. These figures have been constructed so that the slopes of the lines are very similar. Figure B.13 has more scatter than does Fig. B.14, and this is reflected in their r values: $r = 0.990$ for Fig. B.13; $r = 0.999$ for Fig. B.14. But close observation will reveal that although the points in Fig. B.13 show considerable scatter, they very reasonably follow a straight line. The points in Fig. B.14, however, clearly describe a curve, although a straight line has been drawn through them. The lesson is that one should not rely on the correlation coefficient alone, but should also plot the data and examine the graph critically. A good way to do this is by "sighting" along the data points as a carpenter sights along the edge of a board to determine how straight it is.

If we conclude that the data are linearly correlated, the next step is to draw the "best" straight line. This is nearly universally done now by a statistical technique

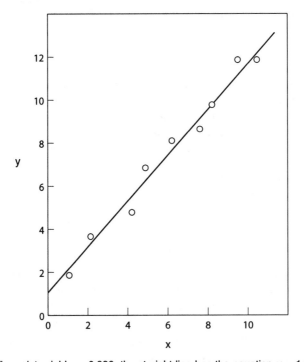

Figure B.13. The points yield $r = 0.990$; the straight line has the equation $y = 1.16x + 1.15$.

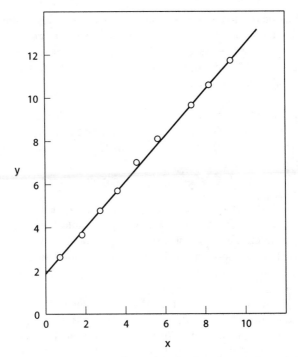

Figure B.14. The points yield $r = 0.999$; the straight line has the equation $y = 1.07x + 2.49$.

called the *method of least squares* or *linear regression analysis*. The line is drawn such that the sum of the squares of the vertical distances of the points from the line is a minimum.[11]

Let the least-squares line be written

$$\hat{y}_i = mx_i + b \qquad (B.109)$$

where m and b are the slope and intercept of the line (not yet known) and $\hat{y}_i$ is the value of y on the least squares line corresponding to x_i. Then we write

$$G = \sum (y_i - \hat{y}_i)^2 \qquad (B.110)$$

where y_i is the experimental value of y for observation i and $\hat{y}_i$ is the corresponding value from the line. Thus the right-hand side expresses the sum of squares of differences of the points from the line. To minimize this sum, we use the methods of calculus, taking the partial derivatives $\partial G/\partial m$ and $\partial G/\partial b$, setting these equal to zero, and solving for the parameters. The results are

$$b = \bar{y} - m\bar{x} \qquad (B.111)$$

$$m = \frac{\sum xy - n\bar{x}\,\bar{y}}{\sum x^2 - n\bar{x}^2} \qquad (B.112)$$

In these equations $\bar{x}$ and $\bar{y}$ are the mean values of these variables, and n is the number of data points. Inasmuch as scientific electronic calculators are capable of generating the parameters m and b of the least-squares regression line, it is unlikely that you will make direct use of Eqs. (B.111) and (B.112). This is how the calculator does it, however.

Example B.20. In Example B.10, the data in Table B.2 were analyzed as a linear correlation. Repeat the analysis using the method of least squares.

Using an electronic calculator, we obtain the following for the least-squares regression line:

$$y = 0.447x + 0.0397$$

In Example B.10 the line was drawn "by eye," and its equation turned out to be $y = 0.453x + 0.0397$. These two results compare quite favorably. The reason for the general preference for the least-squares treatment is that it is objective; any number of scientists applying the least squares method to the same set of data will obtain the same result.

Since the slope and intercept values of the least-squares regression line are themselves estimates of statistical parameters, they possess uncertainties that can be expressed as their standard deviations. We will not go into the evaluation of the standard deviations of the slope and intercept values.

Propagation of Errors. We nearly always subject our raw experimental data to arithmetic operations in order to arrive at a number that is useful to us, as when we convert a titrant volume to a concentration or a weight of sample, or when we operate on a parameter of an equation to give us a rate constant. When we make such calculations we are ultimately interested in the uncertainty (expressed as a standard deviation) of the final calculated result, whereas what we may know are the standard deviations of the quantities that are used in the calculation. We therefore wish to learn how the errors (uncertainties) in the primary quantities are propagated through the calculation into the final result.

Suppose that we let Q represent our final result, which is obtained by carrying out calculations on the two primary quantities x and y; that is, we have

$$Q = f(x, y)$$

Then the equation for the propagation of the uncertainties in x and y into Q, which we will not derive here, is

$$s_Q^2 = \left(\frac{\partial Q}{\partial x}\right)^2 s_x^2 + \left(\frac{\partial Q}{\partial y}\right)^2 s_y^2 \tag{B.113}$$

where the quantities in parentheses are partial derivatives, and s_Q^2, s_x^2, s_y^2 are the variances of the subscripted quantities. We will apply Eq. (B.113) to the basic arithmetic operations.

Sum

$$Q = x + y$$

$$\frac{\partial Q}{\partial x} = 1; \qquad \frac{\partial Q}{\partial y} = 1$$

so, from Eq. (B.113), we have

$$s_Q^2 = s_x^2 + s_y^2 \tag{B.114}$$

Difference

$$Q = x - y$$

$$\frac{\partial Q}{\partial x} = 1; \qquad \frac{\partial Q}{\partial y} - 1$$

$$s_Q^2 = s_x^2 + s_y^2 \tag{B.115}$$

Thus the errors (variances) add for both sums and differences. (We used this result in Example B.19.) This is why the relative error of a difference of two numbers similar in magnitude may be very large.

Product

$$Q = xy$$

$$\frac{\partial Q}{\partial x} = y; \qquad \frac{\partial Q}{\partial y} = x$$

$$s_Q^2 = y^2 s_x^2 + x^2 s_y^2$$

which is equivalent to

$$\frac{s_Q^2}{Q^2} = \frac{s_x^2}{x^2} + \frac{s_y^2}{y^2} \tag{B.116}$$

Quotient

$$Q = \frac{y}{x}$$

Equation (B.116) is again obtained.

The essential result of these demonstrations is that *variances are additive*. For sums and differences, the absolute variances add [Eqs. (B.114) and (B.115)]; for products and quotients, relative variances add [Eq. B.116)]. To find the standard deviation of Q, we first calculate s_Q^2 as in the examples above, and then take its square root.

Example B.21. Suppose that we titrate a solution of acetic acid with 15.00 mL of 0.1000 N NaOH. What is the uncertainty in the weight of acetic acid found if $s_N = 0.0003$ and $s_V = 0.02$ mL?

Since mmol of HOAc $= VN = w/M$, where V is volume of titrant, N is titrant normality (molarity), w is weight of acetic acid in milligrams, and M is the molecular weight of acetic acid, our function is $w = MVN$. Thus

$$s_w^2 = \left(\frac{\partial w}{\partial V}\right)^2 s_v^2 + \left(\frac{\partial w}{\partial N}\right)^2 s_N^2$$

We have $(\partial w/\partial V) = MN$ and $(\partial w/\partial N) = MV$, so

$$s_w^2 = M^2 N^2 s_V^2 + M^2 V^2 s_N^2$$
$$= (60)^2 (0.1)^2 (4 \times 10^{-4}) + (60)^2 (15)^2 (9 \times 10^{-8})$$
$$= 14.4 \times 10^{-3} + 8.1 \times 10^{-3} = 2.25 \times 10^{-2} \text{ mg}^2$$
$$s_w = 0.15 \text{ mg}$$

Since $w = (60)(15)(0.1) = 90$ mg, the relative standard deviation (RSD, or coefficient of variation) is $(100)(0.15)/90 = 0.17\%$.

A practical consequence of the propagation of error treatment is that if one of the uncertainties (say, σ_x^2) is very much larger than the other, then the uncertainty σ_Q^2 will receive its largest contribution from σ_x^2. Any experimental attempts to reduce the error in Q should obviously focus on reducing the error in x, because the error in y makes a negligible contribution to the error in Q.

Significant Figures. In reporting a final numerical result it is necessary to decide how many digits will be retained. This is especially pertinent in modern science because electronic calculators and computers routinely generate numbers having 10 or more digits. There is a temptation to record the entire display, but this is seldom justified. Instead we should retain and report only those digits that have physical significance.

Here is a simple criterion for deciding on how many digits to retain. The final digit should possess some uncertainty, whereas the digit preceding this one should be essentially certain. Some flexibility (within one digit) is acceptable. The number of significant figures in a result is then the total number of digits (exclusive of zeros that are needed solely to establish the position of the decimal point).

In order to use this criterion, we need a means for establishing whether a digit is essentially certain or is uncertain. We have this means at hand in the standard deviation s (or the standard deviation of the mean s_m if it is a mean that we are reporting). Consider, for example, the analytical results reported in Example B.19. For the x series we calculated $\bar{x} = 299.4$, $s_m^x = 1.679$ and for the y series, $\bar{y} = 305.4$, $s_m^y = 1.806$. For both series, therefore, the s_m values indicate variability in the unit place, suggesting that the means are uncertain in the unit place. Accordingly, we would report these results as $\bar{x} = 299$, $s_m^x = 1.7$ and $\bar{y} = 305$, $s_m^y = 1.8$. Incidentally, it is good practice to retain more digits than otherwise may be justified throughout the calculation in order that "rounding errors" not be inadvertently introduced. Then the significant-figure criterion is applied to the final result.

Another guide may be available in experimental practice and experience. For example, much laboratory experience has shown us that very precise titrimetric analysis can routinely be accomplished with precision corresponding to standard deviations in the fourth decimal place of molar concentrations; this is the justification for expressing solution concentrations to the fourth place. Another example occurs in pH measurements, where experience shows that, in careful but nevertheless routine work, the tenth unit is certain and the hundredth unit is uncertain, so we usually write pH values with two decimal places. The experimental procedure itself may determine the significance. For example, on a typical buret the finest graduations are in tenths of a milliliter, and we estimate to the hundredth place; thus we write the volume to two decimal places.

B.6. DIMENSIONS AND UNITS

This subject is not part of pure mathematics, but it fits comfortably into this review, and it makes a nice transition into the physicochemical and biological sciences coursework of the curriculum. Much of this will be familiar material.

Base and Derived Units. The value of a physical quantity is expressed as the product of a numerical value and a unit; thus

$$\text{Physical quantity} = \text{numerical value} \times \text{unit}$$

For example

$$\text{Distance} = 125 \, \text{km}$$

Many systems of units have been used, and several systems are in use today, but in scientific work the standard system of units is the Système International (SI), occasionally varied with a few units from older systems (IUPAC 1993). There are seven SI *base units*, each of these being independent of the others. Table B.9 lists the SI base units. No punctuation is used with symbols, nor are symbols pluralized.

All other units are called *derived units*; these can be obtained by appropriate algebraic combination of the base units. Table B.10 gives a few derived units to illustrate the manner in which they are formed. Of course, in common practice we make wide use of traditional alternatives. For example, we may express area in square centimeters (cm^2) if this is convenient to the problem. Density is usually expressed in grams per milliliter ($g \, mL^{-1}$), and concentration in moles per liter ($mol \, L^{-1}$), which is sometimes written $mol \, dm^{-3}$.

Table B.9. SI base units

Physical Quantity	Symbol for Quantity (Dimension)	Name of SI Unit	Symbol for SI Unit
Length	l	meter	m
Mass	m	kilogram	kg
Time	t	second	s
Electric current	I	ampere	A
Temperature	T	kelvin	K
Amount of substance	n	mole	mol
Luminous intensity	I_V	candela	cd

Table B.10. Some SI derived units

Physical Quantity	Defining Relationship	Derived SI Unit
Area	$l \times l$	m^2
Volume	$l \times l \times l$	m^3
Velocity	Distance per second	$m\,s^{-1}$
Density	Mass per volume	$kg\,m^{-3}$
Concentration	Amount per volume	$mol\,m^{-3}$

A few important physical quantities have special names and symbols for their units; a selection of these is shown in Table B.11. The expression of a derived unit in terms of base units, as illustrated in Table B.10, is obtained from the appropriate physical law or definition. For example, from Newton's law of motion, we have

$$\text{Force} = \text{mass} \times \text{acceleration}$$

and

$$\text{Acceleration} = \frac{\text{velocity}}{\text{time}} = \frac{\text{distance}}{\text{time}^2}$$

Table B.11. Some named derived units

Physical Quantity	SI Unit	SI Symbol	Base Unit Expression
Frequency	hertz	Hz	s^{-1}
Force	newton	N	$m\,kg\,s^{-2}$
Pressure	pascal	Pa	$N\,m^{-2} \equiv m^{-1}\,kg\,s^{-2}$
Energy, heat, work	joule	J	$N\,m \equiv m^2\,kg\,s^{-2}$
Electric charge	coulomb	C	$A\,s$
Electric potential	volt	V	$J\,C^{-1} \equiv m^2\,kg\,s^{-1}\,A^{-1}$
Electric resistance	ohm	Ω	$V\,A^{-1} \equiv m^2\,kg^{-1}\,s^3\,A^2$

so, in terms of SI units

$$N \equiv m\,kg\,s^{-2}$$

Similarly

$$Pressure = \frac{force}{area}$$

so

$$Pascal \equiv N\,m^{-2}$$

Also

$$Work = force \times distance$$

so

$$Joule = N\,m$$

Not all scientists restrict themselves to SI units, and a few quantities are occasionally written in units from older systems. Moreover, the published scientific literature obviously makes use of older units, and so it is essential to be able to interconvert units of the several systems. Table B.12 gives the relationships between the most important of the older units and SI units.

It is often convenient to represent quantities in terms of multiples or submultiples of SI units. Table B.13 gives the prefixes and symbols for these multiplicative operations.

Table B.12. Some older units

Older Unit	SI Equivalent
1 g (gram)	10^{-3} kg
1 mL (milliliter)	10^{-3} L
1 L (liter)	10^{-3} m^3
1 μ (micron)	10^{-6} m
1 Å (angstrom)	10^{-10} m (10^{-8} cm)
1 atm (atmosphere)	101,325 Pa
1 dyn (dyne)	10^{-5} N
1 erg	10^{-7} J
1 cal (calorie)	4.184 J
1 D (debye)	3.336×10^{-30} C m

Table B.13. Submultiple and multiple prefixes

Submultiple	Prefix	Symbol	Multiple	Prefix	Symbol
10^{-1}	deci	d	10	deca	da
10^{-2}	centi	c	10^2	hecto	h
10^{-3}	milli	m	10^3	kilo	k
10^{-6}	micro	μ	10^6	mega	M
10^{-9}	nano	n	10^9	giga	G
10^{-12}	pico	p	10^{12}	tera	T
10^{-15}	femto	f	10^{15}	peta	P
10^{-18}	atto	a	10^{18}	exa	E
10^{-21}	zepto	z	10^{21}	zetta	Z
10^{-24}	yocto	y	10^{24}	yotta	Y

Quantity Algebra. We earlier wrote this equation:

$$\text{Physical quantity} = \text{numerical value} \times \text{unit} \qquad (\text{B.117})$$

We now assert that each of the three quantities in this equation can be treated as an algebraic quantity and manipulated by the rules of algebra. Thus Eq. (B.117) could be written as

$$\frac{\text{Physical quantity}}{\text{unit}} = \text{numerical value} \qquad (\text{B.118})$$

This equation is particularly convenient because, since the right-hand side is a pure number (it has no dimensions), so is the left-hand side. To illustrate this with an example, let us write

$$T = 273.15\,\text{K}$$

in the form of Eq. (B.117). Transforming to the form of Eq. (B.118) gives

$$T/K = 273.15$$

We will call this method of manipulating units *quantity algebra.*[12] It is particularly convenient for designing headings of table columns and for labeling the axes of figures. We will make use of the quantity algebra when converting from one unit to another.

Conversion of Units. We often find it convenient or necessary to convert from one system of units to another. In our study of proportions (Section B.3) as a means of setting up equations we encountered one method for converting units.

Example B.22. Convert an energy change of $125\,\text{kJ mol}^{-1}$ to kcal mol^{-1}.

From Table B.12 we have the essential relationship

$$1 \, \text{cal} = 4.184 \, \text{J}$$

Multiplying each side by 10^3 gives

$$1 \, \text{kcal} = 4.184 \, \text{kJ}$$

Now we form the proportion from statements:

$$\text{Since } 1 \, \text{kcal} = 4.184 \, \text{kJ}$$
$$x \, \text{kcal} = 125 \, \text{kJ}$$

or

$$\frac{1}{x} = \frac{4.184}{125}$$
$$x = 29.9$$

Therefore $125 \, \text{kJ mol}^{-1}$ is equal to $29.9 \, \text{kcal mol}^{-1}$.

Quantity algebra offers a general procedure for the interconversion of units. This is the method—multiply the quantity whose unit must be converted by one or more quotients each being equal to the pure number one, but having the units needed to get the job done.

Example B.23. Convert a wavelength of 560 nm to angstroms.
We know (Table B.13) that $1 \, \text{nm} = 10^{-9} \, \text{m}$, so it follows that $1 \, \text{nm}/10^{-9} \, \text{m} = 1$. Similarly, from Table B.12, $1 \, \text{Å} = 10^{-10} \, \text{m}$, so $1 \, \text{Å}/10^{-10} \, \text{m} = 1$. Therefore we can write

$$560 \, \text{nm} \left(\frac{10^{-9} \, \text{m}}{1 \, \text{nm}} \right) \left(\frac{1 \, \text{Å}}{10^{-10} \, \text{m}} \right) = 5600 \, \text{Å}$$

The method works because each quantity in parentheses is equal to 1, and we know that we can multiply fearlessly by 1. These quantities in parentheses are chosen so that the units that we do not want will cancel, and the units that we want will remain.

Example B.24. The surface tension of water at 25°C is 71.8 erg cm^{-2}. Convert this to SI units:

$$71.8 \, \frac{\text{erg}}{\text{cm}^2} \left(\frac{1 \, \text{J}}{10^7 \, \text{erg}} \right) \left(\frac{1 \, \text{N m}}{1 \, \text{J}} \right) \left(\frac{10^2 \, \text{cm}}{1 \, \text{m}} \right)^2 = 71.8 \times 10^{-3} \, \text{N m}^{-1}$$

This is usually written $71.8 \, \text{mN m}^{-1}$. Note in this multiplication how the unitary multipliers are oriented so as to achieve the desired cancellations. Incidentally, $71.8 \, \text{erg cm}^{-2}$ also equals $71.8 \, \text{dyn cm}^{-1}$, because $1 \, \text{erg} = 1 \, \text{dyn cm}$.

Extensive and Intensive Properties. A physical property whose magnitude is additive is called an *extensive property*; its magnitude depends on the extent (size) of the system. Mass, volume, and energy are examples of extensive properties.

A property whose magnitude is independent of the size of the system is called an *intensive property*. Temperature, pressure, and concentration are intensive properties.

An extensive property can be converted to an intensive property by dividing it by a mass or an amount of substance, thus placing it on a per unit basis. If an extensive property is divided by mass, the adjective *specific* is often used to describe it. Usually the mass unit gram (g) is used, so the specific property refers to the quantity per gram. For example, the volume V is an extensive property, but if V is divided by the mass, we get the *specific volume* (the volume per gram), which is intensive.

If we divide V by the amount of substance in moles, we have V/n, which is called the *molar volume*, and is interpreted as the volume per mole.

Example B.25. The density of acetone is 0.788 at 25°C. Calculate the specific volume and the molar volume of acetone.

The units of density, which are g mL^{-1} (or g cm^{-3}) are not always written out. The specific volume is simply the reciprocal of the density, as we can deduce from its units.

$$\text{Specific volume} = \frac{1 \, \text{mL}}{0.788 \, \text{g}} = 1.269 \, \text{mL g}^{-1}$$

$$\text{Molar volume} = \left(\frac{1.269 \, \text{mL}}{\text{g}}\right)\left(\frac{58.08 \, \text{g}}{1 \, \text{mol}}\right) = 73.7 \, \text{mL mol}^{-1}$$

These two statements have the same meaning:

1. The heat of solution of succinyl sulfathiazole is $12.0 \, \text{kcal mol}^{-1}$.
2. The molar heat of solution of succinyl sulfathiazole is 12.0 kcal.

Dimensional Consistency. We have seen that units can be treated algebraically in that they undergo division and multiplication just as do numerical values. Units have two additional characteristics of great importance when carrying out calculations:

1. In what may appear to be a disagreement with the assertion that units can be treated algebraically, we note that when we add or subtract physical quantities, they must possess the same units, but the units themselves do not add or subtract.

2. When using or deriving physicochemical equations, the left-hand and right-hand sides of the equation must have the same units.

Example B.26. We will use the content of Example B.7 to demonstrate dimensional consistency. Equation (B.32) defined the K_a value:

$$K_a = \frac{[H^+][A^-]}{[HA]}$$

In this equation the square brackets represent concentration in mol L^{-1}, or M for convenience. Thus the units of the right-hand side are $M^2 \, M^{-1}$ or M. It follows that the K_a value has the unit M.

We then wrote the following for the total solute concentration:

$$c_t = [HA] + [A^-]$$

Each concentration on the right has the unit M, so they can properly be added, and c_t also has the unit M. We then derived the following:

$$K_a = \frac{[H^+]^2}{c_t - [H^+]}$$

Clearly this equation is dimensionally consistent, as it has the unit M on each side. Suppose that the superscript 2 had inadvertently been omitted in the numerator of the right-hand side; a quick dimensional check would have detected the error.

Rearrangement to the standard quadratic form gives

$$[H^+]^2 + K_a[H^+] - K_a C_t = 0$$

in which each term has the same units (M^2), so it is dimensionally correct. It may seem that dimensional consistency has been lost because the left side has the units M^2 whereas the right side appears to be dimensionless. Actually, we have no way to assess the dimensionality of the right-hand side because of its numerical value of zero. If this makes us uneasy, we can simply divide both sides of the equation by M^2. Alternatively, we can rearrange to the dimensionally obvious form

$$[H^+]^2 + K_a[H^+] = K_a C_t$$

The quadratic solution is readily seen to be dimensionally consistent:

$$[H^+] = \frac{-K_a \pm \sqrt{K_a^2 + 4 K_a C_t}}{2}$$

Dimensional consistency in equations describing physical systems is a necessary condition for their validity, but it is not a sufficient condition. Incidentally, if approximations are introduced into equations, the approximations must not alter the dimensional consistency.

PROBLEMS

Problems B.1–B.6 pertain to Section B.2; Problems B.7–B.21, to Section B.3; Problems B.22–B.31, to Section B.4; Problems B.32–B.35, to Section B.5; and problems B.36–B.43, to Section B.6.

B.1. Convert these pH values to hydrogen ion concentrations:
   (a) pH $= 4.75$
   (b) pH $= 11.13$
   (c) pH $= 7.19$
   (d) pH $= 2.00$

B.2. Convert these hydrogen ion concentrations to pH values:
   (a) $[H^+] = 3.85 \times 10^{-3}$ M
   (b) $[H^+] = 1.15 \times 10^{-9}$ M
   (c) $[H^+] = 6.46 \times 10^{-8}$ M
   (d) $[H^+] = 1.15$ M

B.3. Convert $\ln x$ to the corresponding Briggsian logarithm.

B.4. How much more acidic is a solution of pH 3.00 compared with a solution of pH 9.00?

B.5. Solve for q in the equation

$$13.52^q = 5.62 \times 10^4$$

B.6. Calculate the product $6,942,821 \times 0.0057384$ by using logarithms. Check the result by direct multiplication on an electronic calculator.

B.7. How many grams of benzoic acid are required to prepare 500 mL of an 0.0025 M solution?

B.8. Ethyl acetate hydrolyzes according to the reaction

$$CH_3COOC_2H_5 + H_2O \rightarrow C_2H_5OH + CH_3COOH$$

How much acetic acid is produced by the hydrolysis of 10.00 g of ethyl acetate?

B.9. Let $R_{A^-} = [A^-]/[HA]$ and $F_{A^-} = [A^-]/([HA] + [A^-])$. Then derive an equation giving R_{A^-} as a function of F_{A^-} (or the reverse).

B.10. Given $[HA] = [A^-]$, calculate the ratios R_{HA}, R_{A^-} and the fractions F_{HA}, F_{A^-}.

B.11. A solution of weak acid is prepared to have a total concentration of 7.50×10^{-4} M, and analysis shows that the ratio $[A^-]/[HA]$ is 0.15. Calculate the individual concentrations $[HA]$ and $[A^-]$.

B.12. Vinegar contains ∼5% acetic acid (i.e., 5 g of acetic acid per 100 ml). The K_a of acetic acid is 1.78×10^{-5}. Calculate the pH of vinegar.

B.13. Repeat Problem B.12 using the approximate solution [Eq. (B.38)].

B.14. Find the value of the intercept on the x axis for the straight line of Eq. (B.39).

B.15. Carry out the algebraic manipulations that give Eqs. (B.49)–(B.51) from Eq. (B.48).

B.16. In this set of data, c is the molar concentration of *trans*-cinnamic acid ($C_6H_5CH{=}CHCOOH$) in acidic solution, and A is a dimensionless measure of light-absorbing ability of the solution called the absorbance. It is anticipated that the data are described by the equation $A = \epsilon b c$, which is called Beer's law, where b is the "pathlength" of light through the solution ($b = 1$ cm in this experiment) and ϵ is called the *molar absorptivity*. Analyze the data:

$10^5 c$ (M)	A
0	0
1.083	0.224
2.165	0.450
3.248	0.679
4.330	0.901

B.17. The noncovalent interaction of cinnamic acid anion with theophylline was studied optically with a pathlength b of 1 cm. These are the data, where we let c be the theophylline concentration.

c (M)	A
0	0.978 (A_0)
0.0111	1.375
0.0125	1.418
0.0143	1.472
0.0167	1.544
0.0200	1.638
0.0250	1.767

We expect the system to be described by

$$\frac{\Delta A}{b} = \frac{BKc}{1 + Kc}$$

where $\Delta A = A - A_0$. Find the equilibrium constant K.

B.18. The equilibrium solubility of a solute usually varies with temperature according to

$$\ln s = -\frac{\Delta H}{RT} + C$$

where s is the solubility corresponding to absolute temperature T, R is the gas constant, C is a constant, and ΔH is the molar heat of solution. These are solubility data for γ-cyclodextrin in water, where s is the mole fraction solubility:

t (°C)	s
25	0.003539
30	0.004456
35	0.005476
40	0.006239
42	0.007583

Find the heat of solution.

B.19. The total solubility S_t of 4,4'-dihydroxybiphenyl varies with the concentration [L] of α-cyclodextrin according to

$$S_t = s_0 + K_{11}s_0[L] + K_{11}K_{12}s_0[L]^2$$

where s_0 is the solubility when $[L] = 0$, and K_{11} and K_{12} are equilibrium constants for the formation of $1:1$ (SL) (substrate : ligand) and $1:2$ (SL$_2$) complexes. Here are data for 25°C:

$10^2[L]$ (M)	$10^4 S_t$ (M)
0	1.98
0.311	2.53
0.412	2.74
0.512	3.13
0.611	3.51
0.709	4.02
0.806	4.39
0.810	4.62
0.902	4.94
0.998	5.74
1.19	6.86

Find K_{11} and K_{12}.

B.20. The rate of hydrolysis of 4-nitrophenyl glutarate at 25° and pH 7 follows a rate law like Eq. (B.52). When the absorbance A is measured as a function of time, the equation is written

$$A_\infty - A_t = (A_\infty - A_0)e^{-kt}$$

where A_t is the absorbance at time t, A_0 at $t = 0$, and A_∞ at $t = \infty$ ("infinity" time, when the reaction is essentially complete). Here are the data; find the rate constant k:

t (s)	A_t	t (s)	A_t
10	0.129	120	0.453
20	0.168	140	0.492
30	0.200	160	0.531
40	0.237	180	0.565
50	0.270	200	0.598
60	0.300	240	0.650
70	0.330	280	0.692
80	0.357	320	0.729
90	0.381	360	0.758
100	0.407	400	0.783
		∞	0.900

B.21. Rearrange this equation to give a linear plotting form

$$y = \frac{1 + ax}{1 + bx}$$

B.22. Consult the set of data in Example B.11. For each pair of adjacent time points, calculate the increment in time (Δt) and the increment in concentration (Δc). Take their quotient $\Delta c/\Delta t$ as a crude estimate of dc/dt. Now plot each $\Delta c/\Delta t$ value against the mean value of c (i.e., $\bar{c} = (c_1 + c_2)/2$] corresponding to the time interval. Interpret the result.

B.23. If $y = a^u$, find dy/dx, where a is a constant and u is a function of x. (*Hint:* Start by taking the logarithm of y.)

B.24. Equation (B.44), a power function, has the form $y = ax^b$.
 (a) Find dy/dx.
 (b) For the special case $b = 2$, evaluate both y and dy/dx when $x = 0.5$, 1, and 2. Compare the x dependencies of y and dy/dx.

B.25. Equation (B.46) is a polynomial, $y = a + bx + cx^2$. Find the first derivative dy/dx and the second derivative d^2y/dx^2.

B.26. Assuming that 48.2 mg of an acid of unknown structure was titrated with 0.0988 M NaOH, the following data (pH as a function of titrant volume V)

were recorded. Find the endpoint volume by the second-derivative technique and calculate the equivalent weight of the acid (for a monoprotic acid, the equivalent weight equals the molecular weight):

V (mL)	pH
1.40	2.74
1.50	2.86
1.60	3.12
1.70	3.60
1.80	6.15
1.90	9.74
2.00	10.40
2.10	10.62
2.20	10.75

B.27. This equation arises in the study of the effect of pH on the rate of hydrolysis of many drugs, where k is an observed rate constant and k_1, k_2, k_3 are constants of the system:

$$k = k_1[H^+] + k_2 + k_3[OH^-]$$

Find the value of pH at which the rate of hydrolysis is a minimum.

B.28. Evaluate this definite integral.

$$y = 24 \int_1^4 x^2 \, dx$$

B.29. Derive an expression giving the time elapsed for the concentration in a first-order reaction to decrease to one-half its initial value. (This time is called the *half-life* of the reaction; it is symbolized $t_{1/2}$.)

B.30. Why is the constant of integration omitted when evaluating a definite integral?

B.31. Write the total differential dw for the function $w = f(x, y, z)$.

B.32. The equilibrium constant K_{11} for the complexation of 4-nitrophenol anion with α-cyclodextrin (in water at 25°C) has been measured by many laboratories; these are the reported values (units are M^{-1}): 2290, 2200, 2500, 2700, 1590, 2439, 1890, 2720, 2143, 2408, 2270, 3550. Calculate the mean, standard deviation, standard deviation of the mean, and the relative standard deviation.

B.33. The acetylation of isopropyl alcohol by acetic anhydride is a second-order reaction:

$$Ac_2O + (CH_3)_2CHOH \rightarrow HOAc + CH_3COOCH(CH_3)_2$$

It is described by this integrated rate equation

$$\log \frac{c_B}{c_A} = \frac{(c_B^0 - c_A^0)kt}{2.303} + \log \frac{c_B^0}{c_A^0}$$

where A is isopropyl alcohol and B is acetic anhydride. These are experimental kinetic data for this reaction:

t (min)	c_A (M)	c_B (M)
0	0.456	0.876
1.50	0.248	0.668
3.13	0.138	0.558
4.50	0.088	0.508
6.10	0.062	0.482
8.00	0.040	0.460
12.10	0.012	0.432

Analyze the data by the method of least squares, and report the value of the second-order rate constant k.

B.34. These values have been reported in the literature for the dipole moment of phenol at 25°C: 1.45, 1.53, 1.54, 1.65, 1.72, 1.86, 1.53, 1.43, 1.64. Calculate the usual statistical parameters, and give 95% confidence limits for the mean.

B.35. Return to Problem B.32 and express the mean with an appropriate number of significant figures.

B.36. The activation energy for the hydrolysis of aspirin in acid solution is 16.7 kcal mol^{-1}. Convert this to kJ mol^{-1}.

B.37. A rate constant for the uncatalyzed hydrolysis of succinylcholine chloride has been reported to be 5.0×10^{-6} h^{-1}. Convert this to s^{-1} (reciprocal seconds).

B.38. Convert a density of 1.86 g mL^{-1} to SI units.

B.39. The tetrahedral covalent radius of carbon is 0.77 Å. Convert this to nanometers.

B.40. R (the gas constant) is equal to 8.314 J K^{-1} mol^{-1}. Convert this to cal K^{-1} mol^{-1}.

B.41. Physicochemical equations often call for taking the logarithm of a quantity having units. It is difficult to conceive of the logarithm of a unit. Describe a way out of this quandary.

B.42. Beer's law for the absorption of light is written $A = \epsilon bc$, where b is pathlength in centimeters, c is molar concentration, and A is absorbance, defined by $A = \log(I_0/I)$, where the I quantities are light intensities. Deduce the units of ϵ, which is called the *molar absorptivity*.

B.43. Both of these equations have been published in the scientific literature. One of them is incorrect. The quantities k_s, k_L, and k_{11} all have the same units. k_{11} is defined $k_{11} = [SL]/[S]\ [L]$. The F quantities are fluorescent intensities. Use dimensional analysis to detect the incorrect equation.

(a) $\dfrac{F}{F_0} = \dfrac{1 + (k_{11}/k_s)K_{11}[L]}{1 + K_{11}[L]} + \dfrac{k_L}{k_s}[L]$

(b) $\dfrac{F}{F_0} = \dfrac{1 + (k_{11}/k_s)K_{11}[L]}{1 + K_{11}[L]} + \dfrac{(k_L/k_s)[L]}{[S](1 + K_{11}[L])}$

NOTES

1. Equation (B.2) is not the standard definition, which requires calculus; rather, it is a consequence of the standard definition.
2. From Eq. (B.1), if $b = b^x$, $x = 1$, so $\log_b b = 1$.
3. From Eq. (B.1), if $a = 1$ and $b = 10$, then $x = 0$, so $\log 1 = 0$.
4. It sometimes happens that b^2 is relatively very large and $4ac$ is relatively very small; but $4ac$ cannot be neglected because then the numerator of Eq. (B.31) would go to zero. In this case an alternative calculational procedure is available; see Connors' *A Textbook of Pharmaceutical Analysis* (1967) (this is the first edition).
5. The equation probably never was truly exact in a physicochemical sense anyway because of the complexity of chemical systems.
6. Computers offer an alternative to manual graphing, but the manual method is better for developing a sense of the physical nature of the data set. This is probably because it requires active participation by the interpreter.
7. Here is the attitude we have adopted. The experimental points have led us to the line as the best interpretation of the dependence of the y values on the x values, so henceforth we base our interpretation on the line and not on the data points.
8. See Daniels and Alberty (1955, p. 323). The reaction yields oxygen and N_2O_4, which exists in equilibrium with NO_2.

$$N_2O_5 \rightarrow N_2O_4 + \tfrac{1}{2}O_2$$
$$N_2O_4 \rightleftharpoons 2NO_2$$

9. Heat and work, however, which are important thermodynamic quantities, are not, in general, state functions.
10. "Student" was the pen name of W. S. Gosset, a British statistician and chemist who worked at Guiness Breweries.

11. It might seem simpler to minimize the sum of the vertical distances themselves, but this sum is zero, because some points are above the line and some are below the line. By squaring the distances, all quantities are converted to positive numbers. It will be seen that this procedure has much in common with the calculation of the variance, Eq. (B.102).

12. The technique is also called "quantity calculus," which seems a bit pompous for such a simple procedure.

ANSWERS TO PROBLEMS

Chapter 1

1.1. $\Delta V = 35.343\,\text{in}^3 = 0.579\,\text{L}$
$w = P\Delta V = 0.579\,\text{L\,atm} = 58.7\,\text{J}$

1.2. $w = -1718\,\text{J}$

1.3. $\Delta U = 0$ and $w = P\Delta V$, so $q = w = P\Delta V$, leading to Eq. (1.15) for q

1.4. $C_p = 18.02\,\text{cal\,mol}^{-1}\,\text{K}^{-1}$

1.5. Specific heat$= 1.74\,\text{J\,g}^{-1}\,\text{K}^{-1}$

1.6. T (final)$= 25°\text{C} + \Delta T = 105°\text{C}$

1.7. Write Eq. (1.26) as $\Delta H = C_p(T_2 - T_1)$, applying it both to water and to iron. Since ΔH (water) $= -\Delta H$ (iron), and T_2 is the same for both, we find $T_2 = 343.36\,\text{K}$ or $70.2°\text{C}$.

1.8. $\Delta H_\text{f} + \Delta H_\text{v} - \Delta H_\text{s} = 0$

Chapter 2

2.1. (a) $(-)$ System becomes more ordered as it crystallizes.

(b) $(+)$ System becomes more random as it vaporizes.

(c) $(-)$ Two particles combine to yield one particle, with decrease in number of microstates.

2.2. Using Trouton's rule, $\Delta H_\text{v} = (21)(353.25) = 7.42\,\text{kcal\,mol}^{-1}$. (The experimental value is $7.35\,\text{kcal\,mol}^{-1}$.)

2.3. $\Delta S_\text{f} = 5040/419.15 = 12.02\,\text{cal\,K}^{-1}\,\text{mol}^{-1}$

2.4. $\Delta S_\text{s} = 17,600/298.15 = 59.0\,\text{cal\,K}^{-1}\,\text{mol}^{-1}$

2.5. $\Delta S = 9.57\,\text{J\,K}^{-1}$ (i.e., $19.14\,\text{J\,K}^{-1}\,\text{mol}^{-1}$)

2.6. $\Delta S = 2.61\,\text{cal\,K}^{-1}\,\text{mol}^{-1}$

2.7. $\Delta S = R\ln(P_1/P_2)$

Chapter 3

3.1. $a = 0.0175\,\text{m}$ (from data in Table 3.1)

3.2. $\Delta\mu = \mu_{(0.05\,\text{m})} - \mu_{(0.005\,\text{m})} = 5.41\,\text{kJ}\,\text{mol}^{-1}$

3.3. $\Delta\mu = -3.44\,\text{kJ}\,\text{mol}^{-1}$

3.4. Making a solution more concentrated yields a positive free-energy change; the process is nonspontaneous. (See Problem 3.2.) In Problem 3.3 the process takes the solution from 1 M (the standard state) to 0.25 M, and this is spontaneous. It is possible for nonideal behavior (activity coefficient effects) to reverse this conclusion, however.

Chapter 4

4.1. From the integrated Clausius–Clapeyron equation, $\Delta H_{\text{vap}} = 9.45\,\text{kcal}$ $\text{mol}^{-1} = 39.5\,\text{kJ}\,\text{mol}^{-1}$.

4.2. $\Delta G° = -1.82\,\text{kcal}\,\text{mol}^{-1} = -7.61\,\text{kJ}\,\text{mol}^{-1}$

4.3. $\Delta H_{\text{vap}} = +8.79\,\text{kcal}\,\text{mol}^{-1}$

4.4. $\Delta G° = 2.303\,\text{RT}\,pK_a$

4.5. $C_6H_5OH \rightleftharpoons H^+ + C_6H_5O^-$
$K_a = a_{H^+}a_{PhO^-}/a_{PhOH}\ (Ph \equiv C_6H_5)$
$\Delta G° = +1.36\,\text{kcal}\,\text{mol}^{-1}$

4.6. $\Delta S° = -16.9\,\text{cal}\,\text{mol}^{-1}\,\text{K}^{-1}$

4.7. We might expect $\Delta S°$ to be positive, because one particle is being transformed into two particles, with (presumably) an increase in number of accessible microstates. Since $\Delta S°$ is negative, however, we may infer that something else, something not apparent in the reaction as written, must be occurring. The most likely possibility is that the ions on the right-hand side of the equation are limiting the motions of solvent (water) molecules via strong ion–dipole interactions. The implication is that, taking into account the solvent, there are more particles, and therefore more accessible microstates, on the left-hand side of the equation.

4.8. $\Delta G° = -5.25\,\text{kcal}\,\text{mol}^{-1}$

Chapter 5

5.1. $x_2 = 0.0000270$, so $x_1 = 1 - x_2 = 0.999973$

5.2. About 12.4 M

5.3. 55.5 M

5.4. $\mu_c^o - \mu_x^o = -RT \ln 55.5$
$$= -2.38 \, \text{kcal mol}^{-1}$$
$$= -9.96 \, \text{kJ mol}^{-1}$$

5.5. $c_i = M_i \rho_1$

5.6. $x_2 = \dfrac{c_2(n_1 M_1 + n_2 M_2)}{1000 \rho (n_1 + n_2)}$

where M_1 and M_2 are molecular weights. [*Suggestion:* Start by writing the mass of solution as $n_1 M_1 + n_2 M_2$; then use ρ to write the volume of solution as $(n_1 M_1 + n_2 M_2)/1000\rho$ in liters.]

Chapter 6

6.1. 45°C

6.2. $C = 2$ and $P = 3$, so $F = 1$; however, the pressure is fixed by experimental design, so there remain no degrees of freedom.

Chapter 7

7.1. $\Delta S_{\text{mix}}^{\text{ideal}} = +1.36 \, \text{cal mol}^{-1} \, \text{K}^{-1} = +5.70 \, \text{J mol}^{-1} \, \text{K}^{-1}$
$\Delta G_{\text{mix}}^{\text{ideal}} = -0.41 \, \text{kcal mol}^{-1} = -1.72 \, \text{kJ mol}^{-1}$

7.2. Alanine: $\Delta \mu^\circ = +4.01 \, \text{kcal mol}^{-1} = 16.8 \, \text{kJ mol}^{-1}$
Phenothiazine: $\Delta \mu^\circ = -5.66 \, \text{kcal mol}^{-1} = -23.7 \, \text{kJ mol}^{-1}$

7.3. $x_B = 0.23$; total pressure $= 34 \, \text{mm}$

7.4. $k^x \, (\text{CHCl}_3) \approx 157 \, \text{mm}$

7.5. Six extractions

7.7. (a) $P_{AB} = c_A/c_B; P_{BC} = c_B/c_C; P_{AC} = c_A/c_C$
   (b) $P_{AB} = P_{AC}/P_{BC}$
   (c) $p_A = P_{AB}V_A/(P_{AB}V_A + V_B + V_C/P_{BC})$

7.8. $P = 0.25; 1.00; 4.00$

Chapter 8

8.1. $B + \text{HOAc} \rightleftharpoons \text{BH}^+\text{OAc}^- \rightleftharpoons \text{BH}^+ + \text{OAc}^-$

8.2. NaCl, $I = 3.0 \, \text{m}$; CaCl_2, $I = 9.0 \, \text{m}$; ZnSO_4, $I = 12.0 \, \text{m}$

8.3. $\gamma_\pm = 0.807$

8.4. $\gamma_\pm = 0.850$; $a_\pm = 0.0085 \, \text{M}$

8.5. $I = 0.65\,\text{M}$

8.6. $C = 0.21\,|z_+z_-|$

Chapter 9

9.1. From $p_1 = x_1 P_1^*$, derive $P_1^* - p_1 = x_2 P_1^*$

9.2. $K_b = 1.23°\,\text{C}$

9.3. $K_f = 3.58°\,\text{C}$

9.4. Take 0.6 g pilocarpine nitrate, 0.3 g boric acid, and dilute to 30 mL ("q.s. ad" is a prescription abbreviation meaning "a quantity sufficient to make;" sterile water is intended in this case).

9.5. $\Delta T_f = 0.469°\,\text{C}$ (the experimental value is $0.470°$); 5.54% dextrose will be isotonic.

Chapter 10

10.1. $x_2 = 0.158$

10.2. At 24°C (e.g.), $c_2 = 3.34 \times 10^{-4}\,\text{M}$. The heat of solution is identical with that obtained in Example 10.2. (Enthalpy changes do not change value when the concentration scale is altered, unlike free-energy and entropy changes.)

10.3. $K_{sp} = 108s^5$; $s = 7.14 \times 10^{-7}\,\text{M}$

10.4. AgI, then AgBr, then AgCl

10.5. $x_2 = 0.0117$ (calculated taking $\phi_1 = 1$) (the experimental value is $x_2 = 0.0142$)

10.6. Log $c_2 = -4.50$ [Eq. (10.29)] or log $c_2 = -4.87$ [Eq. (10.30a)] (the experimental value is log $c_2 = -4.42$)

10.7. $\varphi_2 = 0.55$

Chapter 11

11.1. 67.6 dyn cm^{-1}

11.2. Water on ether: $S = -66$

Ether on water: $S = +44.6$

Ether will spread on water readily; water will not spread on ether.

11.3. $\Delta G = \gamma\,\Delta A = 4\pi\gamma(r_{\text{final}}^2 - r_{\text{initial}}^2)$

$\Delta G = 2.23 \times 10^{-4}\,\text{mJ}$

11.4. (a) $1/n_b = 1/Kn_{max}c_2 + 1/n_{max}$

   (b) $n_b/c_2 = -Kn_b + Kn_{max}$

11.5. $K = 386\,M^{-1}$; $y_{max} = 146\,mg\,g^{-1}$ (we also calculate $\sigma = 105\,\text{Å}^2\,molecule^{-1}$)

Chapter 12

12.1. (a) $pH = 3.60$

   (b) $pH = 3.30$

   (c) $pH = 10.93$

   (d) $pH = 5.32$

   (e) $pH = 11.48$

12.2. $pH = 4.67$

12.3. Dissolve 6.055 g tris in 325.3 mL 0.10 M HCl and dilute to 500 mL.

12.4. (a) Both are $\frac{1}{15}\,M = 0.0667\,M$

   (b) $pH = 6.98$

12.5. At 0 mL, $pH = 11.95$; 2 mL, $pH = 11.45$; 5 mL, $pH = 10.94$; 8 mL, $pH = 10.60$; 12 mL, $pH = 10.12$; 16 mL, 5.76; 18 mL, $pH = 1.84$; methyl red or bromcresol purple

12.7. (a) $K_{eq} = K_a$ (benzoic acid)$/K_a$ (methylamine) $= 2.76 \times 10^6$

   (b) $K_{eq} = K_a$ (phenol)$/K_w = 1.00 \times 10^4$

12.8. (a) pK_1 (COOH); pK_2 (OH)

   (b) pK_1 (COOH); pK_2 (NH$_2$); pK_3 (guanidine)

   (c) pK_1 (aromatic amine); pK_2 (aliphatic amine)

   (d) This is an acidic group, the 7-NH structurally similar to an imide.

12.9. $[H^+]^3 + (K_a + b)[H^+]^2 - (K_a c - K_a b + K_w)[H^+] - K_a K_w = 0$

12.10. (a) $[NH_4^+] + [H^+] = [OH^-] + [Cl^-]$

   (b) $[H^+] = [OH^-] + [H_2A^-] + 2[HA^{2-}] + 3[A^{3-}]$

   (c) $[Na^+] + [H^+] = [OH^-] + [H_2PO_4^-] + 2[HPO_4^{2-}]$

12.11. $pH = 5.31$

12.12. $pH = 7.69$

12.13. (a) $pH = pK_a = 9.25$

   (b) $pH = 5.52$

12.14. $\Delta G^\circ = +13.64\,kcal\,mol^{-1}$

12.15. 0.1689 g of sodium acetate

12.16. $F = R/(R+1)$

12.17. $3.91 \times 10^{-4}\,\text{M}$

12.18. (a) Decrease

(b) Decrease

12.19. $\text{pH} = 1.70$

12.20. $8.528\,\text{g of } NaH_2PO_4 \cdot H_2O \text{ and } 5.424\,\text{g of } Na_2HPO_4$

12.21. $\Delta G^\circ = -19.1\,\text{kcal mol}^{-1} = -79.8\,\text{kJ mol}^{-1}$

Chapter 13

13.1. (a) $ClO_3^- + 3Sn^{2+} + 6H^+ = Cl^- + 3Sn^{4+} + 3H_2O$

(b) $PbO_2 + 2I^- + 4H^+ = Pb^{2+} + I_2 + 2H_2O$

(c) $3OCl^- + 2NH_3 = 3Cl^- + N_2 + 3H_2O$

(d) $2MnO_4^- + 5H_2O_2 + 6H^+ = 2Mn^{2+} + 5O_2 + 8H_2O$

(e) $MnO_4^- + 3CuI + 4H^+ = MnO_2 + 3Cu^{2+} + 3I^- + 2H_2O$

(f) $S_2O_8^{2-} + 2Fe^{2+} = 2SO_4^{2-} + 2Fe^{3+}$

(g) $2NH_2OH + 4Ce^{4+} = N_2O + 4Ce^{3+} + H_2O + 4H^+$

(h) $2RSH + I_2 = RSSR + 2HI$

13.2. $I = 0.150\,\text{M}$

13.3. $\Delta E = -0.59\,\text{V}$

13.4. $pK'_a = 8.02$

13.5. (a) Slope of plot of E_{cell} versus log (Ca^{2+} activity) $= 0.029$, consistent with 0.059/2

(b) $E_{cell} = +0.162\,\text{V}$

13.6. (a) $I = 0.04\,\text{M}$

(b) $\gamma_\pm = 0.458$

13.7. (a) $E_{cell} = -0.548\,\text{V}$

(b) E_{cell} is negative, so reaction is nonspontaneous (proceeds from right to left); copper dissolves. $2Fe^{2+} + Cu^{2+} \rightleftharpoons Cu + 2Fe^{3+}$

13.8. (a) $E_{cell} = +1.44\,\text{V}$

(b) Silver-plated zinc

13.9. $E^\circ = +0.15\,\text{V}; K = 349$

13.10. $pK_{sp} = -10.85$

Chapter 14

14.1. $\beta_{23} = K_{11}K_{21}K_{22}K_{23}$

14.3. Initial slope$= S_t K_{11}\Delta\epsilon_{11}$

14.4. (a) $\frac{\Delta A/b}{[L]} = -K_{11}(\Delta A/b) + S_t K_{11}\Delta\epsilon_{11}$
  (b) $K_{11} = 10.2\,\text{M}^{-1}$; $\Delta\epsilon_{11} = 257\,\text{M}^{-1}\,\text{cm}^{-1}$

14.5. Initial slope $= K_{11a} - K_{11b}$

Appendix B

B.1. (a) $[\text{H}^+] = 1.78 \times 10^{-5}\,\text{M}$
  (b) $[\text{H}^+] = 7.41 \times 10^{-12}\,\text{M}$
  (c) $[\text{H}^+] = 6.46 \times 10^{-8}\,\text{M}$
  (d) $[\text{H}^+] = 1.00 \times 10^{-2}\,\text{M}$

B.2. (a) $\text{pH} = 2.41$
  (b) $\text{pH} = 8.94$
  (c) $\text{pH} = 7.19$
  (d) $\text{pH} = -0.06$

B.3. $\log x = (\ln x)/2.303 = 0.434\ln x$

B.4. One million times more acidic (i.e., 10^6).

B.5. $q = 4.20$

B.7. 0.1526 g benzoic acid

B.8. 6.82 g acetic acid

B.9. $R_{\text{A}^-} = F_{\text{A}^-}/(1 - F_{\text{A}^-})$ or $F_{\text{A}^-} = R_{\text{A}^-}/(1 + R_{\text{A}^-})$

B.10. $R_{\text{HA}} = R_{\text{A}^-} = 1.0$; $F_{\text{HA}} = F_{\text{A}^-} = 0.5$

B.11. $[\text{HA}] = 6.52 \times 10^{-4}\,\text{M}$; $[\text{A}^-] = 0.98 \times 10^{-4}\,\text{M}$

B.12. $\text{pH} = 2.41$

B.13. $\text{pH} = 2.41$

B.14. $-b/m$

B.16. $\epsilon = 2.08 \times 10^4\,\text{M}^{-1}\,\text{cm}^{-1}$

B.17. $K = 10.8\,\text{M}^{-1}$

B.18. $\Delta H = 7.73\,\text{kcal}\,\text{mol}^{-1}$

B.19. $K_{11} = 41\,\text{M}^{-1}$; $K_{12} = 345\,\text{M}^{-1}$

B.20. $k = 4.90 \times 10^{-3}\,\text{s}^{-1}$

B.21. $(y - 1)/x = a - bx$ (there are other possible linear forms also)

B.22. The plot of $\Delta c/\Delta t$ against $\bar{c}$ is reasonably linear, so it has the equation $-\Delta c/\Delta t = k\bar{c}$, with $k = 6.1 \times 10^{-4}\,\mathrm{s}^{-1}$. You have obtained an experimental rate equation, where $\Delta c/\Delta t$ is the rate of reaction and k the rate constant. Compare your value of k with the value calculated in Example B.11.

B.23. $dy/dx = a^u \ln a (du/dx)$

B.24. (a) $dy/dx = abx^{b-1}$
 (b) At $x = 0.5$, $y = a/4$, $dy/dx = a$; at $x = 1$, $y = a$, $dy/dx = 2a$; at $x = 2$, $y = 4a$, $dy/dx = 4a$

B.25. $dy/dx = b + 2cx$; $d^2y/dx^2 = 2c$

B.26. $V_{\text{endpoint}} = 1.83\,\mathrm{ml}$; equivalent weight $= 266.6$

B.27. $\mathrm{pH_{min}} = \frac{1}{2}\mathrm{p}K_w + \frac{1}{2}\log (k_1/k_3)$, where $\mathrm{p}K_w = -\log K_w$ and $K_w = [\mathrm{H^+}][\mathrm{OH^-}]$

B.28. $y = 504$

B.29. $t_{1/2} = \ln 2/k = 0.693/k$

B.30. Because the constant of integration will disappear anyway in the subtraction process

B.31. $dw = \left(\dfrac{\partial w}{\partial x}\right)_{y,z} dx + \left(\dfrac{\partial w}{\partial y}\right)_{x,z} dy + \left(\dfrac{\partial w}{\partial z}\right)_{x,y} dz$

B.32. $\bar{x} = 2392\,\mathrm{M}^{-1}$; $s = 484\,\mathrm{M}^{-1}$; $s_m = 140\,\mathrm{M}^{-1}$; RSD $= 20.2\%$

B.33. The plot of $\log (c_B/c_A)$ against t has $r = 0.981$, intercept$= 0.262$, slope $= 0.107\,\mathrm{min}^{-1}$, from which is obtained $k = 0.585\,\mathrm{M}^{-1}\,\mathrm{min}^{-1} = 9.75 \times 10^{-3}\,\mathrm{M}^{-1}\,\mathrm{s}^{-1}$.

B.34. $\bar{x} = 1.59$, $s = 0.139$, $s_m = 0.046$; confidence limits $(P = 0.05) = 1.59 \pm 0.11$

B.35. $\bar{x} = 2.4 \times 10^3\,\mathrm{M}^{-1}$; $s_m = 1.4 \times 10^2\,\mathrm{M}^{-1}$ (note that each of these quantities possesses two significant figures; the numbers 2.4×10^3 and 2400 are subtly different in this regard)

B.36. $69.9\,\mathrm{kJ\,mol}^{-1}$

B.37. $1.39 \times 10^{-3}\,\mathrm{s}^{-1}$

B.38. $\left(\dfrac{1.86\mathrm{g}}{\mathrm{mL}}\right)\left(\dfrac{10^3\mathrm{mL}}{1\mathrm{L}}\right)\left(\dfrac{1\mathrm{L}}{10^{-3}\mathrm{m}^3}\right)\left(\dfrac{1\mathrm{kg}}{10^3\mathrm{g}}\right) = 1.86 \times 10^3\,\mathrm{kg\,m}^{-3}$

B.39. $(0.77\,\text{Å})\left(\dfrac{10^{-10}\mathrm{m}}{1\,\text{Å}}\right)\left(\dfrac{10^9\mathrm{nm}}{1\,\mathrm{m}}\right) = 0.077\,\mathrm{nm}$

B.40. $\left(\dfrac{8.314\mathrm{J}}{\mathrm{K\,mol}}\right)\left(\dfrac{1\mathrm{cal}}{4.184\mathrm{J}}\right) = 1.987\,\mathrm{cal\,K}^{-1}\,\mathrm{mol}^{-1}$

B.41. Use quantity algebra to generate a pure number, and then take the logarithm of this pure number. For example, the expression $\log K_a$ really should be interpreted as $\log (K_a/M)$. We use the former symbolism in equations for convenience.

B.42. Since A is dimensionless, and $\epsilon = A/bc$, ϵ has the units $L\ mol^{-1}\ cm^{-1}$, or $M^{-1}\ cm^{-1}$.

B.43. Equation **(a)** is incorrect.

BIBLIOGRAPHY

Adamson, A. W., *Physical Chemistry of Surfaces*, Interscience, New York, 1960 (and later editions).

Albert, A., and E. P. Serjeant, *The Determination of Ionization Constants*, 3rd ed., Chapman & Hall, London, 1984.

Amidon, G. L., and N. A. Williams, *Int. J. Pharm.* **11**, 249 (1982).

Anson, F. C., *J. Chem. Ed.* **36**, 394 (1959).

Atkins, P. W., *Physical Chemistry*, 5th ed., Freeman, New York, 1994.

Bates, R. G., *J. Res. Natl. Bur. Stand.* **66A**, 179 (1962).

Brown, H. C., D. H. McDaniel, and O. Häfliger, in *Determination of Organic Structures by Physical Methods*, E. A. Braude and F. C. Nachod, eds., Academic Press, New York, 1955.

Bummer, P. M., in *Remington: The Science and Practice of Pharmacy*, 20th ed., Mack, Easton, PA, 2000, Chapter 20.

Burnette, R. R., and K. A. Connors, *J. Pharm. Sci.* **89**, 1389 (2000).

Callen, H. B., *Thermodynamics*, Wiley, New York, 1960.

Carstensen, J. T., *Theory of Pharmaceutical Systems*, Vol. II, Academic Press, New York, 1973.

Carstensen, J. T., *Pharmaceutics of Solids and Solid Dosage Forms*, Wiley-Interscience, New York, 1977.

Chen, L.-K., D. E. Cadwallader, and H. W. Jun, *J. Pharm. Sci.* **65**, 868 (1976).

Cohen, J. L., and K. A. Connors, *Am. J. Pharm. Ed.* **31**, 476 (1967).

Connors, K. A., *A Textbook of Pharmaceutical Analysis*, Wiley, New York, 1967.

Connors, K. A., *A Textbook of Pharmaceutical Analysis*, 3rd ed., Wiley-Interscience, New York, 1982.

Connors, K. A., *Binding Constants: The Measurement of Molecular Complex Stability*, Wiley-Interscience, New York, 1987.

Connors, K. A., *Chemical Kinetics*, VCH, New York, 1990.

Connors, K. A., *J. Pharm. Sci.* **84**, 843 (1995).

Connors, K. A., *Chem. Rev.* **97**, 1325 (1997).

Connors, K. A., in *Remington: The Science and Practice of Pharmacy*, 20th ed., Mack, Easton, PA, 2000, Chapter 14.

Connors, K. A., and M. J. Jozwiakowski, *J. Pharm. Sci.* **76**, 892 (1987).

Connors, K. A., and J. L. Wright, *Anal. Chem.* **61**, 194 (1989).

Connors, K. A., S.-F. Lin, and A. B. Wong, *J. Pharm. Sci.* **71**, 217 (1982).

Connors, K. A., G. L. Amidon, and V. J. Stella, *Chemical Stability of Pharmaceuticals*, 2nd ed., Wiley-Interscience, New York, 1986.

Daniels, F., and R. A. Alberty, *Physical Chemistry*, Wiley, New York, 1955.

Denbigh, K., *The Principles of Chemical Equilibrium*, 2nd ed., Cambridge Univ. Press, London, 1966.

Evans, A., *Potentiometry and Ion Selective Electrodes*, Wiley, New York, 1987.

Findlay, A., A. N. Campbell, and N. O. Smith, *The Phase Rule and Its Applications*, 9th ed., Dover, New York, 1951.

Florence, A. T., and D. Attwood, *Physicochemical Principles of Pharmacy*, Chapman & Hall, New York, 1981.

Fowkes, F. M., in *Chemistry and Physics of Interfaces*, S. Ross, ed., American Chemical Society, Washington, DC, 1965, p. 1; reprinted in *Ind. Eng. Chem.* (Sept. 1964).

Glasstone, S., *Thermodynamics for Chemists*, Van Nostrand, Princeton, NJ, 1947.

Grant, D. J. W., and T. Higuchi, *Solubility Behavior of Organic Compounds*, Wiley-Interscience, New York, 1990.

Guggenheim, E. A., *Thermodynamics*, 3rd ed., North-Holland, Amsterdam, 1957.

Gupta, P. K., in *Remington: The Science and Practice of Pharmacy*, 20th ed., Mack, Easton, PA, 2000, Chapter 16.

Haleblian, J., and W. McCrone, *J. Pharm. Sci.* **58**, 911 (1969).

Haleblian, J. K., *J. Pharm. Sci.* **64**, 1269 (1975).

Harned, H. S., and B. B. Owen, *The Physical Chemistry of Electrolytic Solutions*, 3rd ed., ACS Monograph 137, Reinhold, New York, 1958.

Hildebrand, J. H., and R. L. Scott, *The Solubility of Nonelectrolytes*, 3rd ed., Dover, New York, 1964.

Hildebrand, J. H., J. M. Prausnitz, and R. L. Scott, *Regular and Related Solutions*, Van Nostrand Reinhold, New York, 1970.

Hill, T. L., *An Introduction to Statistical Thermodynamics*, Addison-Wesley, Reading, MA, 1960.

J. O., Hirschfelder, C. F. Curtiss, and R. B. Bird, *Molecular Theory of Gases and Liquids*, Wiley, New York, 1954.

Israelachvili, J. N., *Intermolecular and Surface Forces*, Academic Press, London, 1985.

IUPAC, *Quantities, Units, and Symbols in Physical Chemistry*, 2nd ed., Blackwell, Oxford, 1993.

Jozwiakowski, M. J., Ph.D. dissertation, Univ. Wisconsin—Madison, 1987.

Khossravi, D., and K. A. Connors, *J. Solution Chem.* **22**, 321 (1993).

Kramer, P. A., and K. A. Connors, *Am. J. Pharm. Ed.* **33**, 193 (1969).

Leo, A., C. Hansch, and D. Elkins, *Chem. Rev.* **71**, 525 (1971).

LePree, J. M., M. J. Mulski, and K. A. Connors, *J. Chem. Soc., Perkin Trans.* **2**, 1491 (1994).

Lin, S.-F., and K. A. Connors, *J. Pharm. Sci.* **72**, 1333 (1983).

Milosovich, G., *J. Pharm. Sci.* **53**, 484 (1964).

Nash, L. K., *Elements of Statistical Thermodynamics*, 2nd ed., Addison-Wesley, Reading, MA, 1974.

Nys, G. G., and R. F. Rekker, *Eur. J. Med. Chem.* **9**, 361 (1974).

Pauling, L., *The Nature of the Chemical Bond*, Cornell Univ. Press, Ithaca, NY, 1960.

Perrin, D. D., B. Dempsey, and E. P. Serjeant, *pK$_a$ Prediction for Organic Acids and Bases*, Chapman & Hall, London, 1981.

Reich, I., R. Schnaare, and E. T. Sugita, in *Remington: The Science and Practice of Pharmacy*, 20th ed., Mack, Easton, PA, 2000, Chapter 11.

Rossini, F. D., *Chemical Thermodynamics*, Wiley, New York, 1950.

Smith, E. B., *Basic Chemical Thermodynamics*, 2nd ed., Clarendon Press, Oxford, 1977.

Staples, B. R., and R. G. Bates, *J. Res. Natl. Bur. Stand.* **73A**, 37 (1969).

Thompson, J. E., *A Practical Guide to Contemporary Pharmacy Practice*, Williams & Wilkins, Baltimore, 1998.

Williamson, A. G., *An Introduction to Non-Electrolyte Solutions*, Wiley, New York, 1967.

Windholz, M., ed., *The Merck Index*, 10th ed., Merck, Rahway, NJ, 1983.

Wyman, J., and S. J. Gill, *Binding and Linkage: Functional Chemistry of Biological Macromolecules*, University Science Books, Mill Valley, CA, 1990.

Yalkowsky, S. H., and J. T. Rubino, *J. Pharm. Sci.* **74**, 416 (1985).

Yalkowski, S. H., and S. C. Valvani, *J. Pharm. Sci.* **69**, 912 (1980).

Yoshioka, M., B. C. Hancock, and G. Zografi, *J. Pharm. Sci.* **83**, 1700 (1994).

Zografi, G., and A. M. Mattocks, *J. Pharm. Sci.* **52**, 1103 (1963).

INDEX